Cytopathology of the Central Nervous System

ASCP Theory and Practice of Cytopathology 3
William Johnston, MD, Series Editor

The ASCP Theory and Practice of Cytopathology Series

Cytopathology of the Uterine Cervix • Volume 1

Cytopathology of the Endometrium: Direct Intrauterine Sampling • Volume 2

Teaching Slide Sets in the ASCP Theory and Practice of Cytopathology Series

Cytopathology of the Uterine Cervix and Endometrium Teaching Slide Set

Cytopathology of the Endometrium Teaching Slide Set

Cytopathology of the Central Nervous System

Sandra H. Bigner, MD

Professor of Pathology
Associate Chief, Division of Cytopathology
and Cytogenetics
Duke University Medical Center
Durham, North Carolina

William W. Johnston, MD, FIAC

Professor of Pathology
Chief, Division of Cytopathology
and Cytogenetics
Codirector, Anatomic Pathology
Duke University Medical Center
Durham, North Carolina

ASCP PRESS

American Society of Clinical Pathologists
Chicago

Publishing Team
Jeffrey Carlson (design/production)
Renee Kastar (marketing)
Karen D. Johnson (editorial)
Joshua Weikersheimer (publishing direction)

Notice

Trade names for equipment and supplies described herein are included as suggestions only. In no way does their inclusion constitute an endorsement or preference by the American Society of Clinical Pathologists. The ASCP did not test the equipment, supplies, or procedures and, therefore, urges all readers to read and follow all manufacturers' instructions and package insert warnings concerning the proper and safe use of products.

Library of Congress Cataloging-in-Publication Data

Bigner, Sandra H.
Cytopathology of the central nervous system/Sandra H. Bigner, William W. Johnston.
p. 208
Includes bibliographical references and index.
ISBN 0-89189-362-8
1. Central nervous system—Cytopathology. I. Johnston, William W. II. Title.
[DNLM: 1. Cytological Techniques. 2. Central Nervous System—cytology. 3. Central Nervous System Diseases—diagnosis. WL 300 B593c 1994]
RC361.B53 1994
616.8'047—dc20
DNLM/DLC 93-2289
for Library of Congress CIP

Printed in Hong Kong

98 97 96 95 94 5 4 3 2 1

Contents

Tables

Figures

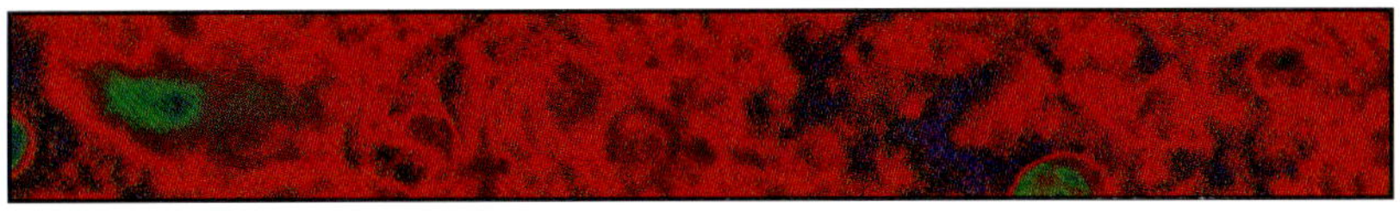

Preface

Cytopathology of the Central Nervous System represents an effort to present the cytologic features of normal cells, non-neoplastic conditions, and primary and secondary neoplasms in cerebrospinal fluid and in brain aspirates. For the benefit of readers unfamiliar with neuroanatomy and neuropathology, we have used gross nervous system pathology and histologic illustrations liberally in addition to descriptions and photographs of cytologic preparations. The basic neuroanatomy, neuropathology, and cytopathology of the central nervous system have changed little during the last several decades. Three significant events, however, have had profound effects on most areas of nongynecologic cytopathology and have changed the practice of central nervous system cytology. These three developments—the widespread use of immunohistochemistry, the AIDS epidemic, and the dawn of the era of molecular biology—are reflected in this monograph.

We have dedicated a chapter to immunohistochemical procedures and have used many images of immunohistochemical preparations throughout the text. This emphasis mirrors the widespread application of immunohistochemical procedures to cerebrospinal fluid and to brain aspirates in a broad spectrum of clinical situations. A second area of expansion is the emphasis on AIDS in the chapter on inflammatory conditions. We have illustrated and discussed a variety of opportunistic organisms that can be detected in the cerebrospinal fluid and brain aspirates from patients with AIDS. In contrast to the impact of immunohistochemistry and AIDS on the practice of central nervous system cytology, the era of molecular biology is only beginning to have an effect. DNA probes are used routinely to detect some types of viruses, and the polymerase chain reaction has been used on central nervous system specimens to detect immunoglobulin gene rearrangements in lymphoma. With the advent of such tools as fluorescence in situ hybridization and rapid progress toward understanding the molecular events that lead to human neoplasia, we predict that the application of molecular biologic methods to central nervous system specimens will increase markedly in the coming years.

CHAPTER ONE

Introduction, Historical Background, and Cytopreparation

The practice of cytopathology of the central nervous system (CNS) applies general principles of cytopathology to a basic knowledge of neuroanatomy, neuropathology, and clinical neurology and neurosurgery. In this text, we have illustrated a spectrum of neoplastic and non-neoplastic diseases manifested in cerebrospinal fluid (CSF) and in stereotactically directed needle aspirates. We have drawn the gross and histologic counterparts of these lesions from basic neuroanatomy and neuropathology to create a comprehensive picture of the cytopathology of the central nervous system.

Historical Background

Malignant neoplastic cells in CSF were first observed by Dufour[12] in 1904, but, for the next 50 years, only scattered similar observations were reported. Papanicolaou's *Atlas of Exfoliative Cytology* (1954)[54] makes no reference to cytopathology of CSF. In the 1950s, interest in CSF cytopathology was revived. In 1951, Platt[56] reported the application of the Papanicolaou staining method[53] to sediments of CSF. In 1954, Spriggs[65] provided the first major literature review and found 66 acceptable cases of tumor cells in CSF. Of these, 19 were primary intracranial or intraspinal tumors and 47 were metastatic tumors. In 1959, Spriggs and Boddington[66] similarly reviewed the 19 previously reported cases of leukemic cells in CSF.

The next major advances occurred in the area of cytopreparatory techniques, allowing better concentration of the sparse cells of CSF than that achieved with the older methods of centrifugation and wet film preparation. In 1956, Seal[62] reported a method of using a bacteriologic membrane filter made by the Millipore Corporation to concentrate the cellular material from specimens of large liquid volume. McCormick and Coleman[39] were among the first to demonstrate malignant neoplastic cells in cerebrospinal fluid prepared by Millipore® filtration; in 1962 they reported neoplastic cells in 12 cases. Similarly, the Nuclepore® filter was developed in 1964[16] and applied to many types of specimens including CSF.[37,59]

Gravity sedimentation of cells onto slides is an alternative to membrane filter usage. This technique was developed by Schonenberg in 1949,[61] modified by means of a sedimentation chamber by Sayk in 1960,[60] and reported in detail in English by Bots et al[8] in 1964 and Kolar and Zeman in 1968.[33]

The 1960s brought contributions from Naylor[48-50] and Kline,[29,30] both of whom reviewed their experience with neoplastic cells in CSF. These observations, concerning the prevalence of cells in CSF from various primary brain tumors, are among the most valuable statistics available today. In this same decade, the cytocentrifuge[10,70] was developed and applied to CSF.[26] It has subsequently become one of the most widely used methods of cytopreparation.

During the last 30 years, the natural history of acute leukemia, particularly childhood acute lymphocytic leukemia, has changed markedly. The longer life spans achieved with systemic chemotherapy make CNS relapse a significant problem. The observations that meningeal infiltrates could occur in patients with neurologically asymptomatic leukemia[51] and that CSF specimens with normal cell counts (<4 cells/mm) might contain leukemia cells[15,51] have made periodic examination of CSF from leukemia patients one of the major roles of many cytopathology laboratories.

During the last 30 years, the natural history of acute leukemia has changed markedly

CSF cytopathology has become an important diagnostic procedure in patients with metastatic tumors, leukemia, lymphoma, and primary brain tumors with suspected meningeal spread, and in patients presenting initially with signs of meningeal disease of obscure etiology. Recent advances in the treatment of malignancies, with new chemotherapeutic agents and new modalities such as bone marrow transplantation, have made periodic examination of CSF indispensable in following up the course of individual patients from CSF relapse through remission.

Within the past decade, fine needle aspiration biopsy has become widely utilized in the United States for a variety of body sites,[6,17,31,32] including intracranial masses. The use of steroids to control edema[43] and the application of computed tomography–guided stereotaxis[7,23,27,41,64] have resulted in low morbidity and mortality rates for this diagnostic procedure. It has been applied successfully to deep gliomas[23] and to tumors in the pineal[55] and suprasellar regions,[73] and in evaluating posterior fossa masses and spinal cord lesions.[23,52,58]

The development of monoclonal antibody technology[35] and the immunohistochemical application of these reagents to histologic and cytopathologic samples have greatly refined morphologic diagnoses. During the last 10 years, immunohistochemistry of CSF and of fine needle aspirates of CNS lesions has gone from a research technique to a routinely utilized diagnostic procedure. Today, lymphoid markers are commonly applied to specimens of CSF and aspirates of intracranial masses to distinguish lymphoma from lymphocytic reactions.[63] Antibodies against glial fibrillary acid protein (GFAP) cytokeratins and carcinoma-associated antigens are used to differentiate gliomas from metastatic carcinoma.[69] As the spectrum of specific antibodies available for tumor identification continues to broaden, an unlimited potential will exist for improving diagnostic accuracy of specimens from the CNS.

Applications of new diagnostic procedures to CNS specimens are emerging

As newer diagnostic approaches are being developed and applied to cytologic preparations, applications of these procedures to CNS specimens are emerging. Some observers have demonstrated an increased ability to diagnose malignancies involving CSF when flow cytometric ploidy analyses are used in addition to routine cytologic examination. DNA and RNA hybridization techniques are being applied to a variety of cytologic specimens to detect viruses, to determine immunoglobulin gene and T-cell receptor gene rearrangements in lymphoma, and to uncover amplification, increased expression, and rearrangements of oncogenes.[68] Although Southern and Northern blotting, slot blots, and dot blots can be successfully applied to specimens derived by cytologic methods, these approaches are limited by the requirement of relatively large sample sizes. New modifications, such as enzymatic amplification of DNA sequences using the polymerase chain reaction (PCR), have made the detection of point mutations and gene rearrangements possible from only a few cells. This approach is beginning to be applied to cytologic specimens. In addition, in situ hybridization is a basic morphologic method that is readily adapted to smears and cytocentrifuged preparations, and this technique makes detection of herpesvirus and cytomegalovirus possible.

Finally, cytogenetic analysis of neoplastic cells derived from CSF has been successful.[11] Almost 50% of malignant gliomas contain amplification and high-level expression of the c-*erb* B gene, which codes for the epidermal growth factor receptor. A small proportion of these tumors contain amplification of N-*myc* or *gli*. As the clinical significance of these amplifications is defined, evaluation of CSF and brain tumor aspirates for oncogene amplification may become an important diagnostic procedure.

Cytopreparation

Cerebrospinal Fluid

Since the cellular component of CSF obtained from the lumbar area is generally scant, an efficient means of concentrating this material is necessary. The oldest method of cytopreparation utilized for CSF is the smear, or wet film, prepared from centrifuged sediment. Due to the sparse cellularity of CSF, these preparations require relatively large volumes of CSF to produce satisfactory results. Although ventricular fluid is often withdrawn in large quantities, smaller volumes of CSF are obtained by lumbar puncture, especially in children or in patients with suspected intracranial masses. Considerable effort, therefore, has been expended during the past 30 years to develop techniques for concentrating the cellular material from small volumes (0.5–1.0 mL) of CSF. The most commonly utilized methods today are membrane filtration and cytocentrifugation.

The relative merits of various means of cytopreparation continue to be debated. One major consideration studied quantitatively by several authors is the potential for cell loss with some of these techniques. Barrett and King[1] achieved the following cell recovery rates: 81% ± 3% with a Millipore® filter; 64% ± 3% with a Gelman filter; 59% ± 3% with a Nuclepore® filter; and 11% ± 1% with a cytocentrifuged preparation. Dyken et al[13] found a 5% to 72% (mean 25%) cell recovery rate by gravity sedimentation and a 1% to 49% (mean 16%) rate by cytocentrifugation. These studies underscore the serious potential for cell loss with both gravity sedimentation and cytocentrifugation as compared to membrane filtration. This problem has been overcome in some laboratories by modifications in cytopreparatory technique. Whitmore et al[71] achieved a 100% cell recovery rate by cytocentrifugation as determined by hemocytometer counts. The combined technique of sedimentation with Millipore® filtration reported by Kolmel[34] increased cell recovery from 30% with sedimentation alone to a maximum of 90% with this forced sedimentation procedure.

Considerations for selection of cytopreparation techniques include the potential for cell loss, clarity of cellular detail, and spectrum of stains offered

The second major consideration when comparing cytopreparatory techniques is the clarity of cellular detail obtained by a particular method. With regard to Millipore® filters, some observers regard the tendency for overstaining and the green background to be serious disadvantages, particularly if the preparations are to be photographed. Although authors vary in their preferences for techniques, the quality of an individual preparation is generally more dependent on preservation of cells in the sample and excellence of execution of a specific cytopreparatory technique than on choice of method.

A third important consideration is the spectrum of stains offered by each technique. Krentz and Dyken[36] stressed the advantage of sedimentation over membrane filtration when dealing with inflammatory or leukemic cells, since Wright-Giemsa stains can be applied to sedimentation preparations. The cytocentrifuge technique also allows use of virtually all types of fixation and staining, including the preparation of cells for immunohistochemistry, immunofluorescence, and in situ hybridization.

Regardless of the specific cytopreparatory technique used, the sparse cellularity of CSF makes laboratory contamination of these specimens a serious potential hazard. General problems include collection of CSF specimens in contaminated tubes, introduction of contaminating organisms into specimens in the laboratory, and spreading of cellular material from other types of specimens by way of instruments or staining fluids during handling of wet specimens. Each specific method of cytopreparation used in a given laboratory should be examined step by step to identify points of potential problems. Several such pitfalls for Millipore® filters are pointed out in the Cytopreparatory Techniques section of this chapter. Contamination of any type of CSF preparation can occur during staining. We advocate that all staining solutions be changed or filtered prior to staining CSF and that these specimens be stained first, before any other type of specimen.

Excellent cellular recovery and preservation can be obtained using any of these techniques if careful attention to detail in cytopreparation is observed. In our laboratory, Millipore® filtration with fixation in 95%

ethanol and staining by a modified Papanicolaou technique is the standard method of preparation of lumbar puncture or ventricular CSF specimens. In addition, we use cytocentrifugation in cases in which Romanowski staining or immunohistochemistry is indicated. The methods utilized in our laboratory for Millipore® filter preparation and cytocentrifugation of CSF are presented in the Cytopreparatory Techniques section of this chapter.

Stereotactic Biopsies

When dealing with tissue fragments or aspirates obtained stereotactically, the choice of preparatory method in a given case is dependent on the size and consistency of the material obtained. These properties are determined by the inherent nature of the disease process as well as the gauge needle used. Fragments may be processed histologically by embedding in paraffin, sectioning, and staining with the histopathologic stain of choice. For immediate diagnosis, they may be frozen on a cryostat and sectioned. Alternatively, they can be imprinted, smeared or squashed on a slide, air dried or wet fixed, and stained with a variety of stains.[42,52] Smaller fragments or liquid specimens can also be smeared or squashed on a slide or prepared as other liquid specimens by membrane filtration or cytocentrifugation.[18,58]

In our laboratory, large tissue fragments are imprinted and then prepared histologically. Smaller fragments are smeared on slides. Thick liquid specimens are centrifuged, and smears are prepared from the button; thin fluid specimens are prepared by Millipore® filtration and cytocentrifugation. In all cases in which needles are used, their barrels are washed with balanced salt solution, and Millipore® filters and cytocentrifuged slides are prepared.

Immunohistochemistry

Immunoperoxidase technique allows identification of many antigenic substances

The immunoperoxidase technique allows identification of a variety of antigenic substances in histologic and cytologic preparations. It has been used most extensively to identify the surface markers of lymphoid populations,[22,40] polypeptide hormones, and structural and matrix proteins.[14,38,45] This method requires a specific antibody directed against the substance in question and a one-[46,47] or two-step[67] bridge linking the antibody to peroxidase. A reaction is then performed with hydrogen peroxide and diaminobenzidine to give a colored precipitate. Recent modifications include the avidin-biotin complex (ABC) method in which a secondary antibody linked to biotin is used in conjunction with avidin linked to peroxidase. A variation of this procedure is the use of avidin linked to alkaline phosphatase.[72] The actual sequence of steps in these immunohistochemical procedures is relatively standard and uncomplicated (see Cytopreparatory Techniques section).

Successful utilization of the immunoperoxidase technique depends on several important factors. First, the primary antibody or antiserum must be specific for the substance in question, and demonstration of this specificity requires careful attention to appropriate positive and negative controls. Second, antigens vary with respect to the fixation methods required to preserve their ability to react with the antiserum.

Some proteins, such as calcitonin and GFAP, react beautifully following formalin fixation and paraffin embedding of histologic sections. Many of the lymphocyte surface markers, however, are best demonstrated with acetone fixation and/or freezing. Third, each antiserum and monoclonal antibody differs in its titer; therefore, the dilution required for optimal preparations varies considerably among laboratories and among different antisera within the same laboratory. Therefore, each reagent must be titrated to determine the appropriate concentration for its use. Finally, the presence of endogenous peroxide in many tissues and nonspecific background staining may render preparations uninterpretable. These problems can be overcome by using appropriate blocking agents and washing steps, but procedures may have to be individualized for various antisera and tissue types. Smear and cytocentrifuge preparations from virtually any body site lend themselves well to immunohistochemical techniques, because almost any type of fixation can be applied to these slides. The biggest obstacle to the routine application of immunohistochemistry to CSF is the difficulty in acquiring a sufficient volume for the multiple slide preparations necessary to run the appropriate controls. Otherwise, CSF specimens can be handled similarly to other cytologic specimens.

As with needle aspirates from other body sites, stereotactically derived brain aspirates lend themselves readily to immunocytochemical techniques. Antibodies against lymphocyte subset markers are useful in distinguishing lymphoma from reactive conditions, and panels of antibodies are helpful in distinguishing metastases from lymphoma and primary brain tumors.[63,69]

In Situ Hybridization

The basic principle of in situ hybridization is the same as that operating in other types of DNA and RNA hybridization: single-stranded DNA and RNA of complementary sequences hybridize through base pairing, forming double-stranded DNA-DNA, DNA-RNA, and RNA-RNA. This method can be used to detect virtually any sequence for which a probe is available. One major limitation is that the method is relatively insensitive, making it useful only if large amounts of target DNA or RNA are present in the cellular sample. A second problem is that the method is not strictly quantitative. Thus, it can readily demonstrate the presence versus the absence of a particular sequence, but it is more limited in distinguishing quantitative differences in the amount of the target gene or transcript. A third consideration is that the most sensitive methods require radiolabelled probes and autoradiography. ^{32}P produces a signal with sufficient strength for development within hours or a few days. The signal is too diffuse, however, to be resolved to single cells. ^{3}H and ^{35}S can be used with an autoradiographic emulsion, and the resultant fine grains produce cellular localization. Unfortunately, these isotopes usually require several weeks of exposure time. Recently, methods have been developed using biotinylated probes. This approach circumvents the need for special facilities for isotope handling and can be executed in less than 24 hours. The major disadvantage is that it is less sensitive than the isotopic methods and at the present time can only detect sequences that are present in large numbers.

In situ hybridization can detect virtually any sequence for which a probe is available

Electron Microscopy

Optimal preparation of specimens for study by electron microscopy requires the following: (1) rapid fixation of well-preserved cells in an appropriate fixative (most commonly glutaraldehyde); (2) viewing of the preparation by light microscopy to select the cells of interest; and (3) removal of the chosen cells for plastic embedding and preparation of ultrathin sections on viewing grids. In our laboratory, we have used smears from sputum,[25] cytocentrifuged fine needle aspirates, and filtered CSF,[28] followed by immediate immersion in 3% glutaraldehyde and Papanicolaou staining. The cells of interest were identified and marked with a diamond pen. The coverslip was then removed, the specimen was destained and embedded in Epon®, and ultrathin sections were prepared. This method has been reported previously[25] and is outlined in detail in the Cytopreparatory Techniques section. Our laboratory has no experience with preparation of cytologic specimens for scanning electron microscopy, but Becker et al[3] have reported a method using Papanicolaou-stained specimens.

Cell Culture

Observation of the morphology of cultured cells is an important component in studying their behavior. Although visualization of the unstained, living cells is the most practical method for day-to-day observation, the need occasionally arises for more permanent morphologic preparations.

Two general cytopreparatory methods have been reported for this purpose. First, cultured cells can be grown on sterile slides or coverslips, followed by washing, fixing, and staining, by a number of methods varying from formalin fixation and hematoxylin and eosin (H&E) staining[9] to air drying and Wright-Giemsa staining. We have found that fixation in 95% ethanol followed by Papanicolaou staining yields crisp cellular detail for evaluation of overall growth pattern[4] and nuclear detail.[5,57] Alternatively, cells can be trypsinized, centrifuged, or cytocentrifuged and stained. This technique yields cells that are similar to the rounded-up cells seen in effusions.[2,24]

Cell cultures provide a means of demonstrating morphologic characteristics for correlation

Regardless of the specific method used, cytologic preparations of cultured cells provide a means of demonstrating their morphologic characteristics for correlation with their other biologic and functional characteristics. In addition, cultured cells are useful as controls for a variety of special procedures such as immunohistochemistry and in situ hybridization since infinite quantities of identical cellular preparations can be obtained.

Cytopreparatory Techniques

1.1 Millipore® Filtration

Excellent recovery and display of cells in CSF can be obtained if Millipore® filters are properly prepared and stained. The following technique has proven to be very satisfactory and reproducible.

A wall vacuum may be used, but it must be monitored with a gauge to ensure that the pressure does not exceed 100 mm Hg negative pressure. An alternate approach is to use a vacuum pump such as the one marketed by the Millipore Corporation.[19,44] A side-arm Erlenmeyer flask, set in a shallow tray to catch the residue, is an adequate filtration funnel holder; however, for a laboratory doing a large number of filters, a three-place manifold is more practical.[19,44]

Procedure

1. Using an indelible ballpoint pen, write the last three digits of the specimen number twice on the filter border (type SM 47-mm, 5-μm, pore-size filter).
2. Immerse the filter into a Petri dish of 95% ethyl alcohol and let it expand for at least 10 seconds.
3. Insert the frit apparatus into the filtration funnel holder (either flask or manifold), place the pre-expanded filter on the frit, and secure it with the companion funnel.
4. With the vacuum off, pour balanced salt solution into the funnel to establish a reservoir of about 5 cm in depth.
5. Apply vacuum pressure and add the CSF to the reservoir of balanced salt solution.
6. Rinse the CSF collection vial with balanced salt solution and add to the reservoir. Do not let the reservoir depth drop below 1 cm.
7. Fix the cells by adding, from a plastic squeeze bottle, a fine jet of 95% ethyl alcohol around the inside of the funnel and continue filtration.
8. Break the vacuum when a shallow pool (⅛ inch) remains over the filter and allow the filter to fix for at least 30 seconds. Be absolutely sure that the liquid is always covering the filter, as cells will be destroyed if the filter is permitted to air dry.
9. Remove the funnel and, using Millipore® forceps, remove the filter and immediately submerge in the Petri dish of 95% ethyl alcohol.
10. Fix the filter in 95% ethyl alcohol for 15 to 20 minutes before staining.
11. The filter and frit apparatus should be soaked and washed in a soapy solution containing Clorox®. To provide good circulation of stains and solutions through the filters during staining, the filters should not be clipped to 3 x 1-in microslides. Instead, they should be taken through the staining sequence with a special holder (Gelman) clipped to a polypropylene mount with a 42-mm diameter circle cut out or resuspended from applicator sticks with a Bulldog clip on the border of the filter. We prefer to use the polypropylene mount, which can then be placed in a regular staining rack.

The two most common errors in this procedure are (1) allowing the reservoir of fluid to completely drain, which results in air drying, and (2) using a vacuum that is too strong or leaving the vacuum on too long, which distorts the cells.

All solutions must be filtered or replaced before staining CSF specimens

Cross-contamination is a serious potential problem when dealing with membrane filter preparations of CSF. We recommend that all solutions in the staining set-up be filtered or replaced before staining any CSF specimens. They can then be stained together before any other types of specimens are stained.

1.2 Shandon® Centrifugation

The Shandon® cytocentrifuge can be used for preparing CSF for cytopathologic evaluation. The following idiosyncrasies related to the operation of the original model of this instrument must be counteracted to ensure good preparations: (1) cells are inherently lost into the filter paper that is part of the filtration assembly; (2) only material in the horizontal cylinder of the filter apparatus ever reaches the slide; and (3) the cytocentrifuge has a cover lock that prohibits removal of the head shield from the rotor for a minimum of 30 seconds following completion of the spinning, thereby increasing the chances for air drying to occur. Although the Cytospin II® has largely overcome these limitations, the following procedures (developed by Gary Gill, Johns Hopkins Hospital) address these problems and can be applied to the older model.

Procedure

1. Load the rotor as follows:
   a. Wet the area around the hole in the blotter with 1 or 2 drops of balanced salt solution.
   b. Assemble and align the specimen chamber, blotter, and slide.
   c. Seat the assembly in the rotor. To minimize cell loss, it is absolutely essential that the assembly be properly seated. Press chamber, blotter, and slide to the bottom of the rotor. Press chamber assembly flat against blotter and slide, making sure that the whole assembly is flat against the outside rotor wall. It is best to look down onto the top of the completed assembly to make sure that everything is properly aligned and flat.
   d. The specimen chamber (horizontal cylindrical portion) holds 20 drops and must be completely filled for proper operation. Using a Pasteur pipette, place 2 drops of balanced salt solution into the horizontal chamber by holding the tip of the pipette at the base of the cone. Add up to 18 drops of CSF behind the balanced salt solution. If a quantity of 18 drops of CSF is not available, fill the remainder of the chamber with balanced salt solution. If the specimen is to be alcohol fixed and Papanicolaou stained, add 1 to 2 drops of 95% ethyl alcohol behind either the 18 drops of specimen or the second round of drops of balanced salt solution. If the CSF specimens are to be air dried for Romanowski staining, do not add the 95% ethanol to the specimen chamber but rather fill the horizontal cylinder with specimen and balanced salt solution only.
   e. If the material does not move to the slide and blotter assembly, seat a dropper bulb into the cone and squeeze. This applies sufficient air pressure to force the specimen so that absorption can begin.
   f. Press a closure cap on each specimen chamber.
   g. Check to make sure the assembly is properly seated.
   h. Set the head shield in place.
   i. Centrifuge at 1,500 rpm for 5 to 7 minutes.
2. Remove the slides from the cytocentrifuge as follows:
   a. For air-dried slides: Remove each assembly from rotor, discard filter paper, and rapidly wave slide to dry.

b. For alcohol-fixed (95% ethyl alcohol) slides: Remove the slide from the cytocentrifuge as rapidly as possible. Since the head shield is locked in place for 30 seconds, air drying may occur unless you break that connection. The most satisfactory procedure to perform is as follows: (1) unplug the cytocentrifuge from the wall socket, which releases the head shield as soon as the tachometer indicates that spinning has stopped; and (2) remove the head shield and each filter assembly in turn. Immediately place the slide in a Coplin jar of 95% ethyl alcohol and discard the filter paper.

3. Slides can be stained by either the Papanicolaou or the Romanowski method.

Important steps to minimize cell loss in the cytocentrifuge include: (1) wetting the area around the hole in the blotter with 1 or 2 drops of balanced salt solution; (2) properly seating the assembly; and (3) completely filling the horizontal cylindrical portion of the chamber.

1.3 Imprints and Smears

Crisp imprints of tissue fragments can be made by blotting the tissue to remove blood and fluid. The tissue is then lightly touched many times quickly to the surface of a clean glass microscopic slide. The slide is rapidly immersed in 95% ethanol for Papanicolaou staining or air dried for Romanowski staining. For smear preparations of needle aspirates, the material is expressed onto a frosted slide and smeared with the needle before rapid ethanol immersion. Alternately, the expressed material can be squashed between two slides and pulled, as in the preparation of bone marrow or peripheral blood slides.

Cyst fluids or needle washings are processed by Millipore® filtration as described for CSF.

1.4 Modified Papanicolaou Stain

All Millipore® filters and alcohol-fixed microslides prepared in our laboratory are stained with the modified Papanicolaou technique developed by Gill.[20,21] The formulae for preparing the stains are given below. The working solutions of these stains are also commercially available from Poly-Sciences and Lerner Laboratories.

1.4A Preparation of Stains

Hematoxylin.—Combine the following ingredients together in a magnetic mixer at room temperature and stir for 1 hour:

Distilled water	730 mL
Ethylene glycol	250 mL
Hematoxylin, anhydrous, certified (C.I. [color index] No 75290)	2.0 g
Sodium iodate	0.2 g
Aluminum sulfate $(Al_2SO_4)_3$ + 18 H_2O	17.6 g
Glacial acetic acid	20.0 mL

This stain can be used immediately after preparation and is stable for over a year. The staining times may need to be adjusted for freshly prepared stain, but 2 minutes in the hematoxylin is adequate for stains that are 1 week old or more. The stain is a progressive staining hematoxylin and requires no differentiation.

SCOTT'S TAP WATER SUBSTITUTE.—The bluing agent used in the staining sequence is Scott's tap water substitute. To prepare a liter of this agent, dissolve the following:

Magnesium sulfate ($MgSO_4$)	10 g
Sodium bicarbonate	20 g
Tap water	1 L

1.4B Preparation of Counterstains

The percentage dye content must be considered when preparing counterstains

In preparing the counterstains, orange G (OG-6) and eosin polychrome (EA), the percentage dye content must be taken into consideration. The percentage dye content is printed on the label of the dye containers. The formulae that follow call for 100% dye content, and the commercially available dyes contain impurities. The orange G dye may be only 80% actual dye, whereas the light-green yellowish or eosin Y may be 65% or 85%. It is essential to calculate the amount of dye stuff needed to achieve 100% content.[21] For example, if a commercial preparation of orange G is 85% actual dye/g of dye stuff and the formula calls for 9.05 g of orange G, it will require 10.6 g of dye stuff to yield 9.05 g of dye.

ORANGE G STAIN.—Prepare a 0.2 M orange G (C.I. No 16230) aqueous stock solution by dissolving 9.05 g of orange G in distilled water up to 100 mL in a volumetric flask. To prepare a working orange G solution, combine the following ingredients:

0.2 M orange G aqueous stock solution	20 mL
Phosphotungstic acid	1.0 g
95% Ethyl alcohol	970 mL
Glacial acetic acid	10 mL

The staining solution should be filtered before use.

EOSIN POLYCHROME (EA) STAIN.—Prepare the following aqueous stock solutions by dissolving the dyes in distilled water at 70 °C to 80 °C in 100-mL volumetric flasks. Be sure to correct for dye content.

0.05 M Light green SF yellowish stock solution (C.I. No 42095)	3.96 g
0.30 M Eosin Y (C.I. No 45380)	20.80 g

To prepare a working EA solution, combine the following ingredients:

0.05 M Light green SF yellowish stock solution	10 mL
0.30 M Eosin Y stock solution	20 mL
Phosphotungstic acid	2.0 g
95% Ethyl alcohol	700 mL
Absolute methyl alcohol	250 mL
Glacial acetic acid	20 mL

The staining solution should be filtered before use.

1.4C Procedure for Staining Millipore® Filters

The filters should be dipped gently in each container of solution and drained well before moving on to the next container.

Tap water	10 dips
Tap water	10 dips
Hematoxylin	2 minutes
Tap water	10 dips
Tap water	10 dips
HCl	1 minute or until filter becomes yellow
Tap water	10 dips
Tap water	10 dips
Scott's tap water substitute	1 minute or until filter becomes blue
Tap water	10 dips
95% Ethyl alcohol	1 minute
95% Ethyl alcohol	1 minute
Modified OG-6	1 minute
95% Ethyl alcohol	1 minute
95% Ethyl alcohol	1 minute
Modified EA	8 minutes
95% Ethyl alcohol	4 minutes
95% Ethyl alcohol	2 minutes
95% Ethyl alcohol	1 minute
Absolute isopropyl alcohol	1 minute
Absolute isopropyl alcohol	1 minute
Xylene	1 minute
Xylene	1 minute
Xylene	At least 15 minutes (until coverslipped)

Each rack of slides should be drained and blotted between each staining dish. They should be blotted on clean paper towels before going from the last dish of 95% ethyl alcohol into the container of absolute alcohol.

All tap water containers should be changed between each rack of slides. Dip the filters very gently to avoid loss of cells during staining. In instances in which minutes are stated in the formula, do not dip the racks but rather place them in the container of the solution for the specified period. Hematoxylin should be changed at the end of each month or sooner if the solution becomes purple. Orange G and EA should be changed every 2 weeks.

Tap water containers should be changed between each slide rack

1.4D Procedure for Slides

To prepare slides, perform the following steps:

Tap water	10 dips
Tap water	10 dips
Hematoxylin	2 minutes
Tap water	10 dips
Tap water	10 dips
Hematoxylin	2 minutes
Tap water	10 dips
Tap water	10 dips

Scott's tap water substitute	1 minute
Tap water	10 dips
Tap water	10 dips
95% Ethyl alcohol	10 dips
95% Ethyl alcohol	10 dips
Modified OG-6	1 minute
95% Ethyl alcohol	10 dips
95% Ethyl alcohol	10 dips
95% Ethyl alcohol	10 dips
Absolute ethyl alcohol	10 dips
Absolute ethyl alcohol	10 dips
Absolute ethyl alcohol	10 dips
Xylene	10 dips
Xylene	10 dips
Xylene	At least 15 minutes (until coverslipped)

1.5 Romanowski Stain

Romanowski is for differential staining in hematology

The air-dried, cytocentrifuged preparations of CSF are stained with the Diff-Quik® stain manufactured by Harleco. This stain is for differential staining in hematology and gives results similar to that seen with a Wright-Giemsa stain. The three-part fixation and staining operation is fast, simple, and provides delicate staining of the blood cells present.

1.6 Coverslips for Millipore® Filters

Millipore® filters (47-mm size) must be cut in half and trimmed before mounting on a 3 x 1-in microslide. It is also important to replace the xylene retained in the pores of the filters with mounting medium so that the filters do not dry out. The following procedure has proven satisfactory in our laboratory.

1. Pour a small amount of mounting medium (Permount®, Kleermount®, or Eukit®) into an aluminum foil milk-testing dish.
2. Remove the stained and cleared filter from the staining holder or Bulldog clip and place it cell-side-up on a small piece of paper towel.
3. Using clean scissors, trim the border away from the cellular area of the filter, making sure that you retain the accession number on the filter.
4. Cut the filter in half between the two sets of numbers and immerse these cut filters in the milk-testing dish.
5. Let the filters soak in the mounting medium for a minimum of 5 minutes.
6. Using Millipore® forceps, lift the filter out of the mounting medium and let it drain until just a drop of mounting medium clings to the filter.
7. Gently place the filter on a 3 x 1-in microslide, being careful to avoid trapping any air bubbles under the filter. (It is most satisfactory to roll the filter onto the slide.)
8. Place a 50 x 24-mm No 1 coverslip over the filter without using any extra mounting medium, and, again if possible, avoid trapping any air bubbles.

9. Place the slide flat on a tray, and the mounting medium will gradually fill in under the coverslip.
10. Dip the scissors into xylene and carefully wipe with gauze to remove any cells that might have come off the filter.
11. Dispose of the milk-testing dish and mounting medium.

It is best to let the filters cure for a few hours before examining them under the microscope. This allows the mounting medium to settle and the coverslip to be more firmly in place for ease in dotting.

Let the filters cure before microscopic examination

After the filters have been examined microscopically, it is best to place them in an oven set to 70 °C drying for 24 hours and then file them horizontally for a month before they are placed in a vertical slide file. If they are filed too soon, the mounting medium will ooze out from the slides and cause them to stick together.

1.7 Electron Microscopy

1. Prepare smear or Cytospin® slides with immediate fixation in 3% glutaraldehyde for 15 to 30 minutes.
2. Stain with Papanicolaou stain.
3. Select appropriate cells for electron microscopy and mark slide with diamond pen.
4. Remove coverslip with xylol.
5. Rehydrate in graded alcohols (100%, 95%, 75%, and 35%) for 3 minutes each.
6. Wash in sucrose buffer for 3 minutes, three times. Refix with 4% glutaraldehyde for 5 minutes. Rinse with sucrose buffer.
7. Postfix in 1% osmium tetroxide for 30 minutes.
8. Stain with buffered uranyl acetate for 10 minutes.
9. Dehydrate in graded alcohols (35%, 70%, 95%, and 100% two times) for 3 minutes each.
10. Immerse in propylene oxide for 3 minutes, two times.
11. Flood slide with 50/50 propylene oxide/Epon® for 10 minutes. Then flood slide with pure Epon® for 3 minutes, three times. Place in an oven set to 60 °C for 12 hours.
12. Strip Epon® film from slide with hot water.
13. Excise area of interest, re-embed in a propolymerized block, and place in oven set to 90 °C for 30 minutes.
14. Cut thin sections on an ultramicrotome and stain with uranyl acetate and lead citrate.

1.8 Avidin-Biotin Complex Immunoperoxidase Staining

1. Prepare at least one test slide, one negative control slide, and one positive control slide. These slides can be smears or cytocentrifuged slides. The type of fixative and time of fixation are variable and depend largely on the stability of the antigen. We generally use acetone at 4 °C until ready for use.
2. To block endogenous peroxidase, incubate for 30 minutes at room temperature in methanol with 0.3% hydrogen peroxide (2 mL of 30% H_2O_2 in 200 mL of methanol).

3. Rinse in 0.01 M Dulbecco's phosphate-buffered saline (PBS), pH 7.2 to 7.4, for 5 minutes, two times.
4. To reduce nonspecific background staining, incubate with 10% normal serum diluted in PBS for 30 minutes at room temperature. This serum should be from the same species as the secondary antiserum (eg, normal goat serum [NGS]).
5. If the cellular material covers only a small portion of the slide, encircle it with a ring of petroleum jelly. Incubate with primary antiserum (rabbit) diluted with 10% NGS for 18 hours at 4 °C (final 2 hours at room temperature); alternately incubate for 2 hours at 37 °C. (We generally have found the longer incubation to produce better results.) The dilution of the primary antiserum varies considerably among antisera. The order of magnitude is generally 1:1,000 to 1:10,000.
   The best negative control is the primary antiserum that has been absorbed with the purified antigen. If this absorbed control is not available, normal serum from the species in which the primary antiserum was prepared can be substituted. For monoclonal antibodies, an irrelevant antibody of the same isotype is used.
6. Rinse in PBS for 5 minutes, two times.
7. Incubate with a biotinylated secondary antiserum (Zymed), goat anti-mouse Ig 1:40, diluted with 5% NGS for 30 minutes at 37 °C.
8. Rinse in PBS for 5 minutes, two times.
9. Block endogenous peroxidase for 1 minute at room temperature with methanol containing 0.3% H_2O_2.
10. Rinse in PBS for 5 minutes, two times.
11. Incubate with 1:300 dilution of horseradish peroxidase-streptavidin (Zymed).
12. Rinse in PBS for 5 minutes, two times.
13. Treat with 0.02% 3-amino-9-ethyl carbazole and 0.01% H_2O_2 for 10 minutes.
14. Rinse in water.
15. Counterstain in hematoxylin or methyl green for about 30 seconds.
16. Rinse in water.
17. Dip in ammonia water (2 drops of concentrated ammonia in about 200 mL) if using hematoxylin (optional).
18. Rinse in water.
19. To dehydrate, place in 95% ethanol for 2 to 3 minutes, two times; 100% ethanol for 2 to 3 minutes, two times; xylene for 10 to 15 minutes; and xylene until petroleum jelly is dissolved.
20. Mount with Permount®.

References

1. Barrett DL, King EB: Comparison of cellular recovery rates and morphologic detail obtained using membrane filter and cytocentrifuge techniques. *Acta Cytol* 20:174–180, 1976.
2. Bean MA, Hajdu SI: Cytologic characterization of human tumor cells from monolayer cultures. In: Fogh J, ed. *Human Tumor Cells In Vitro.* New York, NY, Plenum Press, 1975, pp. 333–358.

3. Becker SN, Wong JY, Marchiondo AA, Davis CP: Scanning electron microscopy of alcohol-fixed cytopathology specimens. *Acta Cytol* 25:578–584, 1981.

4. Bigner DD, Bigner SH, Ponten JN, Westermark B, Mahaley MS Jr, Ruoslahti E, Herschman H, Eng LF, Wikstrand CJ: Heterogeneity of genotypic and phenotypic characteristics of fifteen permanent cell lines derived from human gliomas. *J Neuropathol Exp Neurol* 40:201–229, 1981.

5. Bigner SH, Bullard DE, Pegram CN, Wikstrand CJ, Bigner DD: Relationship of in vitro morphologic and growth characteristics of established human glioma–derived cell lines to their tumorigenicity in athymic nude mice. *J Neuropathol Exp Neurol* 40:390–409, 1981.

6. Bodo M, Dobrossy L, Sinkovics I, Tarjan G, Daubner K: Fine-needle biopsy of thyroid gland. *J Surg Oncol* 12:289–297, 1979.

7. Boethius J, Collins VP, Edner G, Lewander R, Jajicek J: Stereotactic biopsies and computer tomography in gliomas. *Acta Neurochir* 40:223–232, 1978.

8. Bots GTAM, Went LN, Schaberg A: Results of a sedimentation technique for cytology of cerebrospinal fluid. *Acta Cytol* 8:234–241, 1964.

9. Bullard DE, Bigner SH, Bigner DD: The morphologic response of cell lines derived from human gliomas dibutyryl adenosine 3':5'-cyclic monophosphate. *J Neuropathol Exp Neurol* 40:231–246, 1981.

10. Dore CF, Balfour BM: A device for preparing cell spreads. *Immunology* 9:403–405, 1965.

11. Dosik H, Rodriguez J, Verma RS: Cytogenetic studies of blast cells in the cerebrospinal fluid in meningeal leukemia. *Cancer Genet Cytogenet* 12:89–91, 1984.

12. Dufour H: Miningite sarcomateuse diffuse avec envahissement de la moelle et des racines. Cytologie positive et speciale du liquide cphalo-rachidien. *Rev Neurol* 12:104–106, 1904.

13. Dyken PR, Shirley S, Trefz J, El Gammal T: Comparison of cytocentrifugation and sedimentation techniques for CSF cytomorphology. *Acta Cytol* 24:167–170, 1980.

14. Eng LF, Rubinstein LJ: Contribution of immunohistochemistry to diagnostic problems of human cerebral tumor. *J Histochem Cytochem* 26:513–522, 1978.

15. Evans DIK: CSF in acute childhood leukaemia: cytocentrifuge studies. *Arch Dis Child* 49:496, 1974.

16. Fleischer RL, Price PB, Symes EM: Novel filter for biological materials. *Science* 143:249–250, 1964.

17. Frable WJ: Thin-needle aspiration biopsy: a personal experience with 469 cases. *Am J Clin Pathol* 65:168–182, 1976.

18. Frederiksen P, Knudsen V, Reske-Nielsen E: Diagnostic aid of aspiration biopsy cytology in brain lesions. *Neurochirurgia* 22: 229–235, 1979.

19. Gill GW: Exfoliative Cytology. Application Report 24. Bedford, MA, Millipore Corporation, 1969.

20. Gill GW, Frost JK, Miller KA: A new formula for a half-oxidized hematoxylin solution that neither overstains nor requires differentiation. *Acta Cytol* 18:300–311, 1974.

21. Gill GW, Miller KA: *Laboratory Cytopathology Techniques for Specimen Preparation.* Baltimore, MD, Division of Cytopathology, Department of Pathology, The Johns Hopkins University School of Medicine, 1973.

22. Goodson JD, Strauss GM: Diagnosis of lymphomatous leptomeningitis by cerebrospinal fluid lymphocyte cell surface markers. *Am J Med* 66:1057–1059, 1979.

23. Hahn JF, Levy WJ, Weinstein MJ: Needle biopsy of intracranial lesions guided by computerized tomography. *Neurosurgery* 5:11–15, 1979.

24. Hajdu SI, Bean MA, Fogh J, Hajdu EO, Ricci A: Papanicolaou smear of cultured human tumor cells. *Acta Cytol* 18:327–332, 1974.

25. Hamilton CW, Bigner SH, Wells SA Jr, Johnston WW: Metastatic medullary carcinoma of the thyroid in sputum: a light and electron microscopic study. *Acta Cytol* 27:49–53, 1983.

26. Hansen HH, Bender RA, Shelton BJ: The cytocentrifuge and cerebrospinal fluid cytology. *Acta Cytol* 18:259–262, 1974.

27. Heath RG, John S, Foss O: Stereotaxic biopsy: a method for the study of discrete brain regions of animals and man. *Arch Neurol* 4:291–300, 1961.

28. Johnston WW, Ginn FL, Amatulli JM: Light and electron microscopic observations on malignant cells in cerebrospinal fluid from metastatic alveolar cell carcinoma. *Acta Cytol* 15:365–371, 1971.

29. Kline TS: Cytological examination of the cerebrospinal fluid. *Cancer* 15:591–597, 1962.

30. Kline TS: Cytology of nervous tissue. In: Minckler J, ed. *Pathology of the Nervous System*, vol 1. New York, NY, McGraw-Hill Book Co, 1968, pp. 234–240.

31. Kline TS: Fine-needle aspiration biopsy: past, present, future. *Arch Pathol Lab Med* 104:117, 1980.

32. Kline TS, Neal HS: Needle aspiration biopsy: a critical appraisal. Eight years and 3267 specimens later. *JAMA* 239:36–39, 1978.

33. Kolar O, Zeman W: Spinal fluid cytomorphology: description of apparatus, technique and findings. *Arch Neurol* 18:44–51, 1968.

34. Kolmel HW: A method for concentrating cerebrospinal fluid cells. *Acta Cytol* 21:154–157, 1977.

35. Koprowski H, Steplewski A, Herlyn D, Herlyn M: Study of antibodies against human malignant melanoma produced by somatic cell hybrids. *Proc Natl Acad Sci* 75:3405–3409, 1978.

36. Krentz MJ, Dyken PR: Cerebrospinal fluid cytomorphology: sedimentation vs. filtration. *Arch Neurol* 26:253–257, 1972.

37. McAlpine LL, Ellsworth B: A modified membrane filter technic for cytodiagnosis. *Am J Clin Pathol* 52:242–244, 1969.

38. McComb RD, Jones TR, Pizzo SV, Bigner DD: Specificity and sensitivity of immunohistochemical detection of factor VIII/von Willebrand factor antigen in formalin-fixed paraffin-embedded tissue. *J Histochem Cytochem* 30:371–377, 1982.

39. McCormick WF, Coleman SA: A membrane filter technique for cytology of spinal fluid. *Am J Clin Pathol* 38:191–197, 1962.

40. Mann RB, Jaffe ES, Braylan RC, Eggleston JC, Ransom L, Kaizer H, Berard CW: Immunologic and morphologic studies on T-cell lymphoma. *Am J Med* 58:307–313, 1975.

41. Maroon JC, Bank WO, Drayer BP, Rosenbaum AE: Intracranial biopsy assisted by computerized tomography. *J Neurosurg* 46:740–744, 1977.

42. Marshall LF, Adams H, Doyle D, Graham DI: The histological accuracy of the smear technique for neurosurgical biopsies. *J Neurosurg* 39:82–88, 1973.

43. Marshall LF, Jennett B, Langfitt TW: Needle biopsy for the diagnosis of malignant glioma. *JAMA* 228:1417–1418, 1974.

44. *Millipore Catalogue and Purchasing Guide.* Bedford, MA, Millipore Corporation, 1979.

45. Nadji M: The potential value of immunoperoxidase techniques in diagnostic cytology. *Acta Cytol* 24:442–447, 1980.

46. Nakane PK, Kawaoi A: Peroxidase-labeled antibody: a new method of conjugation. *J Histochem Cytochem* 22:1084–1091, 1974.

47. Nakane PK, Pierce GB Jr: Enzyme-labeled antibodies: preparation and application for localization of antigens. *J Histochem Cytochem* 14:929–931, 1966.

48. Naylor B: Cytologic study of intracranial fluids. *Acta Cytol* 5:198–202, 1961.

49. Naylor B: An exfoliative cytologic study of intracranial fluids. *Neurology* 11:198–202, 1961.

50. Naylor B: The cytologic diagnosis of cerebrospinal fluid. *Acta Cytol* 8:141–149, 1964.

51. Nies BA, Malmgren RA, Chu EW, Del Vecchio PR, Thomas LB, Freireich EJ: Cerebrospinal fluid cytology in patients with acute leukemia. *Cancer* 18:1385–1391, 1965.

52. Ostertag CB, Mennel HD, Kiessling M: Stereotactic biopsy of brain tumors. *Surg Neurol* 14:275–283, 1980.

53. Papanicolaou GN: New procedure for staining vaginal smears. *Science* 95:438–439, 1942.

54. Papanicolaou GN: *Atlas of Exfoliative Cytology.* Cambridge, MA, Harvard University Press, 1954.

55. Pecker J, Scarabin JM, Vallee B, Brucher JM: Treatment in tumors of the pineal region: value of stereotaxic biopsy. *Surg Neurol* 12:341–348, 1979.

56. Platt WR: Exfoliative-cell diagnosis of central nervous system lesions. *Arch Neurol Psychiatry* 66:119–144, 1951.

57. Preissig SH, Pegram CN, Bigner DD: Cytopathologic characteristics of permanent cell lines derived from anaplastic gliomas. *Acta Cytol* 23:412–419, 1979.

58. Quencer RM: Needle aspiration of intramedullary and intradural extramedullary masses of the spinal canal. *Radiology* 134:115–126, 1980.

59. Reynaud AJ, King EB: A new filter for diagnostic cytology. *Acta Cytol* 11:289–294, 1967.

60. Sayk J: *Cytologie der Cerebrospinal Flussigkeit; Ergebnisse Vergleichender Untersuchungen.* Jena Gustav Fischer, 1960, pp. 42–43.

61. Schonenberg H: Eine einfache methode zur herstellung gut differenzierbarer liquorzellpraparate. *Dtsch Med Wochenschr* 74:881, 1949.

62. Seal SH: A method for concentrating cancer cells suspended in large quantities of fluid. *Cancer* 9:866–868, 1956.

63. Sherman ME, Erozan YS, Mann RB, Kumar AAJ, McArthur JC, Royal W, Uematsu S, Nautar HJW: Diagnosis of lymphoma by CT-guided stereotactic brain biopsy. *Acta Cytol* 34:722, 1990.

64. Spiegel EA, Wycis HT, Marks M, Lee AJ: Stereotaxic apparatus for operations on the human brain. *Science* 106:349–350, 1947.

65. Spriggs AI: Malignant cells in cerebrospinal fluid. *J Clin Pathol* 7:122–130, 1954.

66. Spriggs AI, Boddington MM: Leukaemic cells in cerebrospinal fluid. *Br J Haematol* 5:83–91, 1959.

67. Sternberger LA, Hardy PH Jr, Cuculis JJ, Meyer HG: The unlabeled antibody enzyme method of immunohistochemistry preparation and properties of soluble antigen-antibody complex (horseradish peroxidase-antihorseradish peroxidase) and its use in identification of spirochetes. *J Histochem Cytochem* 18:315–333, 1970.

68. Szporn AH, Clarke H, Stranchen J, Fasy TM, Gribetz A, Deligdisch L, Heller D, Dottino P: Primary "liquid lymphoma": effusion cytology and diagnosis by gene rearrangement studies. *Acta Cytol* 34:724–725, 1990.

69. Vick WW, Wikstrand CJ, Bullard DE, Kemshead J, Coakham HB, Schlom J, Johnston WW, Bigner DD, Bigner SH: The use of a panel of monoclonal antibodies in the evaluation of cytologic specimens from the central nervous system. *Acta Cytol* 31:815–824, 1987.

70. Watson P: A slide centrifuge: an apparatus for concentrating cells in suspension onto a microscope slide. *J Lab Clin Med* 68:494–501, 1966.

71. Whitmore EL, Hochberg F, Wolfson L, Royalty J, Taft PD: Quantitative cytocentrifugation in the evaluation of cerebrospinal fluid (CSF). *Acta Cytol* 26:847–850, 1982.

72. Yam LT, English MC, Janckila AJ, Ziesmer S, Li CY: Immunocytochemistry of cerebrospinal fluid. *Acta Cytol* 31:825–833, 1987.

73. Zaharopoulos P, Wong JY: Cytology of common primary midline brain tumors. *Acta Cytol* 24:384–390, 1980.

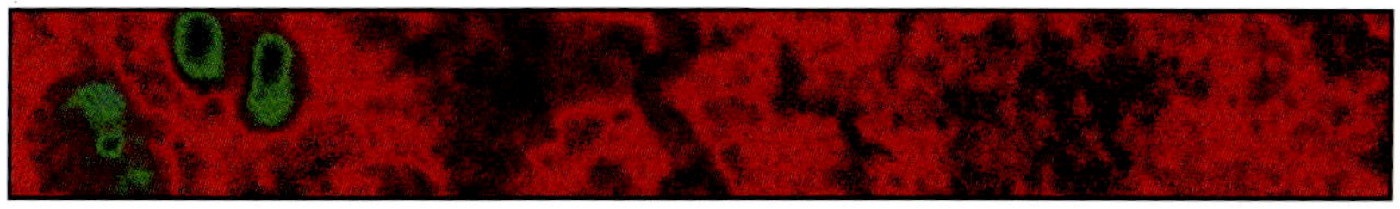

CHAPTER TWO

Neuroanatomy, Normal Cells, and Contaminants in CSF

The subarachnoid space (SAS) is a fluid-filled cavity that covers the brain and spinal cord and communicates with the internal ventricles of the brain (Figure 2.1). It is bound externally by a fine arachnoid membrane and internally by the pial surface of the brain, and normally contains only blood vessels and strands of connective tissue (Image 2.1). Cerebrospinal fluid (CSF) is produced by the choroid plexus, which is located in the floors of the lateral ventricles (Figure 2.2) and roofs of the third and fourth ventricles. The CSF travels from the lateral ventricles through the third ventricle and the cerebral aqueduct and into the fourth ventricle (Figure 2.3) and passes out of the ventricular system at the base of the brain and into the SAS by means of the foramina of Luschka and Magendie (Figure 2.4).

Cerebrospinal Fluid

Although CSF is theoretically acellular, small numbers of lymphocytes and occasional monocytes are seen in most CSF samples (Image 2.2). Counts of less than 5 to 10 cells per mm^3 are considered to be normal in the adult based on evaluations of samples from patients in whom no neurologic disorder was found, as well as from patients with seizures and those undergoing myelography. Slightly higher cell counts may be

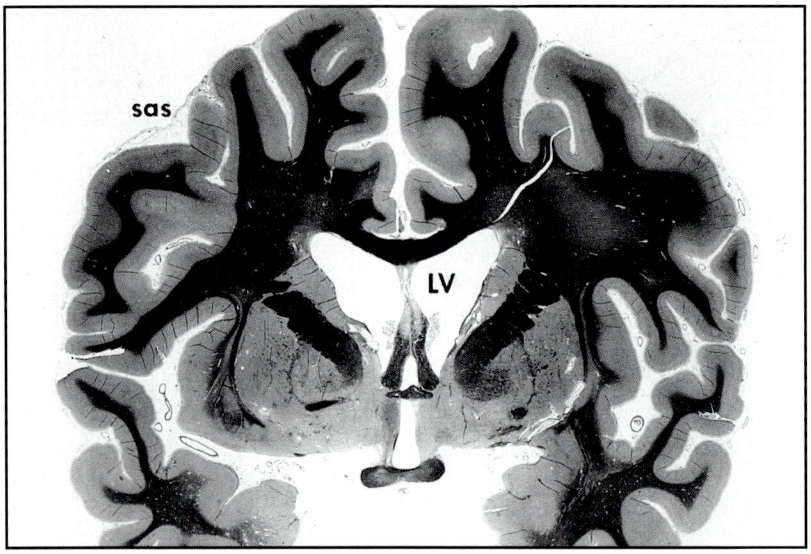

Figure 2.1
Coronal section of a normal brain demonstrates the subarachnoid space (sas). The lateral ventricles (LV) are lined by the ependyma and contain the choroid plexus (H&E, Luxol fast blue, 7X).

seen in neonates, although opportunities to examine fluid from neurologically uninvolved individuals in this age group occur infrequently.

Lumbar puncture fluid is obtained from the spinal SAS (Figure 2.5). The SAS is lined externally by the arachnoid membrane, which is composed of a single layer of flat, meningothelial cells (Image 2.1). The arachnoid membrane of normal individuals sometimes contains focal proliferations of these cells, which are termed meningothelial rests (Image 2.3). Groups of meningothelial cells also comprise the tips of the arachnoid granulations, which are protrusions from the SAS into the dural sinuses.

Lumbar puncture fluid is obtained from spinal SAS

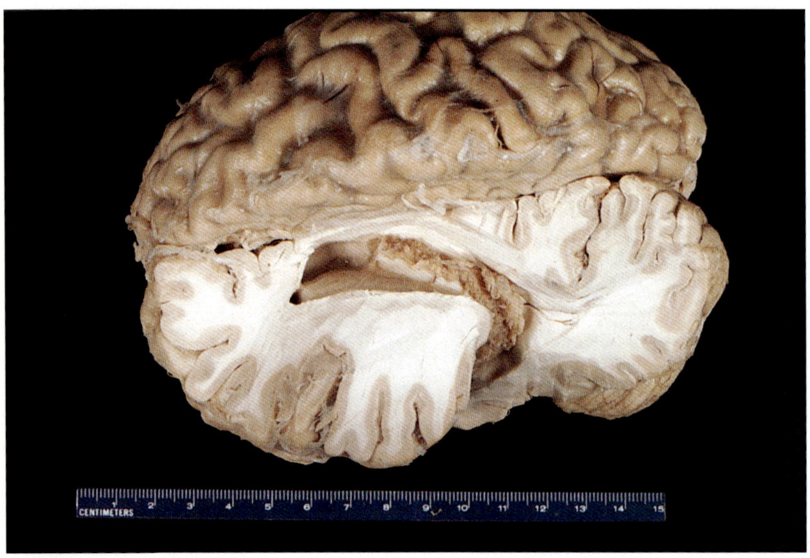

Figure 2.2
Brain dissected at autopsy to reveal the choroid plexus (arrow) in the floor of the lateral ventricle.

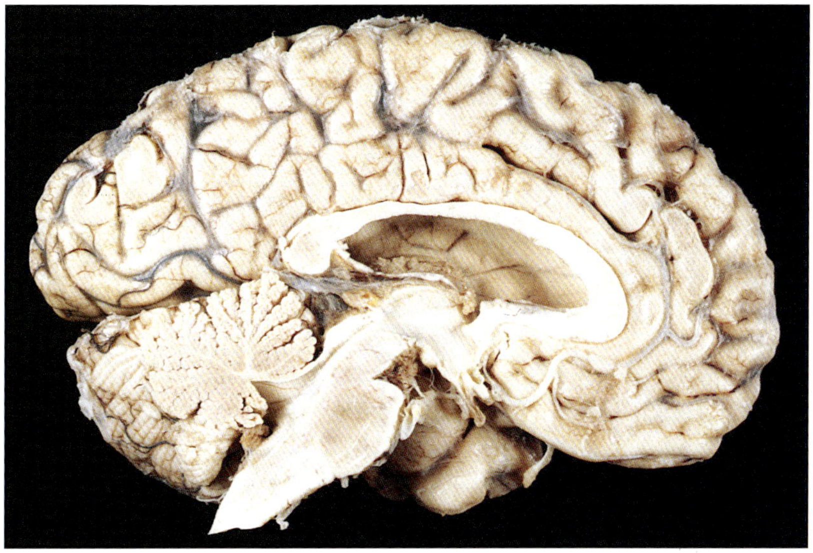

Figure 2.3
Midsagittal section of a normal brain showing the lateral ventricle viewed from its medial aspect. Cerebrospinal fluid travels from the lateral ventricle, through the foramen of Monro, into the third ventricle, through the cerebral aqueduct, and into the fourth ventricle (arrows).

Meningothelial cells in CSF are not in themselves diagnostic of meningioma

Fragments composed of meningothelial cells are occasionally seen in CSF from normal individuals, and they are probably derived from either meningothelial rests or arachnoid granulations (Image 2.4). Rarely they are seen in moderate numbers, raising the possibility of a meningioma. Image 2.5 illustrates such a situation in which numerous groups of meningothelial cells were seen, but no meningioma was found after careful followup studies. This case emphasizes that the presence of meningothelial cells in CSF is not in itself diagnostic of meningioma in the absence of a clinically

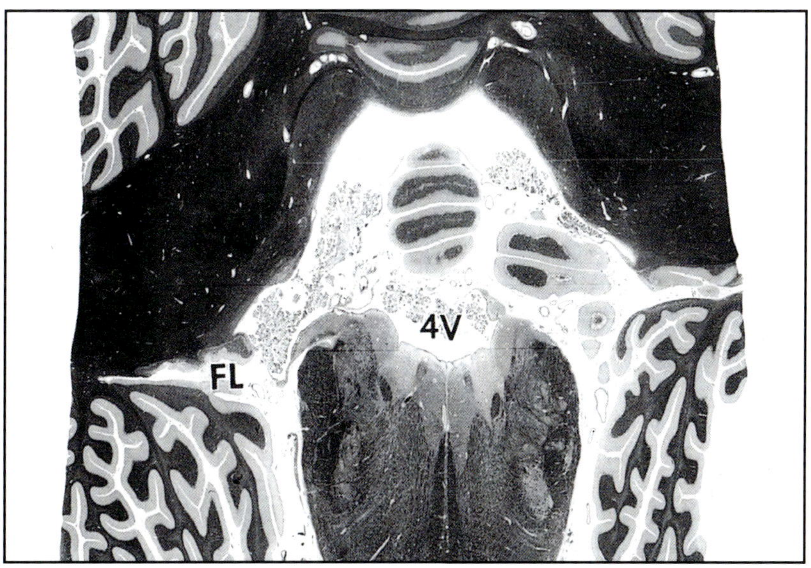

Figure 2.4
The two lateral foramina of Luschka (FL) connect the fourth ventricle (4V) with the SAS (H&E, Luxol fast blue, 7X).

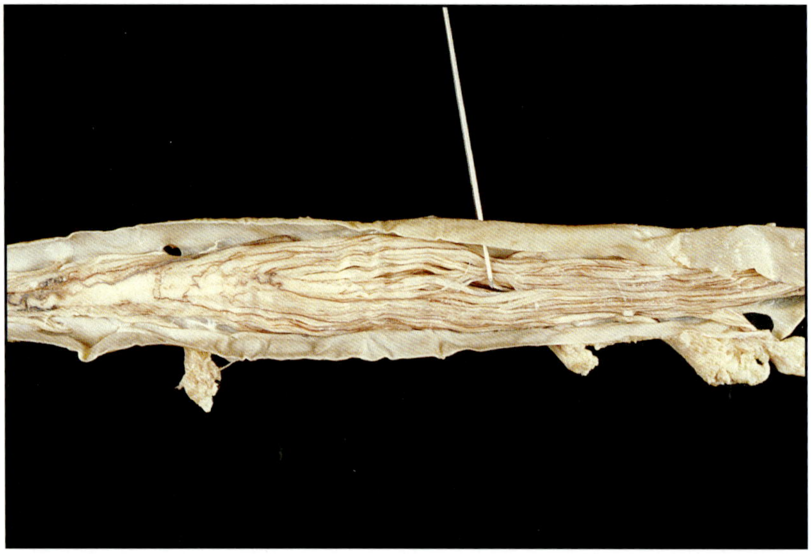

Figure 2.5
Cerebrospinal fluid is aspirated by placing a needle between the spinous processes of the lumbar vertebrae to penetrate the dura and enter the subarachnoid space below the end of the spinal cord, where it contains only nerve roots.

detectable mass. Non-neoplastic cellular elements, such as squamous cells presumably from the skin, may be found occasionally[6]; and sometimes fragments of capillaries, striated muscle, and adipose and fibrous tissue are carried in from subcutaneous tissue or muscle.[8]

Choroid plexus and ependymal cells have ready access to CSF

Cells from the choroid plexus (Figure 2.2 and Image 2.6) and the cuboidal or columnar ependymal cells that line the ventricles (Image 2.7) are normal brain elements that have ready access to CSF.[1,6] They occasionally occur singularly or in papillary clusters in CSF obtained by lumbar puncture from normal individuals (Image 2.8). It is not usually possible to determine morphologically whether a given cell is ependymal or choroidal in origin, although an autopsy study utilizing scanning electron microscopy concluded that the majority of cells found in CSF are derived from the choroid plexus.[7] Other central nervous system parenchymal components are only rarely seen in CSF sampled by lumbar puncture from normal patients. Trojanowski et al[13] applied an antibody against glial fibrillary acidic protein to a series of lumbar puncture–derived CSF samples and confirmed the absence of astrocytic elements.

Starch particles from surgical gloves are a frequent contaminant of CSF. Although these refractile, angulated bodies can usually be readily identified on routine preparations, their Maltese cross configuration, when viewed with polarized light, allows positive identification (Image 2.9). Reinhartz et al[10] have demonstrated that these particles may be engulfed by macrophages, and care must be taken to avoid confusing these structures with *Cryptococcus neoformans*.

Another contaminant of lumbar puncture–derived CSF is the chondrocyte (Image 2.10), which is probably derived from the intervertebral disc.[5,12] Since the pyknotic, basophilic nucleus superficially resembles a macronucleolus, these cells may be mistaken for neoplastic cells. The presence of these cells in CSF, however, has no known pathologic significance.

Ventricular Fluid

Ventricular fluid is obtained by introducing a needle or cannula through a burr hole in the skull and cerebral hemisphere until the ventricular cavity is reached. The needle, therefore, traverses the SAS, cerebral cortex, white matter, and finally the ependyma (Figure 2.6). Fragments from any of these structures may be found in ventricular fluid. Cerebral cortex is composed of neurons and glia in a fibrillary matrix (Image 2.11). When seen in ventricular fluid, the neurons with their prominent nucleoli may be alarming, as they could be confused with malignant cells (Image 2.11c). Fragments of white matter with small glial nuclei (Image 2.11d) are less likely to be mistaken for tumor cells.

Ependymal and/or choroidal cells are frequently seen in ventricular samples. When they are present in large numbers, it may be impossible to distinguish these normal ependymal-choroidal cells from choroid plexus papillomas (see Chapter Eight). Wilkins and Odom[15] have shown that these fragments are especially common in the ventricular fluid samples from hydrocephalic children. Image 2.12 shows numerous fragments of choroid plexus in a ventricular fluid from an infant with hydrocephalus. Capillaries and fragments of normal brain were also seen in this sample.

Corpora amylacea may exfoliate into ventricular fluid

Preissig and Buhaug[9] have reported one case in which ventricular fluid from an elderly man with ventriculitis contained amorphous round corpora amylacea, the polysaccharide bodies that concentrate around the ventricles and pial surface of elderly individuals (Image 2.13). Images 2.13b and 2.13c show similar structures in a ventricular fluid from a man with necrotizing herpetic encephalitis. These two cases suggest that breakdown of the ependymal lining is necessary for corpora amylacea to be released into ventricular fluid. Although contamination of ventricular fluid with these structures is rare, awareness that corpora amylacea may

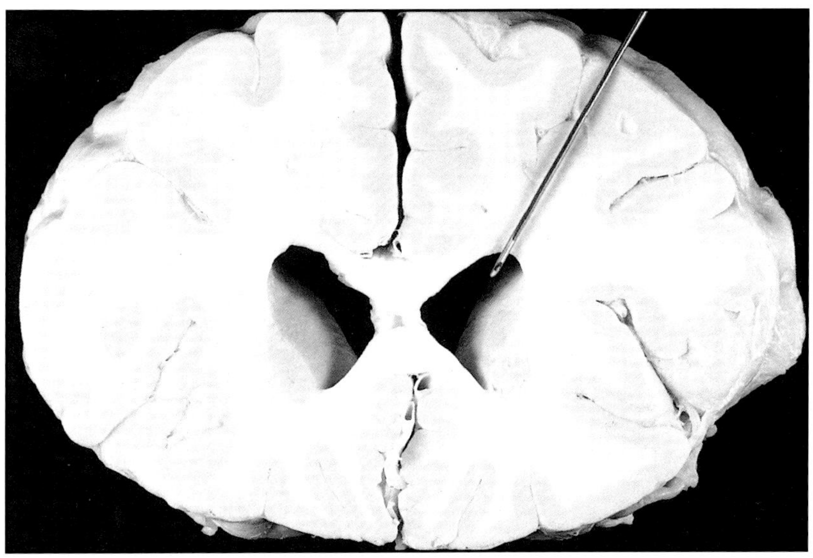

Figure 2.6
Coronal section depicted through the frontal lobes of a brain at autopsy. A ventricular needle or cannula must penetrate the subarachnoid space, grey matter, white matter, and ependyma before reaching the ventricular cavity.

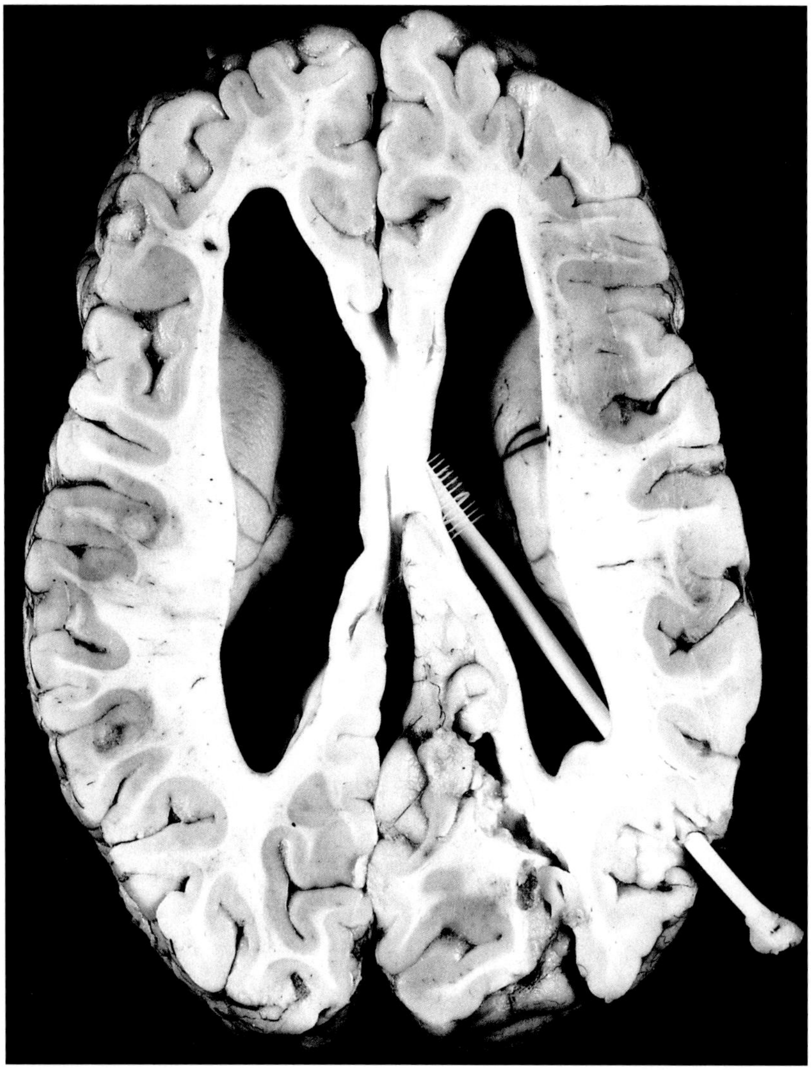

Figure 2.7
Horizontal section of a brain at autopsy from a patient with a ventriculoperitoneal shunt.

exfoliate into ventricular fluid can prevent confusing them with the yeast forms of *C neoformans*.

Tumor cells may disseminate into cavities by means of ventricular shunts

When ventriculoperitoneal, ventriculopleural, or ventriculoatrial shunts (Figure 2.7) are implanted for treatment of hydrocephalus, cells that are present in the ventricular fluid may be found in the peritoneal or pleural cavities. Numerous reports describe dissemination of tumor cells into the body cavities by this means.[3,4,11,14] We have seen an ascitic fluid specimen, from a girl with an optic nerve glioma and a ventriculoperitoneal shunt, that showed no tumor cells; however, the fluid did contain abundant fragments of normal choroid plexus (Image 2.14).[2]

Image 2.1
The subarachnoid space (SAS) is lined externally by the arachnoid membrane and internally by the pia, with a loose fibrovascular stroma (H&E, Luxol fast blue, 250X).

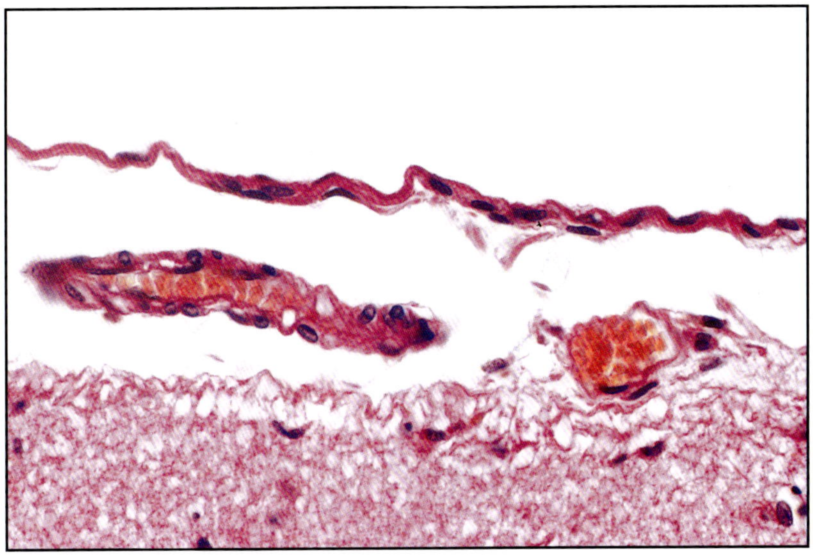

Image 2.2
Normal CSF containing a few lymphocytes (a through c) and macrophages (d through f). The leukocytic derivation of these cells is confirmed by reactivity with panleukocyte antibody 2D1 (a and d, Papanicolaou; b and e, Romanowski; c and f, Immunoperoxidase reaction with panleukocyte antibody 2D1; all 1,000X).

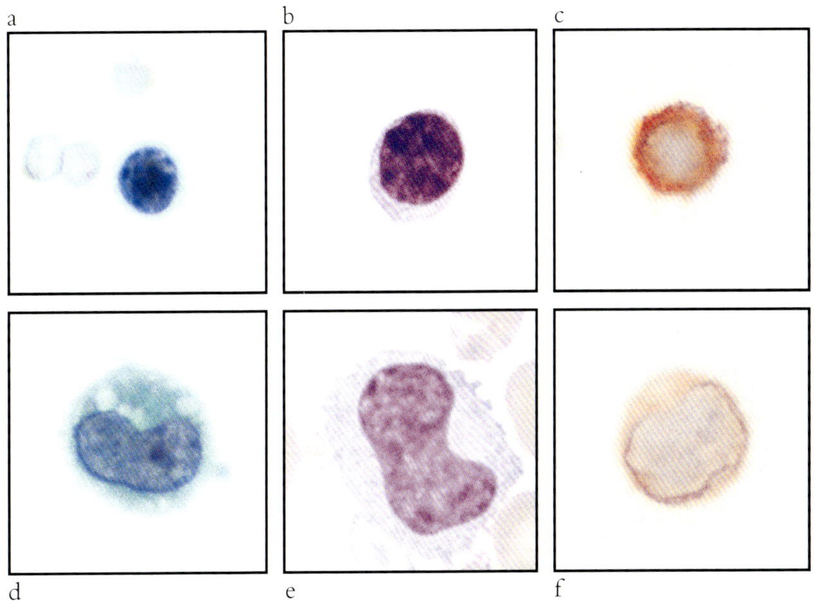

Image 2.3
Histologic section of the arachnoid membrane in an individual without neurologic disease showing a focal accumulation of meningothelial cells constituting a meningothelial rest (H&E, 400X).

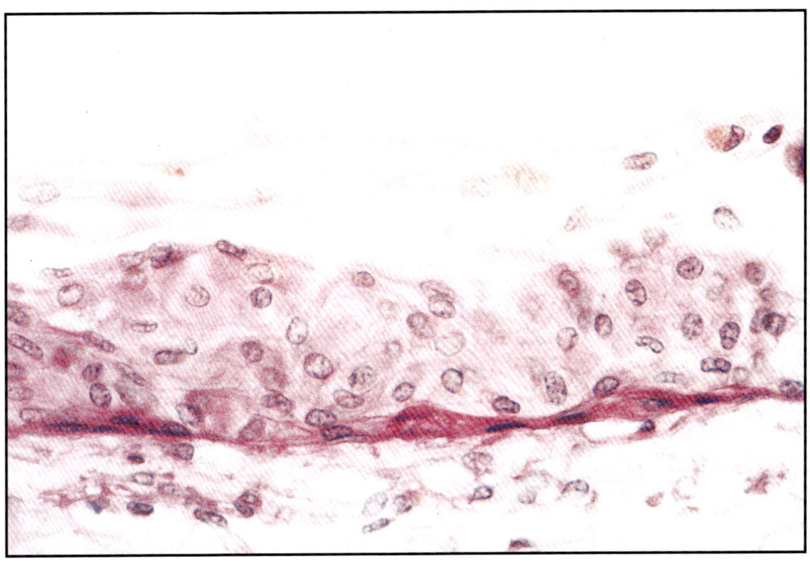

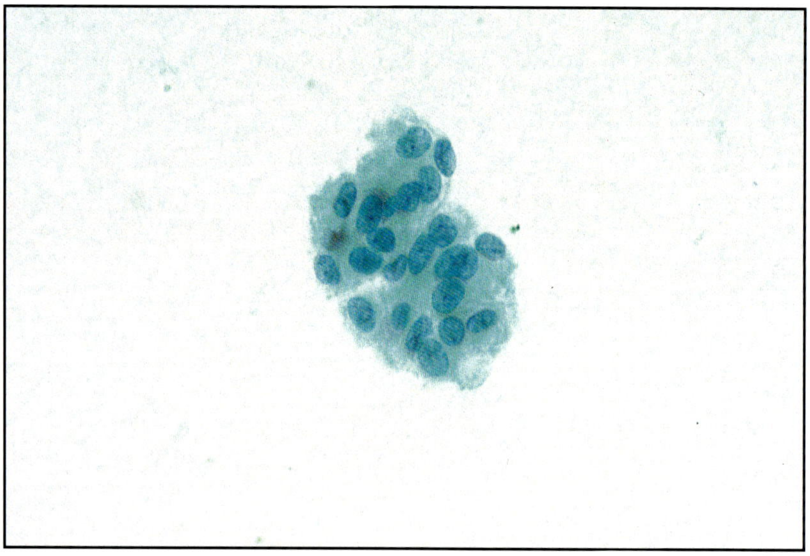

Image 2.4
A cluster of plump cells with oval nuclei found in lumbar puncture–derived CSF in an individual without neurologic symptoms. These cells are probably meningothelial cells (Papanicolaou, 400X).

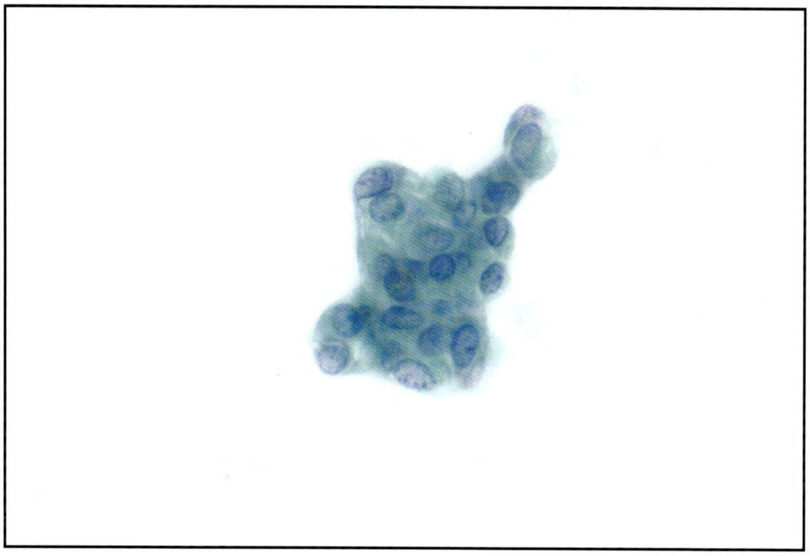

Image 2.5
Clusters of meningothelial cells seen in a sample of CSF from a 35-year-old man. Since no meningioma was found in long-term followup, these cells were probably derived from meningothelial rests or arachnoid granulations (Papanicolaou, 400X).

a b

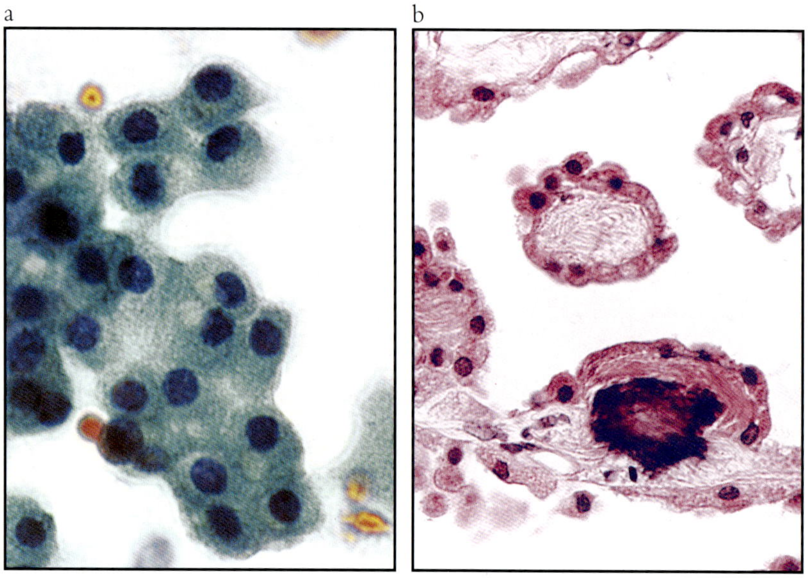

Image 2.6
Cells from the choroid plexus in imprint (a) and histologic section (b) obtained at autopsy (a, Papanicolaou, 1,000X; b, H&E, 400X).

Image 2.7
Ependymal cells line the ventricular cavities in imprint (a) and histologic section (b) obtained at autopsy (a, Papanicolaou, 1,000X; b, H&E, 400X).

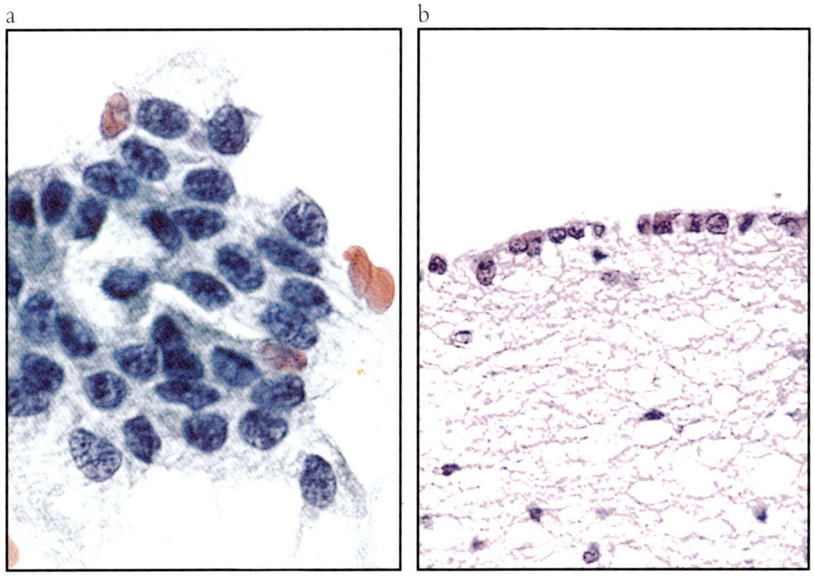

Image 2.8
Benign ependymal/choroidal cells obtained by lumbar puncture from a patient without central nervous system tumor (Papanicolaou, 1,000X).

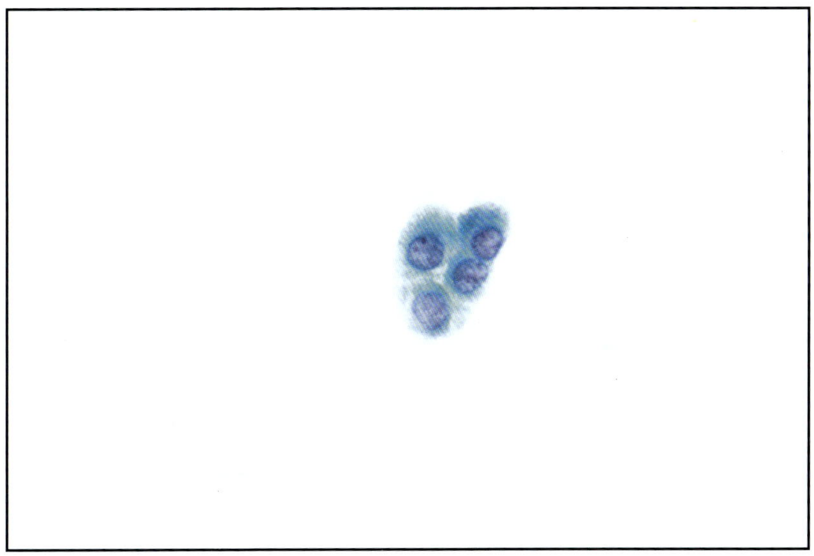

Image 2.9
Particles of glove powder in CSF showing variations in configuration (a through c). A Maltese cross configuration is noted (d) (a through c, Papanicolaou, 400X; d, Papanicolaou, 400X, polarized light).

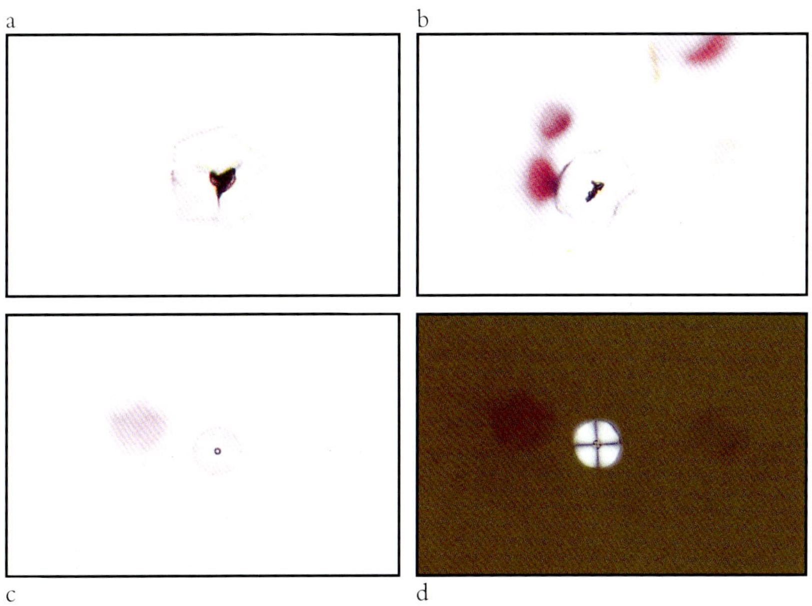

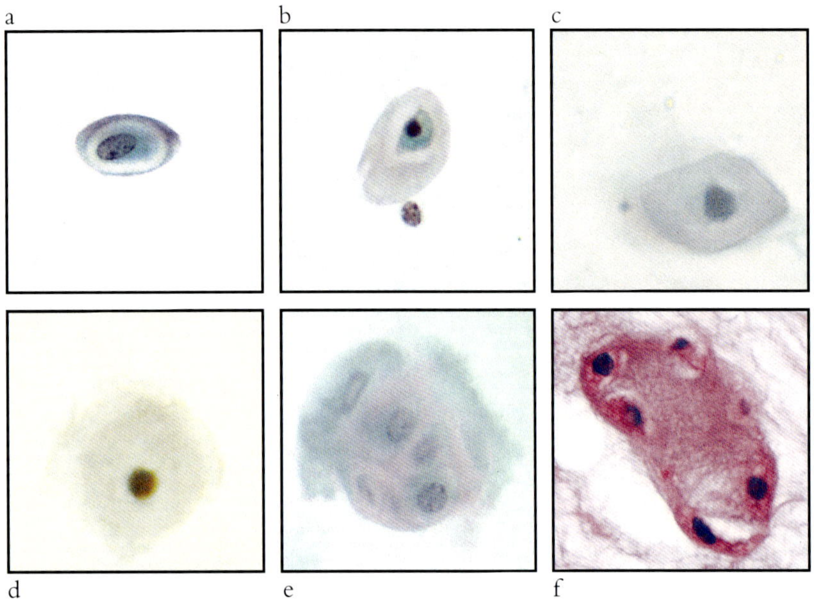

Image 2.10
Chondrocytes exhibiting subtle variations in morphology and occurring singly (a through d) or in fragments (e) are seen in occasional samples of lumbar puncture–derived CSF. Surgically removed herniated nucleus pulposus demonstrates the histologic counterpart of these cells (f) (a through e, Papanicolaou, 400X; f, H&E, 400X).

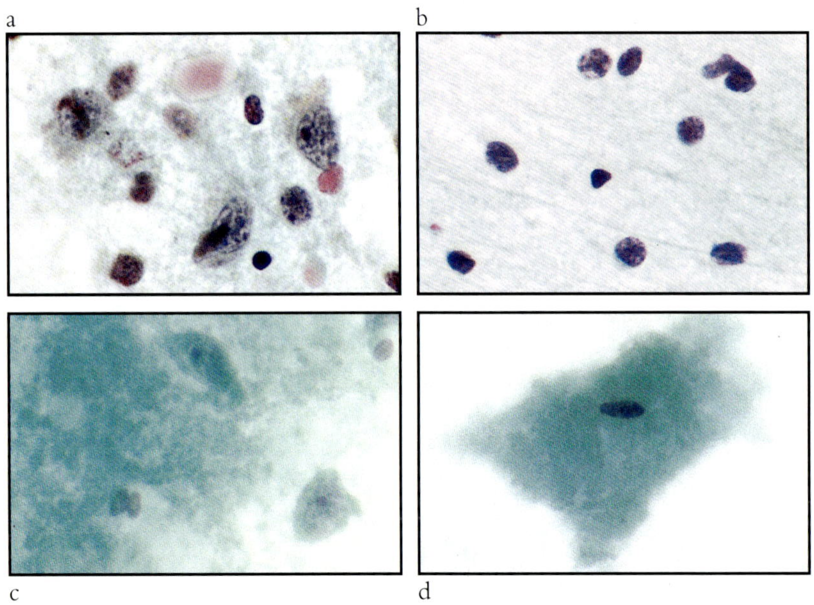

Image 2.11
Imprints of normal cerebral cortex that contains neurons (a) (note corpora amylacea) and of normal white matter that contains glia (b). Fragments of cerebral cortex (c) and fibrillary white matter containing glial nuclei (d) are seen in a ventricular fluid specimen from a 25-year-old woman with a history of medulloblastoma (all, Papanicolaou, 400X).

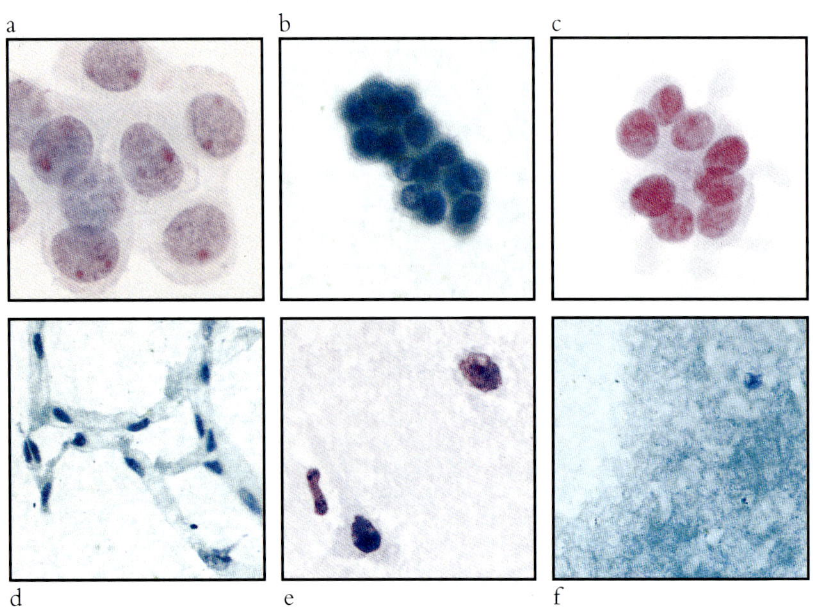

Image 2.12
Ventricular fluid specimen from a 4-month-old male infant with hydrocephalus contains numerous choroid plexus cells (a through c) as well as capillaries (d) and fragments of grey matter (e) and white matter (f) (a and e, Papanicolaou-stained Cytospin®; b, d, and f, Papanicolaou-stained Millipore® filter; c, Romanowski-stained Cytospin®; all 400X).

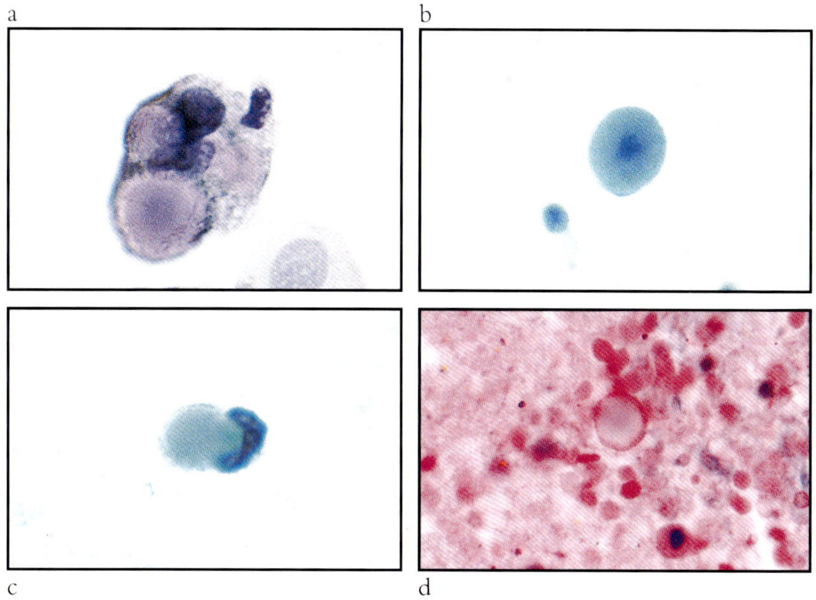

Image 2.13
Corpora amylacea in a macrophage is seen in ventricular fluid specimen from a 60-year-old man with ventriculitis (a). Corpora amylacea is seen in a ventricular fluid specimen from a 59-year-old man with angioimmunoblastic lymphadenopathy who developed herpetic encephalitis (b and c). Corpora amylacea is seen in the necrotic subependymal area of his brain at autopsy (d) (a through c, Papanicolaou, 400X; d, H&E, 400X).

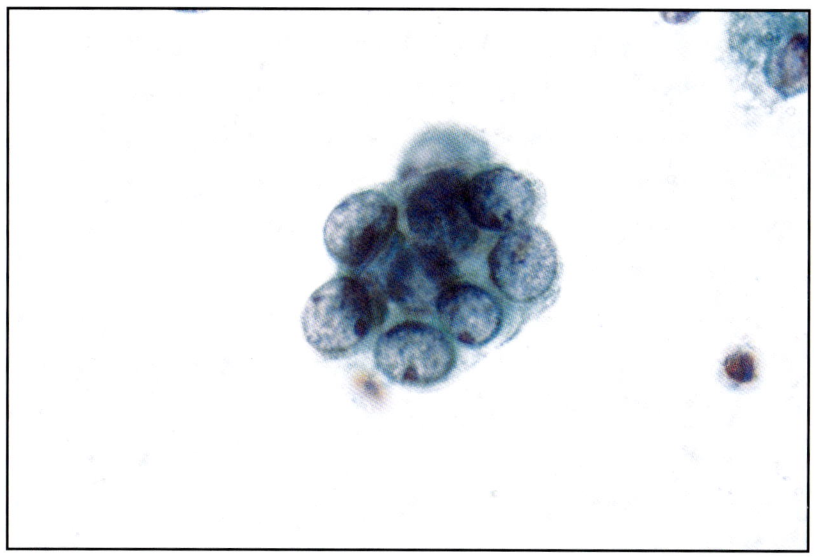

Image 2.14
Fragments of choroid plexus are noted in an ascitic fluid specimen from a patient with a ventriculoperitoneal shunt (Papanicolaou, 1,000X).

References

1. Bigner SH, Johnston WW: The cytopathology of cerebrospinal fluid. A review, part I: non-neoplastic conditions, lymphoma and leukemia. *Acta Cytol* 25:335–353, 1981.
2. Bigner SH, Elmore PD, Dee AL, Johnston WW: The cytopathology of reactions to ventricular shunts. *Acta Cytol* 29:391–396, 1985.
3. Brust JCM, Moiel RH, Rosenberg RN: Glial tumor metastases through a ventriculopleural shunt. *Arch Neurol* 18:649–653, 1968.
4. Haimovic IC, Sharer L, Hyman RA, Beresford HR: Metastasis of intracranial germinoma through a ventriculoperitoneal shunt. *Cancer* 48:1033–1036, 1981.
5. Leiman G, Klein C, Berry AV: Cells of nucleus pulposus in cerebrospinal fluid: a case report. *Acta Cytol* 24:347–349, 1980.
6. McGarry P, Holmquist ND, Carmel SA: A postmortem study of cerebrospinal fluid with histologic correlation. *Acta Cytol* 13:48–52, 1969.
7. Mathios AJ, Nielsen SL, Barrett D, King EB: Cerebrospinal fluid cytomorphology: identification of benign cells originating in the central nervous system. *Acta Cytol* 21:403–412, 1977.
8. Naib ZM: *Exfoliative Cytopathology*, 2nd ed. Boston, MA, Little, Brown and Co, 1976, pp. 443–455.
9. Preissig SH, Buhaug I: Corpora amylacea in cerebrospinal fluid: a source of possible diagnostic error. *Acta Cytol* 22:511–514, 1978.
10. Reinhartz T, Lijovetzky G, Levij IS: Intracellular starch granules in cytologic material. *Acta Cytol* 22:36–37, 1978.
11. Russell DC, Rubenstein LJ: *Pathology of Tumors of the Nervous System*, 5th ed. Baltimore, MD, Williams and Wilkins Co, 1989, pp. 439–441.
12. Takeda M, King DE, Choi HY, Gomi K, Lang WR: Diagnostic pitfalls in cerebrospinal fluid cytology. *Acta Cytol* 25:245–250, 1981.
13. Trojanowski JQ, Atkinson B, Lee VM: An immunocytochemical study of normal and abnormal human cerebrospinal fluid with monoclonal antibodies to glial fibrillary acidic protein. *Acta Cytol* 30:235–239, 1986.
14. Wakamatsu T, Matsuo T, Kawano S, Teramoto S, Matsumura H: Glioblastoma with extracranial metastasis through ventriculopleural shunt. *J Neurosurg* 34:697–701, 1971.
15. Wilkins RH, Odom GL: Ependymal-choroidal cells in cerebrospinal fluid: increased incidence in hydrocephalic infants. *J Neurosurg* 41:555–560, 1974.

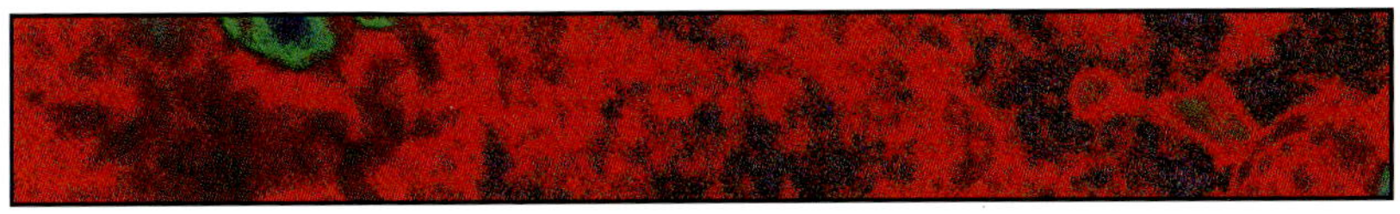

CHAPTER THREE

Inflammatory Conditions

A variety of infectious agents, including bacteria, spirochetes, viruses, fungi, and parasites, can involve the central nervous system (CNS).[3] Infections occurring primarily in the subarachnoid space (SAS) produce meningitis, a condition that can be diagnosed more readily by cerebrospinal fluid (CSF) examination than can lesions that involve mainly the brain parenchyma (Figure 3.1). The presence of increased numbers of inflammatory cells in a sample of CSF, particularly a component of polymorphonuclear leukocytes or enlarged and atypical lymphocytes, suggests that an infectious process may be present. Although higher cell counts are more likely to occur if the disorder involves predominantly the SAS, meningeal infections cannot be reliably distinguished from meningeal infiltrates secondary to primary parenchymal disease of the brain or spinal cord. The composition of the cellular infiltrate may suggest that the process in an individual patient is likely to be infectious rather than a reaction to a noninfectious disorder and that a bacterial, viral, or fungal etiology is the likely origin. Nevertheless, diagnosis of an infection requires demonstration of the responsible organism either by direct visualization, culture, or antibody titer.

Bacterial Infections

The most typical cellular presentation of acute bacterial meningitis is an infiltrate composed predominantly of polymorphonuclear leukocytes. This pattern is not specific for this disorder, however, since an acute inflammatory infiltrate can also be seen in CSF from patients with acute

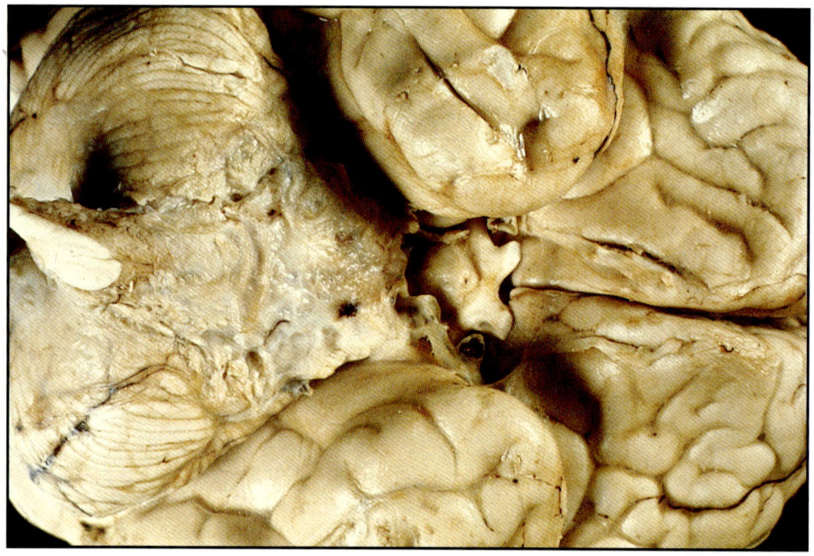

Figure 3.1
A brain at autopsy of a patient with acute bacterial meningitis. Grossly, a thick exudate covers the ventral part of the brain stem.

cerebral infarctions and occasionally in the early stages of viral and fungal infections. Bacterial meningitis may be caused by a number of organisms including *Neisseria meningitidis*, *Diplococcus pneumoniae*, and *Hemophilus influenzae*, as well as other gram-negative rods. These organisms elicit an inflammatory response composed primarily of polymorphonuclear leukocytes that can be readily identified on Papanicolaou- or Wright-stained preparations (Image 3.1). Bacteria may be seen with the Papanicolaou stain, but exact identification requires Gram stain and culture. *Mycobacterium tuberculosis* typically produces an infiltrate composed primarily of lymphocytes[6] in CSF. Although the bacillary forms of this organism are not demonstrable by the Papanicolaou stain, granulomas are rarely identified in the CSF of patients with tuberculous meningitis. In these cases, acid-fast stains may be performed on the original slides or filters to render a rapid, specific diagnosis.

Exact identification of bacteria requires Gram stain and culture

When bacteria primarily involve the brain, parenchymal-circumscribed abscesses are produced (Figure 3.2). These lesions consist of necrotizing acute inflammation surrounded by fibrosis (Image 3.2). This response is especially characteristic of *Staphylococcus aureus*. Since these lesions are not in direct contact with the SAS, only a few inflammatory cells are seen in the CSF. If these lesions are not treated, they may rupture into the ventricles, which is usually rapidly fatal. Similarly, *M tuberculosis* may produce circumscribed parenchyma and tuberculomas (Figure 3.3), and fungi may produce mycetomas. Since these parenchymal lesions do not involve the SAS, fine needle aspiration biopsy is a more practical means of investigating them than is CSF cytology.

Viral Infections

Viral infections frequently involve both the brain parenchyma and the SAS. Viral meningoencephalitis is most often produced by the

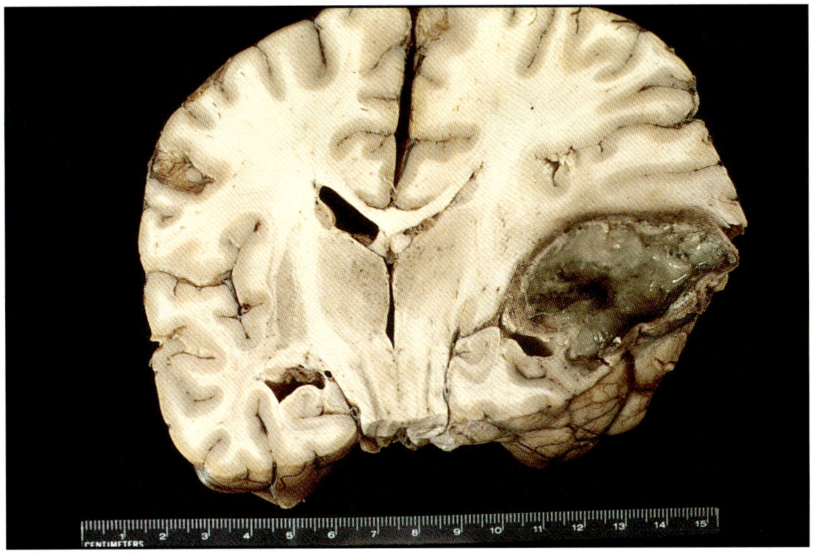

Figure 3.2
Coronal section of a brain at autopsy showing a large, circumscribed abscess cavity with central necrosis located in the temporal lobe.

Specific viral agents may be identified by immunohistochemistry, immunofluorescence, or in situ hybridization

enterovirus group, which includes coxsackievirus, echovirus, and poliovirus. These agents elicit a nonspecific CSF infiltrate composed of lymphocytes and macrophages, and they do not produce identifiable cellular inclusion bodies. Specific viral agents may, however, be identified using immunohistochemistry, immunofluorescence,[7] or in situ hybridization with nucleotide probes. Images 3.3a through 3.3d show cells in the CSF from a patient with enterococcal meningoencephalitis. Images 3.3e and 3.3f show the spinal cord lesions from this patient at autopsy. Enterococci were demonstrated by electron microscopy. In

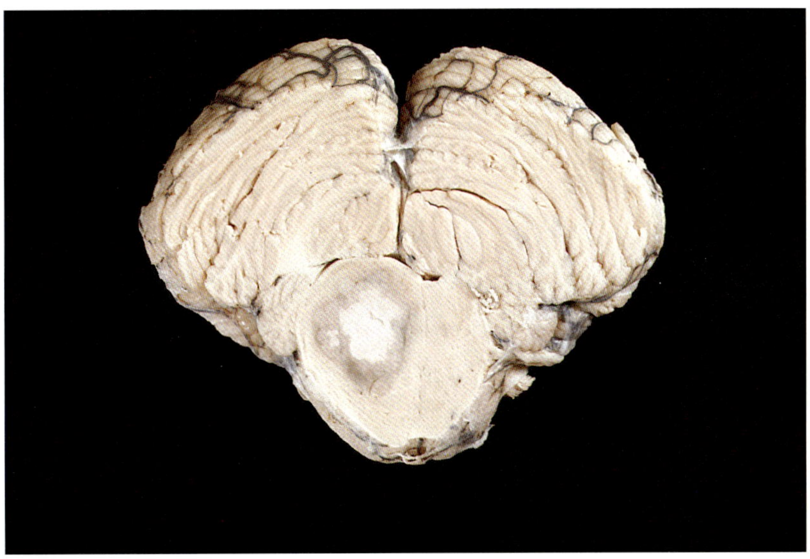

Figure 3.3
A brain at autopsy showing a tuberculoma, which is a chalky, well-circumscribed solid granulomatous mass produced by tubercle bacilli.

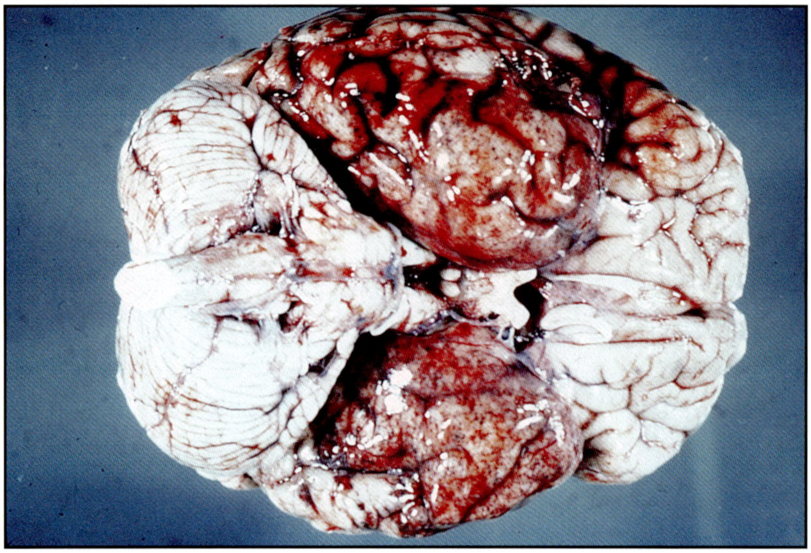

Figure 3.4
A brain at autopsy showing hemorrhagic necrosis of the temporal lobes produced by herpes simplex encephalitis.

viral meningoencephalitis, the inflammatory cells are often numerous and may be enlarged with prominent nucleoli. These cytologic features may lead to confusion with the malignant hematopoietic cells of lymphoma or leukemia.[4,10,19,21] Phenotypic studies of these reactive cells are particularly helpful, because mixtures of T and B lymphocytes are inevitably demonstrated in contrast to a monoclonal population that is present in cases of malignant lymphoma.

Herpes simplex encephalitis is, fortunately, a rare form of CNS infection (Figure 3.4). Viral culture and antibody titers require too much time to be of practical value in diagnosing this condition, and often craniotomy must be undertaken to establish its etiology. A simple and noninvasive means for diagnosing this condition was discovered when Gupta et al[11] observed cells with typical herpetic intranuclear inclusions in the CSF of two patients with documented herpes simplex encephalitis. We have seen one case of herpes zoster encephalitis in which degenerate inclusion-bearing cells were seen in CSF during life and misinterpreted as adenocarcinoma (Image 3.4).[3] At autopsy, inclusions were seen in neurons, astrocytes, and choroid plexus and ependymal cells. Herpetic viral particles were demonstrated by both electron microscopy and viral cultures. This diagnostic pitfall of confusing herpetic inclusions with carcinoma can be avoided by following the principle of not basing a diagnosis of malignancy on degenerate cells.

Do not base a diagnosis of malignancy on degenerate cells

Other viral-associated infections that produce inclusions in brain parenchyma include rabies, cytomegalic inclusion disease, subacute sclerosing panencephalitis, and the JC virus and SV 40-PML virus of progressive multifocal leukoencephalitis (PML). Cells containing the characteristic nuclear inclusions of these viruses can be demonstrated in open biopsy and needle biopsy specimens of the parenchymal lesions, and inclusion-bearing cells are occasionally identified in CSF.[14]

Fungal Infections

Cryptococci are the most frequent cause of fungal meningitis

Cryptococcus neoformans is the most frequent cause of fungal meningitis (Figure 3.5). This organism usually enters the body through the respiratory system and disseminates to the CNS hematogenously.[9] Although cryptococcal meningitis may be a complication of immunosuppression, as is seen in recipients of organ transplants, patients with lymphoma and leukemia, and patients with acquired immunodeficiency syndrome (AIDS), it occasionally occurs in otherwise healthy individuals. In the immunosuppressed patient, in particular, very little cellular reaction may occur, and the CSF may contain multitudes of organisms (Images 3.5a and 3.5b). In some cases, however, a brisk inflammatory reaction may occur (Images 3.5c and 3.5d). The predominant cells are usually lymphocytes, although occasionally polymorphonuclear leukocytes or macrophages are more numerous (Image 3.6). The organisms frequently appear morphologically as round yeast forms of variable diameter that produce thin-necked buds (Image 3.5f).[1,18] Commonly the organisms have a refractile appearance, possibly due to mounting medium that is trapped between the capsule of the organism and the coverslip.[13] Organisms with this presentation can be mistaken for particles of glove powder that are also refractile (see Image 2.9). Cryptococci often possess a thick, mucopolysaccharide capsule that stains readily with mucicarmine, alcian blue, and colloidal iron stains. Organisms without a prominent capsule are sometimes encountered, however, and these structures may be difficult to distinguish from partially lysed erythrocytes or even bubbles of air or water trapped under the coverslip (Images 3.5e and 3.5f). The presence of true buds is useful in distinguishing the organisms from these other structures.

Cryptococci must also be distinguished from other types of budding yeasts such as *Blastomyces dermatitidis* and *Histoplasma capsulatum*,

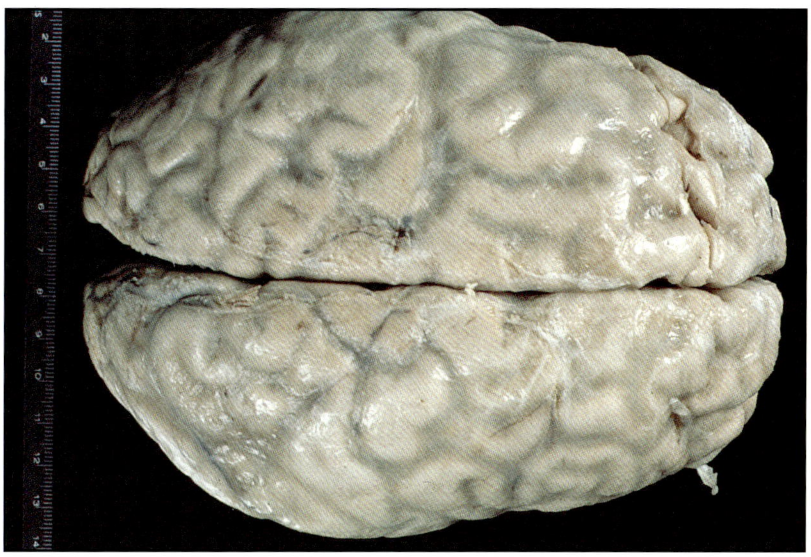

Figure 3.5
A brain at autopsy showing cryptococcal meningitis. Grossly, the meninges have a gelatinous appearance due to the mucopolysaccharide capsules of the organism.

which occur only rarely in CSF. In addition to the thin-necked buds and mucopolysaccharide capsule that are characteristic of *Cryptococcus*, this organism usually displays a wide range of diameters within an individual specimen. In contrast, *Blastomyces* is uniformly large with diameters of 8 to 12 µm and *Histoplasma* is uniformly small, generally 1 to 5 µm. In addition to cytologic diagnosis of cryptococcal meningitis, the organism may be identified by its growth characteristics in culture and by demonstration of cryptococcal antigen by radioimmunoassay.

Aspergillus, *Penicillium*, *Nocardia*, and the Phycomycetes may involve the central nervous system, especially in the immunosuppressed host and in patients with diabetes. The lesions that are largely confined to the brain parenchyma are typically multifocal and may be hemorrhagic or infarcted. Since the SAS is only secondarily involved, fungal hyphae are seldom, if ever, identified in CSF. Needle aspiration and open biopsy are the most practical means of diagnosing fungal infections of the brain parenchyma (see Chapter Eight). Image 3.7 shows broad nonseptate hyphae in a needle aspiration biopsy specimen from a patient with cerebral mucormycosis.[2] Image 3.8 illustrates the slender branching hyphae of *Nocardia* from the brain of a patient with AIDS.

AIDS

CNS disorders associated with AIDS include AIDS encephalopathy, opportunistic infections, and neoplasia

Three types of CNS disorders are seen in patients with AIDS. The first, AIDS encephalopathy, results directly or indirectly from infection of cells within the brain or spinal cord by the human immunodeficiency virus (HIV). Histologically, the lesions consist of glial nodules, chronic inflammation, gliosis, and sometimes multinucleated giant cells. The CSF from these patients usually contains only a nonspecific chronic inflammatory infiltrate, although rarely multinucleated giant cells may be encountered.

The second group of abnormalities consists of opportunistic infections that are most frequently produced by *C neoformans*, *Toxoplasma gondii*, mycobacteria, *Candida*, and viruses such as cytomegalovirus (CMV) and the viruses of PML. Although these organisms or their characteristic cellular inclusions can frequently be demonstrated by open brain biopsy or by needle aspiration of the cerebral lesions,[12] their manifestations in CSF are usually nonspecific with the exception of inclusion-bearing cells in CSF in cases of CMV infections (Image 3.9) and rare examples of *Toxoplasma* infections (Image 3.10). Among these infections, cryptococcal meningitis is the only process in which examination of CSF yields a specific diagnosis in a high percentage of cases.

The third disorder involving the CNS of patients with AIDS is neoplasia, which is most frequently lymphoma. Examination of the CSF often reveals the characteristic malignant cells of lymphoma both in patients with AIDS with primary CNS lymphoma and in patients with systemic lymphomal CNS metastases. Since the majority of these lymphomas are of the B-cell type, immunohistochemical markers are often helpful in establishing this diagnosis.

Image 3.11 shows CSF from a 34-year-old woman who was HIV positive and developed a cerebral infarct. This fluid contains a mixed inflammatory infiltrate with atypical lymphocytes and numerous immunoblasts. This mixed morphologic pattern along with the absence of clinical evidence for lymphoma suggest that this reaction is either part of AIDS encephalopathy or a reaction to a viral infection. The immunohistochemical pattern, consisting of a mixture of T and B cells with T-cell predominance, also supports a reactive process.

Parasites

Cerebral cysticercosis, produced by the larvae of *Taenia solium*, is a common disease in Central America. While the organism itself is not seen in CSF, a pleocytosis frequently occurs. Although predominance of eosinophils may indicate a parasitic infection,[15] Wilber et al[20] have demonstrated eosinophilia in only two out of five cases of cerebral cysticercosis. They stress that an infiltrate of atypical lymphocytes is equally likely as eosinophilia, and that these lymphoid cells may be confused with lymphoma. Plasma cells, which are often a part of the cellular response, may at times be both numerous and immature and may mimic a malignant plasmacytosis.[16]

Other CNS parasitic infections include schistosomiasis, paragonimiasis, fascioliasis, toxocariasis, trichinellosis, ascariasis, echinococcosis, and onchocerciasis.[15] Although CSF eosinophilia has been reported with these infections, the organisms have not been identified in CSF. Two parasitic CNS infectious agents found in patients in Southeast Asia and generally associated with an intense eosinophilia are *Angiostrongylus cantonensis*[22] and *Gnathostoma spinigerum*.[5] The former organism was identified in the CSF from eight patients with this infection,[22] but the latter has not been isolated in CSF. *Entamoeba histolytica* may involve the brain and has been reported in CSF by Duma et al.[8]

Lyme Disease

Awareness of Lyme disease is important to avoid misdiagnosis of lymphoma

Lyme disease is a CNS disorder manifested by headache and painful neuritis and caused by a tick-borne spirochete. Patients develop a pleocytosis in CSF composed of immunoblasts, plasma cells, and foamy macrophages. Although this cytologic picture is nonspecific, awareness of this clinical disorder is important, not only in raising the suspicion of this diagnosis, but also in avoiding an erroneous diagnosis of lymphoma. Although individual cells can be alarming,[17] the mixed nature of the infiltrate and the polyclonal immunologic pattern are helpful in establishing the reactive nature of these infiltrates.

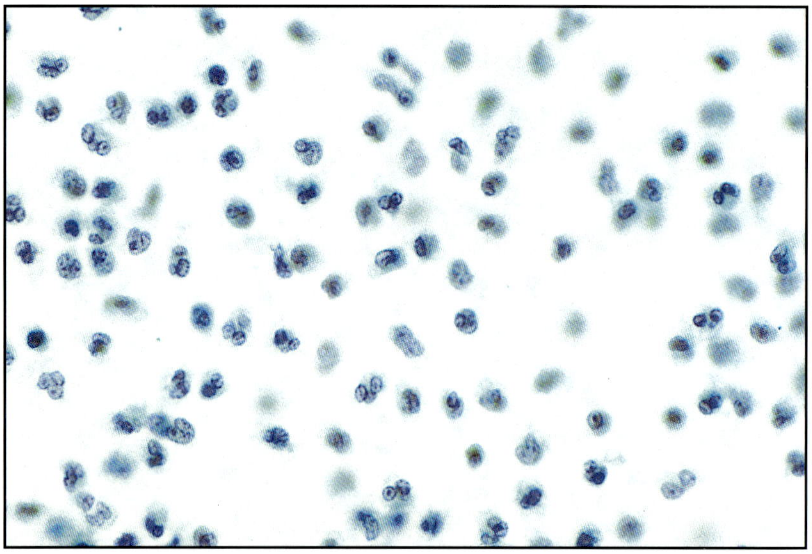

Image 3.1
Polymorphonuclear leukocytes in CSF from a patient with acute bacterial meningitis (Papanicolaou-stained filters, 1,000X).

a b

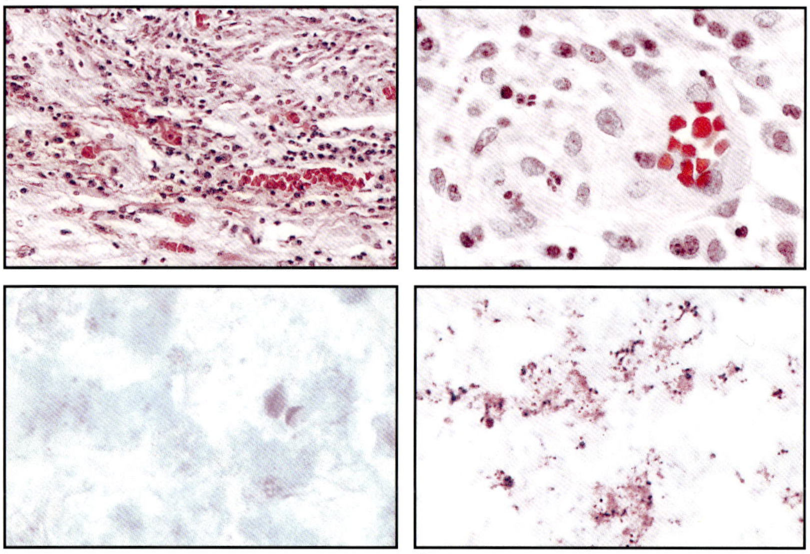

c d

Image 3.2
Histologic section of an abscess showing an outer fibrotic wall (a). Histologic section showing an internal region of granulation tissue, macrophages, and polymorphonuclear leukocytes (b). An aspirate from this abscess cavity showing amorphous necrotic debris within which bacteria could barely be seen with the Papanicolaou stain (c). Gram stain demonstrating gram-positive cocci (d) (a, H&E, 200X; b, H&E, 400X; c, Papanicolaou, 1,000X; d, Gram stain, 1,000X).

a b c

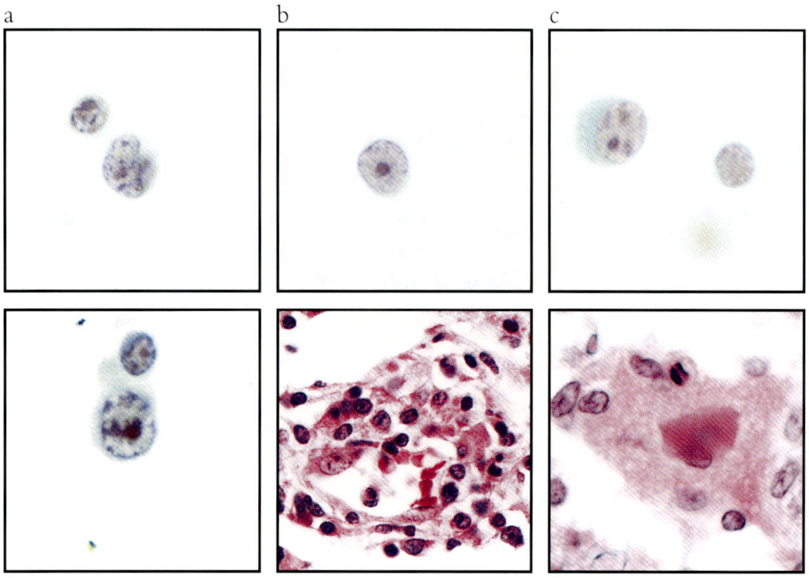

d e f

Image 3.3
Enterococcal meningoencephalitis. Lymphocytes and macrophages with clumped chromatin and prominent nucleoli appear in the CSF of a 28-year-old man (a through d). At autopsy, the brain and spinal cord showed perivascular lymphocytic infiltrates (e) and inflammatory cells surrounding dead anterior horn cells, which is called neurophagia (f). This latter feature is typical of the enterococci that were seen by electron microscopy (a through d, Papanicolaou, 1,000X; e, H&E with Luxol fast blue, 250X; f, H&E with Luxol fast blue, 400X).

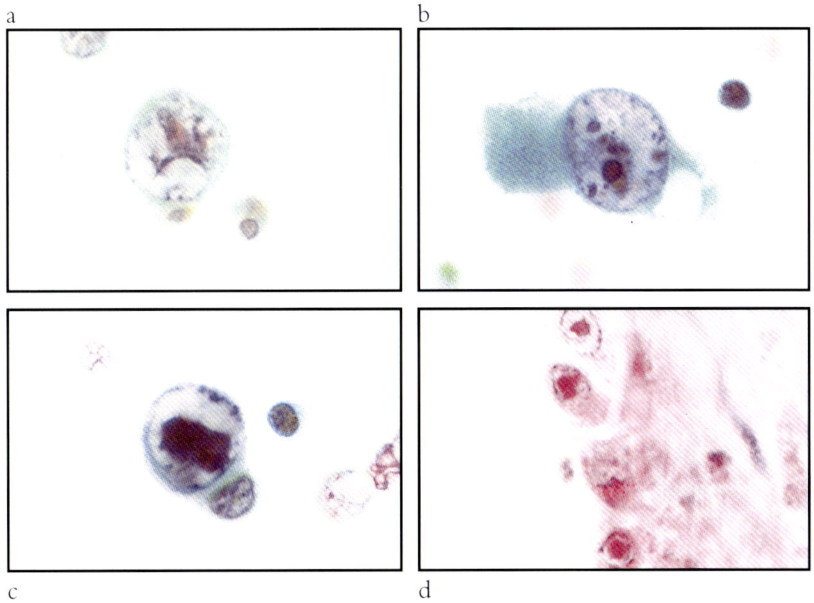

Image 3.4
Herpes zoster meningoencephalitis. Atypical herpetic-infected cells in CSF mimicking carcinoma (a and b). Cell with large intranuclear herpetic inclusion (c). At autopsy, ependymal cells containing herpetic inclusions (d) (a through c, Papanicolaou, 1,000X; d, H&E, Luxol fast blue, 600X).

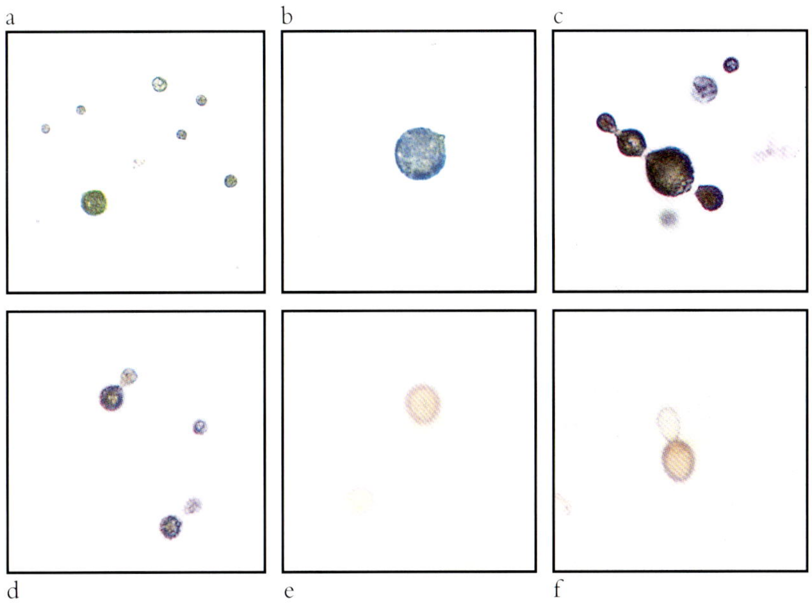

Image 3.5
Cryptococcus neoformans frequently presents in CSF as yeast forms with refractile centers. In cases with little inflammation, the multitude of organisms may be overlooked and regarded as artifacts (a). Small budding protrusions help to identify these structures as yeast forms (b). A brisk inflammatory response is seen, including atypical lymphocytes (c and d). Cryptococcal organisms with inconspicuous capsules (e and f). The presence of thin-necked buds (f) helps to distinguish these organisms from erythrocytes (all, Papanicolaou; a, 400X; b through f, 1,000X).

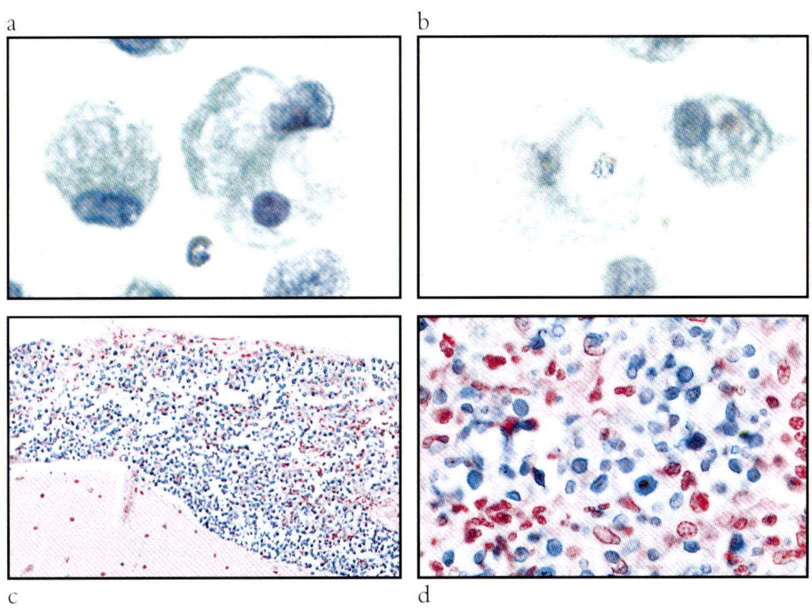

Image 3.6
Cryptococcus neoformans in CSF. Seas of foamy macrophages are seen, many of which contain yeast forms (a and b). At autopsy, this alcian blue stain demonstrates that the subarachnoid space is filled with cryptococcal organisms (c and d) (a and b, Papanicolaou, 1,000X; c and d, Alcian blue; c, 100X; d, 400X).

a b

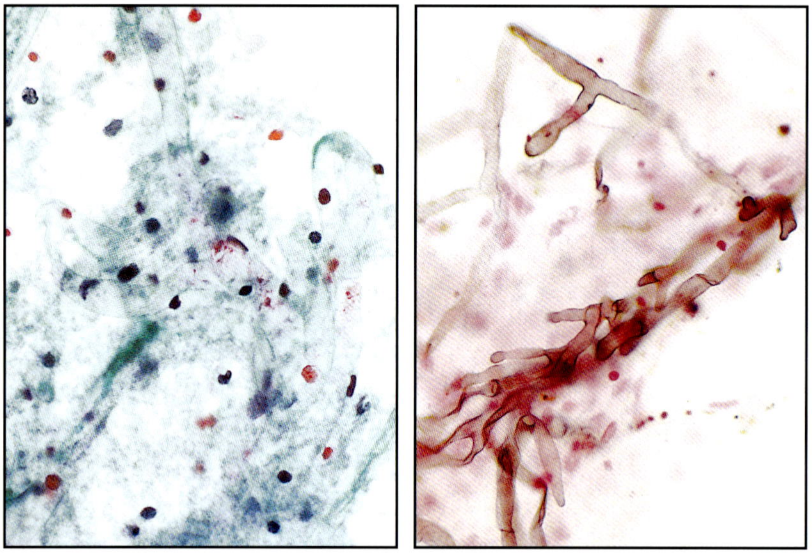

Image 3.7

Broad, nonseptate hyphae of a phycomycete obtained by needle aspiration biopsy (a and b) (a, Papanicolaou, 600X; b, Methenamine silver, 600X).

c d

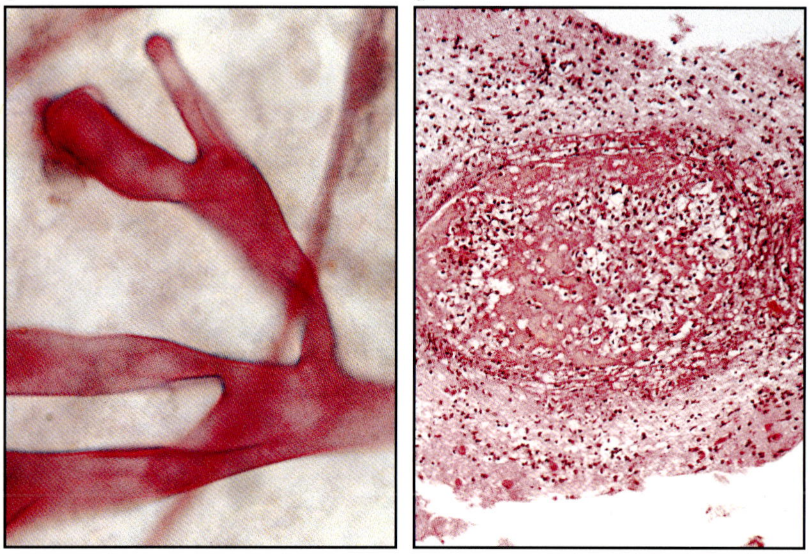

Broad, nonseptate hyphae of a phycomycete obtained by needle aspiration biopsy (c). A cell block prepared from this aspirate contains thrombosed blood vessels with hyphae growing within vessel walls and lumina (d) (c, Periodic acid-Schiff, 1,000X; d, H&E, 100X).

e f

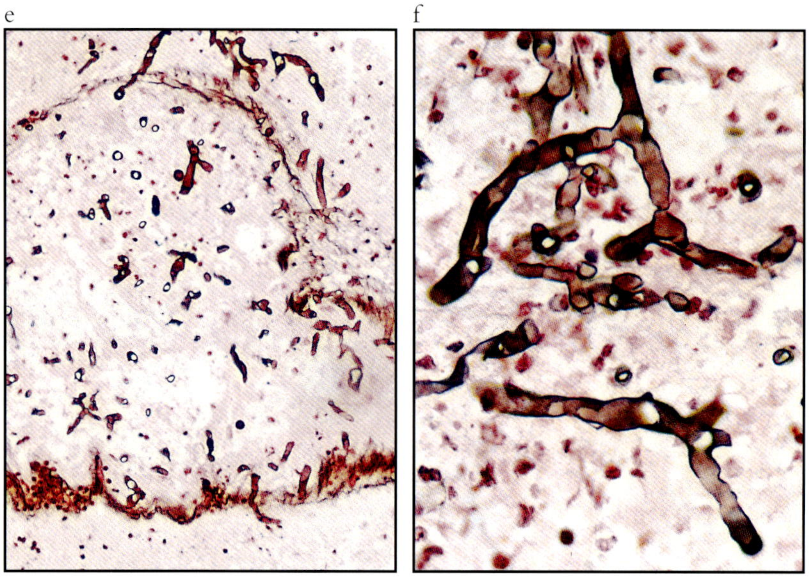

A cell block prepared from this aspirate contains thrombosed blood vessels with hyphae growing within vessel walls and lumina (e and f) (both, Methenamine silver, e, 200X; f, 400X).

Image 3.8
Ring-enhancing lesion in an HIV-positive 35-year-old man. Computed tomographic (CT) scan (a). Aspirate of the lesion showing slender, gram-positive hyphae of *Nocardia* (b) (b, Papanicolaou, 1,000X).

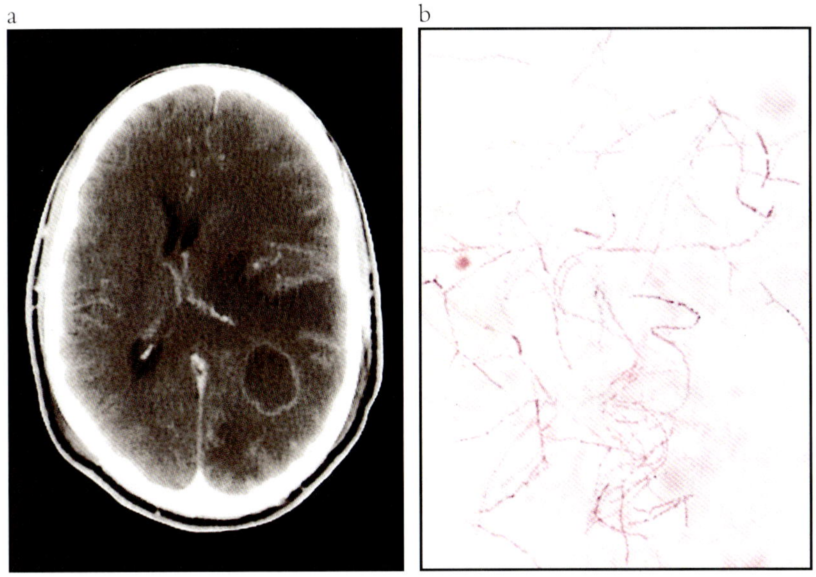

Image 3.9
Specimen of CSF from a patient with AIDS. Specimen shows an inflammatory reaction (a) and cellular enlargement and intranuclear inclusions typical of cytomegalovirus (CMV) (b). This diagnosis was confirmed histologically (c) using an antibody against CMV (d) (Courtesy of Prabodh Gupta, MD) (a and b, Papanicolaou, 400X; c, H&E, 400X; d, Immunoperoxidase, 400X).

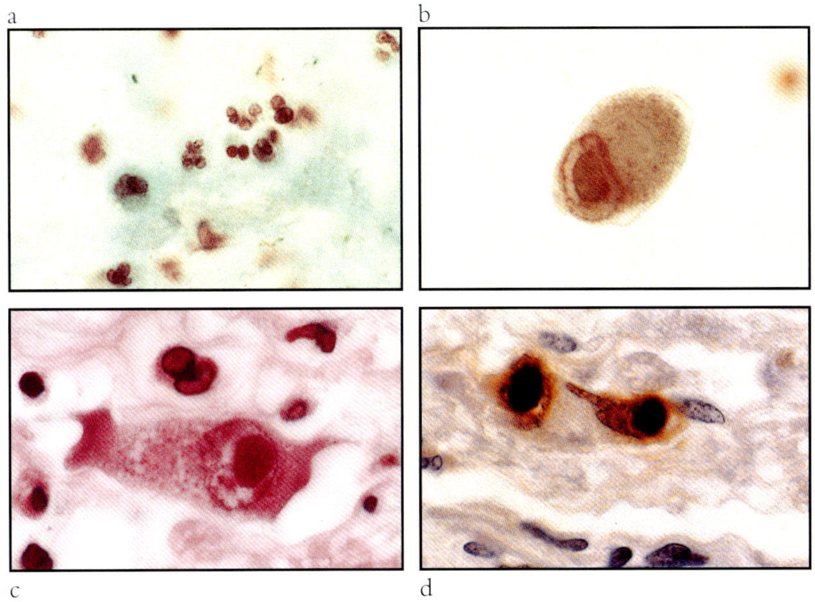

Image 3.10
Toxoplasma in CSF from an immunosuppressed patient with non-Hodgkin's lymphoma (a, Papanicolaou, 1,000X; b and c, Romanowski, 1,000X) (Courtesy of Edmund Cibas, MD).

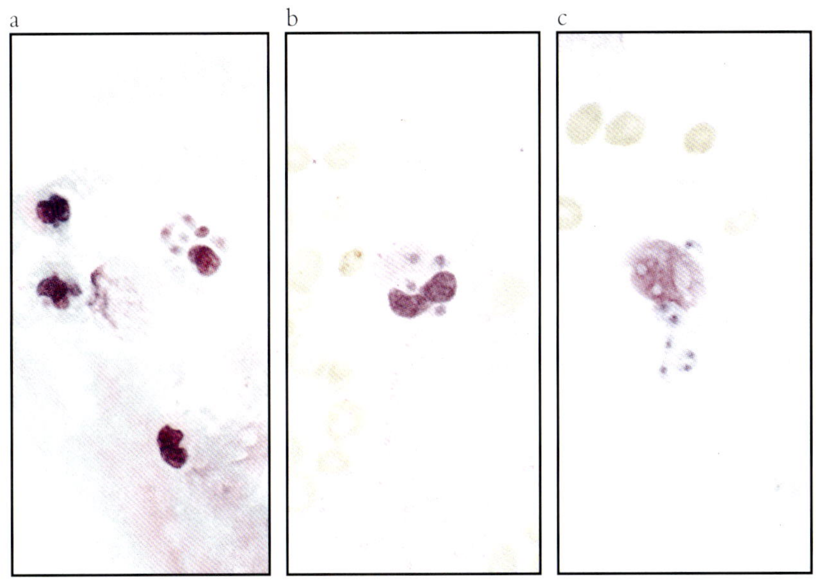

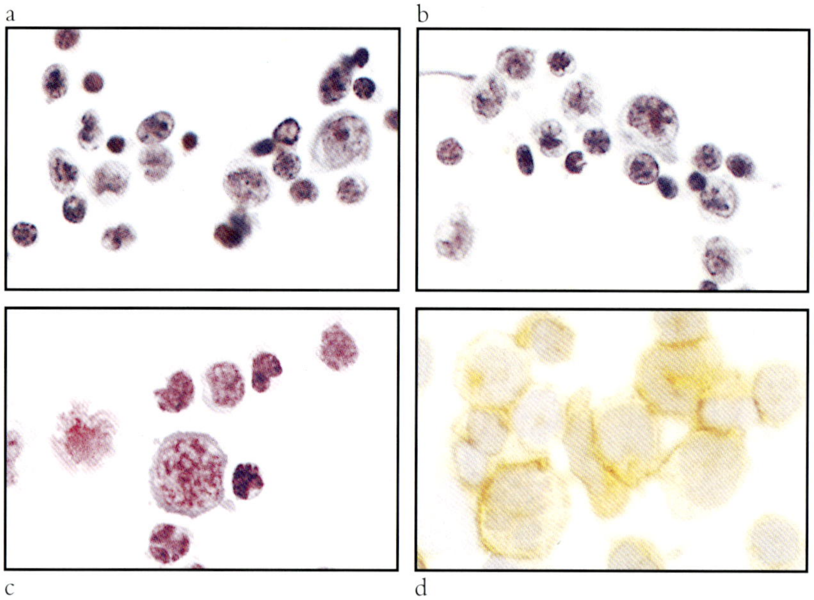

Image 3.11
CSF from a patient with AIDS. Highly reactive lymphocytes of variable size and morphology (a through c). Immunohistochemistry using a pan T antibody shows T-cell predominance, supporting the interpretation that this is a reactive process (d) (a and b, Papanicolaou; c, Romanowski; d, Immunoperoxidase; all, 400X).

References

1. Bigner SH: Cytologic diagnosis of cryptococcal meningitis. *ASCP Cytopathology Check Sample*, vol. 11. Chicago, IL, American Society of Clinical Pathologists, 1983.
2. Bigner SH, Burger PC, Dubois PJ, Nashold BS, Moore JO, Johnston WW: Diagnosis of cerebral mucormycosis by needle aspiration biopsy: a case report. *Acta Cytol* 26:699–704, 1982.
3. Bigner SH, Johnston WW: The cytopathology of cerebrospinal fluid, I. Non-neoplastic conditions: lymphoma and leukemia. *Acta Cytol* 25:335–353, 1981.
4. Borowitz MJ, Bigner SH, Johnston WW: Diagnostic problems in the cytologic evaluation of cerebrospinal fluid for lymphoma and leukemia. *Acta Cytol* 25:665–674, 1981.
5. Bunnag T, Comer DS, Punyagupta S: Eosinophilic myeloencephalitis caused by *Gnathostoma spinigerum*: neuropathology of nine cases. *J Neurol Sci* 10:419–434, 1970.
6. Cumings JN: Clinical pathology in general practice: the cerebrospinal fluid in diagnosis. *Br Med J* 1:449–451, 1954.
7. Den Hartog Jager WA: *Color Atlas of CSF Cytopathology.* Philadelphia, PA, JB Lippincott Co, 1980, pp. 9–10.
8. Duma RJ, Ferrell HW, Nelson EC, Jones MM: Primary amebic meningoencephalitis. *N Engl J Med* 281:1315–1323, 1969.
9. Fetter BF, Klintworth GK, Hendry WS: *Mycoses of the Central Nervous System.* Baltimore, MD, Williams and Wilkins Co, 1967, p. 131.
10. Gondos B, King EB: Cerebrospinal fluid cytology: diagnostic accuracy and comparison of different techniques. *Acta Cytol* 20:542–547, 1976.
11. Gupta PK, Gupta PC, Roy S, Banerji AK: Herpes simplex encephalitis, cerebrospinal fluid cytology studies: two case reports. *Acta Cytol* 16:563–565, 1972.
12. Hinnanti K, Perchick A, Koslow M, Burstein DE: Cytologic findings in brain biopsy crush preparations from 16 patients with AIDS or AIDS risk factors. *Acta Cytol* 32:774, 1988.
13. Johnston WW: Mycoses in cytopathology. In: Wied GL, Koss LG, Reagan JW, eds. *Compendium on Diagnostic Cytology*, vol. 3, no. 1. Tutorial Proceedings. Chicago, IL, Tutorials of Cytology, 1974, pp. 285–293.
14. Katz RL, Alappattu C, Glass PJ, Bruner JM: Cerebrospinal fluid manifestations of the neurologic complications of human immunodeficiency virus infection. *Acta Cytol* 33:233–244, 1989.
15. Kuberski T: Eosinophils in the cerebrospinal fluid. *Ann Intern Med* 91:70–75, 1979.
16. Peter A: The plasma cells of the cerebrospinal fluid. *J Neurol Sci* 4:227–239, 1967.
17. Razavi-Encha F, Fleury-Feith J, Gherandi R, Bernaudin JF: Cytologic features of cerebrospinal fluid in Lyme disease. *Acta Cytol* 31:439–440, 1987.

18. Saigo P, Rosen PP, Kaplan MH, Solan G, Melamed MR: Identification of *Cryptococcus neoformans* in cytologic preparations of cerebrospinal fluid. *Am J Clin Pathol* 67:141–145, 1977.

19. Szecsi S: Neue beitrage zur cytologie des liquor cerebrospinalis: Uber art und herkunft der zellen. *Z Gesamte Neurol Psychiatr* 6:537–588, 1911.

20. Wilber RR, King EB, Howes EL Jr: Cerebrospinal fluid cytology in five patients with cerebral cysticercosis. *Acta Cytol* 24:421–426, 1980.

21. Woodruff KH: Cerebrospinal fluid cytomorphology using cytocentrifugation. *Am J Clin Pathol* 60:621–627, 1973.

22. Yii C-Y: Clinical observations on eosinophilic meningitis and meningoencephalitis caused by *Angiostrongylus cantonensis* on Taiwan. *Am J Trop Med Hyg* 25:223–249, 1976.

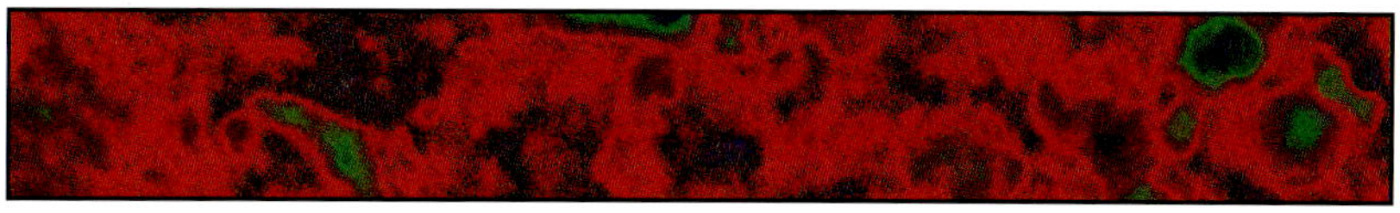

CHAPTER FOUR

Non-neoplastic Disorders

A variety of destructive lesions may involve the parenchyma of the brain and spinal cord and be reflected in cerebrospinal fluid (CSF) as quantitative and qualitative changes in the normal cellular components. The most common nonspecific response to injury is an increase in the number of lymphocytes and monocytes. Lymphocytes enlarge with increased amounts of cytoplasm and display reactive nuclear changes such as chromatin clumping and nucleolar prominence. When these features are pronounced, these cells acquire the morphology of immunoblasts (Image 4.1). Monocytes frequently become macrophages, phagocytizing cellular debris including fragments of blood and myelin (Image 4.2).

Some authors have suggested that the reactive cells in CSF are derived from "pia-arachnoid cells"[6,14] rather than from lymphoid and hematopoietic elements. Evidence supporting the inflammatory origin of these cells is their expression of panleukocyte antigens (Image 4.3) and the observation by phase-contrast microscopy that the monocytoid cells can convert to macrophages.[11]

Another response to injury is the appearance of cell types, not normally seen in CSF, the most common of which is the polymorphonuclear leukocyte. These cells may accumulate in CSF in any acute process and do not necessarily indicate the presence of an infectious agent. Within brain parenchyma, these cells fill vascular lumina and presumably traverse vessel walls to appear in the tissue. Possible routes for these cells to reach CSF are by migration from underlying brain tissue into the subarachnoid space (SAS), by migration through disrupted ependyma into the ventricular cavities, or by entering CSF directly from vessels in the SAS or in the choroid plexus.

Many of these changes seen in non-neoplastic conditions are nonspecific. It is important to recognize these conditions, however, to prevent confusing them with neoplastic processes. This pitfall can be avoided if one is aware of the cellular changes in CSF associated with the more common non-neoplastic conditions.[4,12]

Infarction

Infarction is produced by vascular occlusion and is characterized by necrosis of the brain in the distribution of the occluded vessel (Figure 4.1). Infarcts produced by atherosclerosis and thrombosis are usually pale with little hemorrhage, whereas embolic infarcts, or those caused by venous occlusion, may be hemorrhagic (Figure 4.2). In early infarctions, polymorphonuclear leukocytes are the first cells to respond followed by macrophages, which become filled with necrotic debris (Image 4.4). In the late stages, infarcts are reduced to shrunken cavities that contain blood vessels and macrophages and are rimmed by reactive astrocytes (Images 4.5 and 4.6). The type of infiltrate seen in CSF reflects the populations seen in the underlying brain parenchyma and is, therefore, dependent on the type of infarct (anemic or hemorrhagic) as well as on the time that has elapsed since the initial injury. Image 4.7 shows foamy macrophages and polymorphonuclear leukocytes in CSF from a patient with a subacute infarct.

Infarcts can be confused with tumors clinically and radiographically

Although the clinical presentation of cerebral infarction is typically more acute than that of brain neoplasms, infarcts can sometimes be confused with tumors clinically and radiographically. Needle aspirates may be obtained to confirm the diagnosis (Image 4.8), but these samples may be highly cellular and can be mistaken for metastatic adenocarcinomas or gliomas if the possibility of infarction is not considered. Immunohistochemistry is often helpful since the inflammatory nature of these cells is

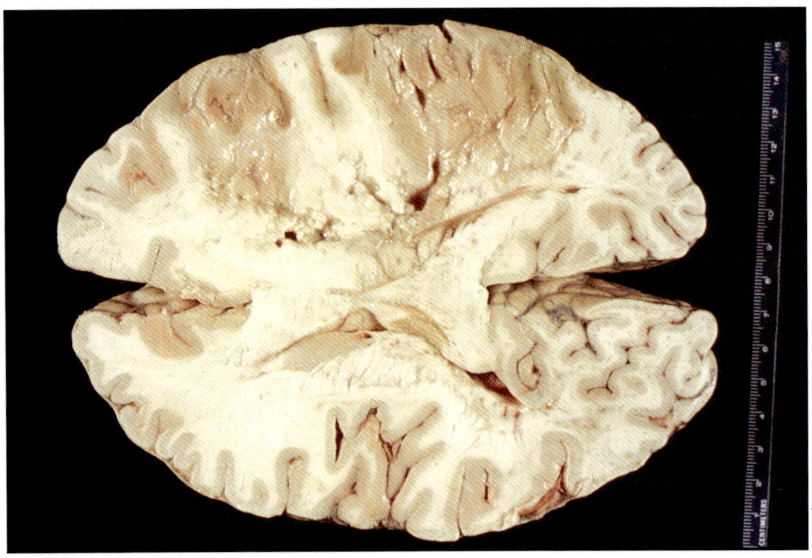

Figure 4.1
Horizontal section of a brain at autopsy showing a large area of early infarction characterized by swelling and softening.

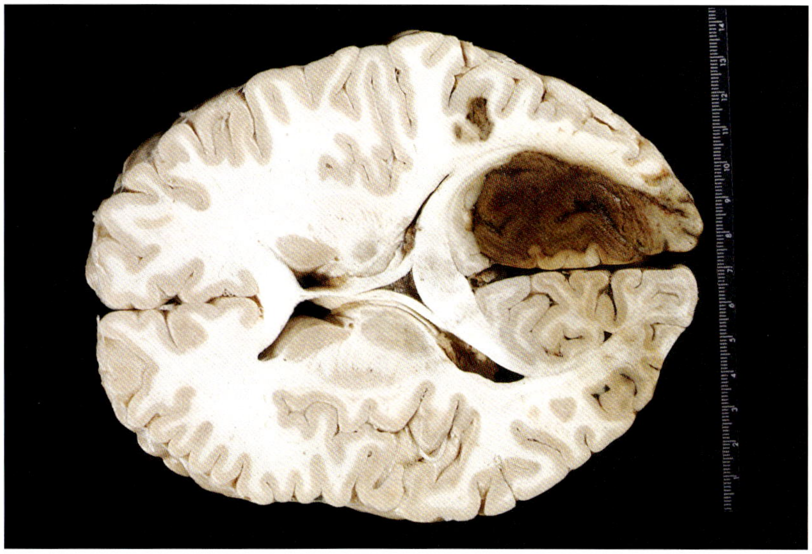

Figure 4.2
Hemorrhagic infarct of the occipital lobe secondary to an embolus.

readily demonstrated by using antipanleukocyte antibodies, although they fail to react with anticarcinoma antibodies (Image 4.8).

Hemorrhage

The cytologic presentation of hemorrhage consists of erythrocytes, erythrophagocytosis, and hemosiderin-laden macrophages

Hemorrhage into the SAS may result from trauma, ruptured aneurysm, spontaneous intracerebral hemorrhage (hypertension or coagulopathy), hemorrhagic infarct, arteriovenous malformation, or tumor (Figure 4.3). Regardless of the cause, the cytologic presentation consists first of intact erythrocytes followed by erythrophagocytosis (Image 4.9) and hemosiderin-laden macrophages (Image 4.10). In most instances, no clues to the cause of the hemorrhage exist, although Koss[5] illustrated an unusual case of endometriosis involving the meninges in which hemorrhage and endometrial cells were seen in CSF. Red blood cells in CSF may also result from a "traumatic" lumbar puncture in which a vessel is punctured and peripheral blood contaminates the CSF. The immediate specimen will be red, and numerous intact erythrocytes will be seen. A repeat lumbar puncture within several days will reveal xanthochromic fluid, and erythrophagocytosis will be present just as in subarachnoid hemorrhages from other causes.

Intraventricular Shunts

Specimens of CSF derived from intraventricular shunts frequently contain a variety of unusual cell types including multinucleated giant cells of the foreign body type, macrophages, and reactive ependymal cells (Image 4.11).[2] This constellation of findings is often associated with a clinical history of shunt malfunction, suggesting that the changes in

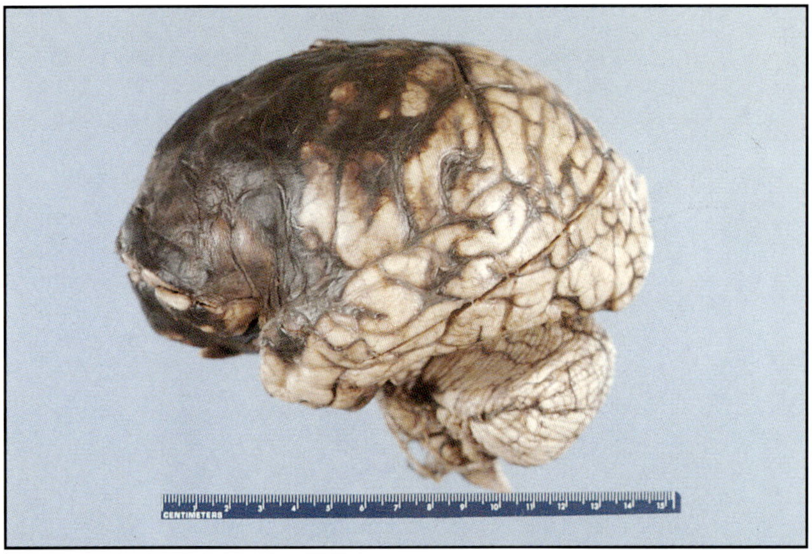

Figure 4.3
Brain of a patient with severe head trauma showing discoloration due to massive hemorrhage within the subarachnoid space (SAS).

the CSF may reflect a granulomatous foreign body reaction that is obstructing the shunt lumen (Image 4.11d). The hypercellularity of these samples and the presence of giant cells can lead to an erroneous diagnosis of granulomatous inflammation due to tuberculosis or sarcoidosis if the relevant history is not available. Since many patients with intraventricular shunts have a history of brain neoplasms, these changes should not be confused with recurrent tumor.

Basilar Skull Fractures

Another traumatic condition that may present a confusing array of findings in CSF is a basilar skull fracture. If the meninges are torn, contents of the nasal sinuses may pass directly into the SAS. In the CSF, a mixture of debris, ciliated columnar cells, squamous cells, bacteria, and *Candida* may be seen (Image 4.12).[1]

Degenerative and Demyelinating Diseases and Other Disorders of Unknown Etiology

The cellular components in CSF from patients with demyelinating diseases are variable, depending on the specific diagnosis and the phase and extent of the disease. In multiple sclerosis, for example, the cell counts and constitution may be normal during quiescent phases of the disease. Immunophenotyping of the lymphocyte populations generally reveals T-cell predominance with mature T cells expressing either the helper or suppressor phenotype.[7] Some observers have described a decreased suppressor/helper cell ratio in both CSF and peripheral blood of patients with multiple sclerosis during exacerbation due to an absolute decrease in the number of suppressor cells.[10] Other studies, however, have failed to demonstrate differences in suppressor/helper cell ratios between CSF from patients with multiple sclerosis and patients with other central nervous system (CNS) disorders such as Guillain-Barré syndrome and CNS infection.[9] Rarely, in acute, rapidly progressive cases other cell types, including polymorphonuclear leukocytes and macrophages, may be seen.

In most cases of Guillain-Barré syndrome, the CSF is acellular, but when inflammatory cells are present, a lymphocytic response predominates. The picture is similar to that seen in viral meningoencephalitis with a polyclonal lymphocytic population with T-cell predominance. For the other diseases in which demyelination is a component, the nature and extent of cellular elements in CSF reflect the nature of the infiltrate within the parenchyma of the brain and spinal cord.

The CSF from patients with dementia is usually normal

Dementia is a devastating clinical disorder characterized by memory loss, disorientation, and confusion. The most common causes of dementia are senile dementia, Alzheimer's disease, and normal pressure hydrocephalus. Less common etiologies are Jakob-Creutzfeldt disease and Pick's disease. Despite the severe functional deficiencies produced by these diseases and their striking histologic abnormalities, the CSF from these patients is usually normal since the lesions are mainly in the brain parenchyma. Parkinson's disease and Huntington's chorea produce disturbances in movement and coordination due to lesions in the basal ganglia. Although Wertlake et al[14] described atypical cells in the CSF from a patient with parkinsonism, we have not observed any characteristic changes associated with either of these disorders.

Image 4.13 shows reactive lymphocytes in CSF from a 59-year-old woman with a granulomatous angiitis of the temporal lobe. This type of lymphocytic response may be the only manifestation in CSF of granulomatous lesions within the brain. Image 4.14 shows macrophages in CSF from a 23-year-old man with a history of leukemia who developed a necrotizing leukoencephalopathy secondary to therapy. The nonspecific reaction in this case illustrates the cell types encountered in a broad spectrum of non-neoplastic conditions that involve destruction of brain tissue. We have seen similar reactions in CSF obtained during craniotomy or in the postoperative period.

Storage Diseases

Macrophages may have foamy cytoplasm due to ingestion of lipids or glycoproteins. Although this morphologic cell type is a nonspecific finding associated with any destructive process involving myelin, in some cases it is reflecting an abnormality in myelin metabolism. Foamy macrophages, for example, have been reported in Tay-Sachs disease,[13] where they presumably contain ganglioside. Oehmichen[8] cited a case of the Hunter-Hurler syndrome that showed similar cells in CSF. Garcia-Riego et al[3] reported a case of Sanfilippo disease in which Buhot cells appeared in CSF. These macrophages with basophilic cytoplasmic inclusions were easily seen with May-Grunwald-Giemsa stain but were barely visible with Papanicolaou stain.

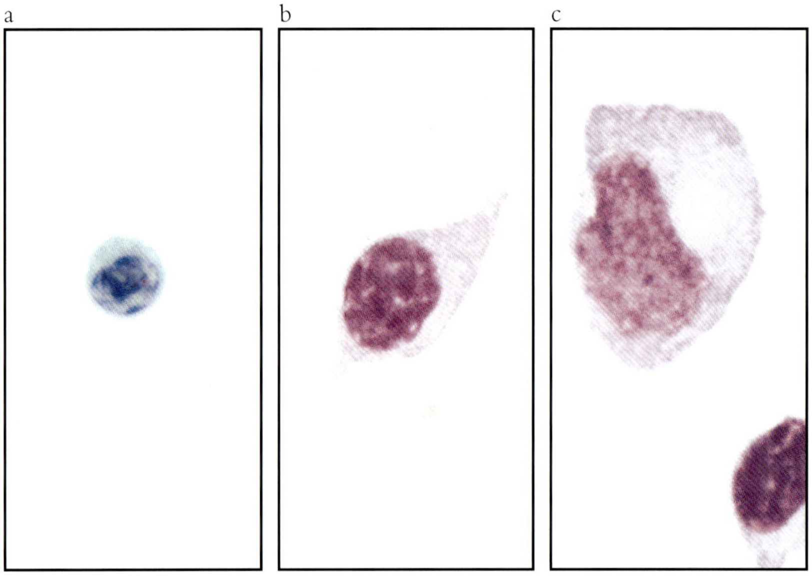

Image 4.1
Reactive cell types in CSF. Reactive lymphocytes are larger and possess more cytoplasm than normal lymphocytes (a and b). Large reactive immunoblast (c) (a, Papanicolaou; b and c, Romanowski; all, 1,000X).

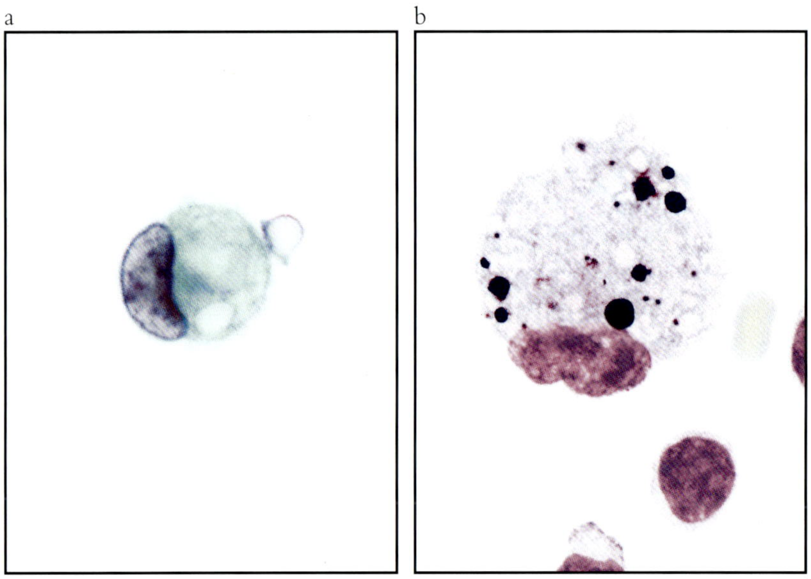

Image 4.2
Macrophages in CSF (a, Papanicolaou; b, Romanowski; both, 1,000X).

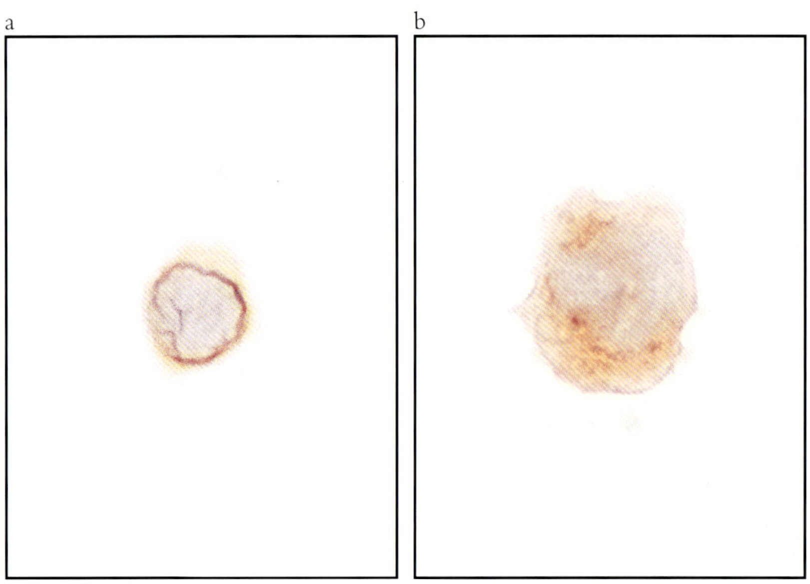

Image 4.3
Reactive lymphocytes (a) and macrophages (b) in CSF stain positively with panleukocyte antibody 2D1 (both, Panleukocyte antibody 2D1, 1,000X).

Image 4.4
Histologic appearance of a subacute cerebral infarct. Within 1 to 2 weeks, a cystic cavity begins to form as seas of macrophages engulf and carry away necrotic debris (both, H&E; a, 100X; b, 400X).

a b

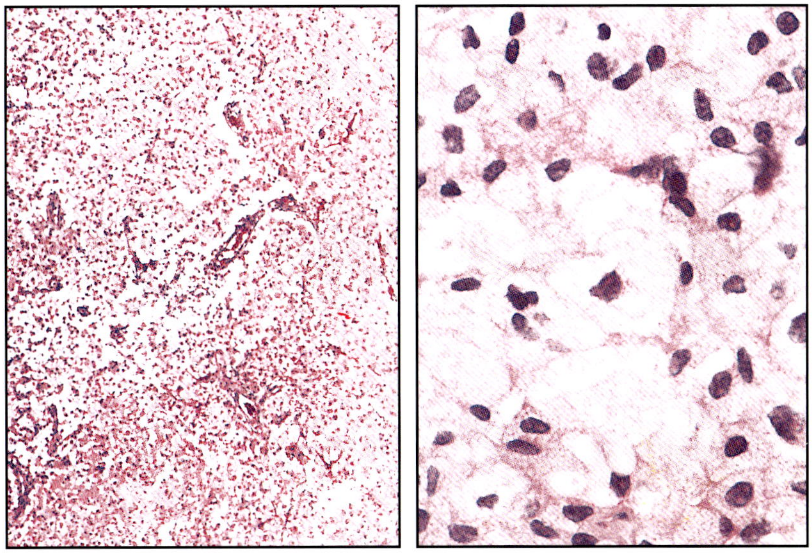

Image 4.5
An old, chronic infarct appearing grossly as a shrunken cavity in this brain at autopsy.

a

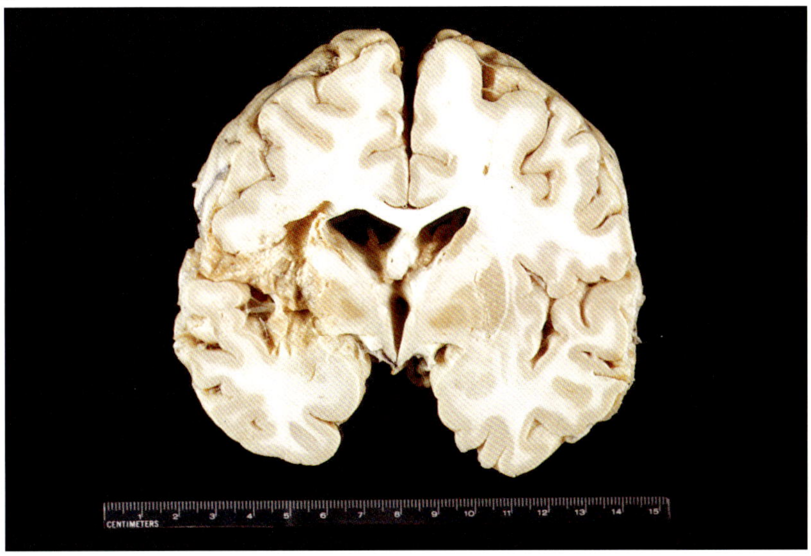

Histologic appearance of this chronic infarct (H&E, Luxol fast blue, 7X).

b

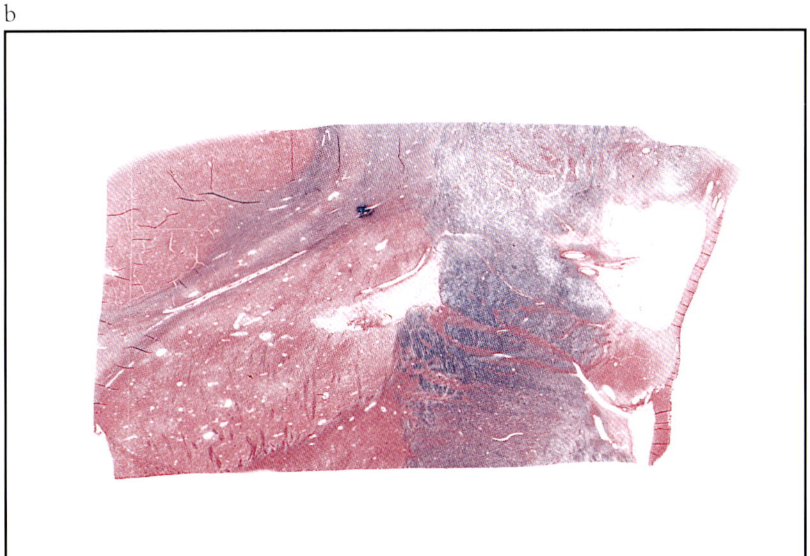

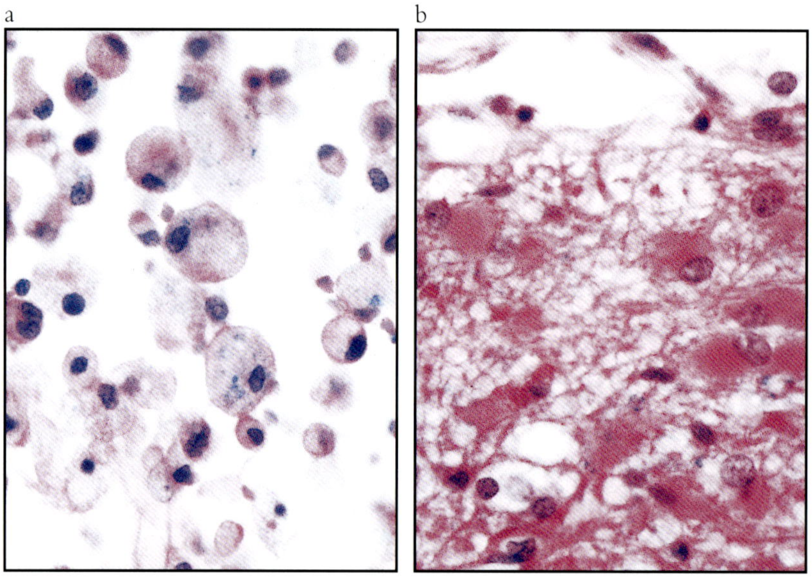

Image 4.6
Histologic appearance of a cavity of a chronic infarct containing macrophages (a) and surrounded by a rim of reactive astrocytes (b) (both, H&E, 400X).

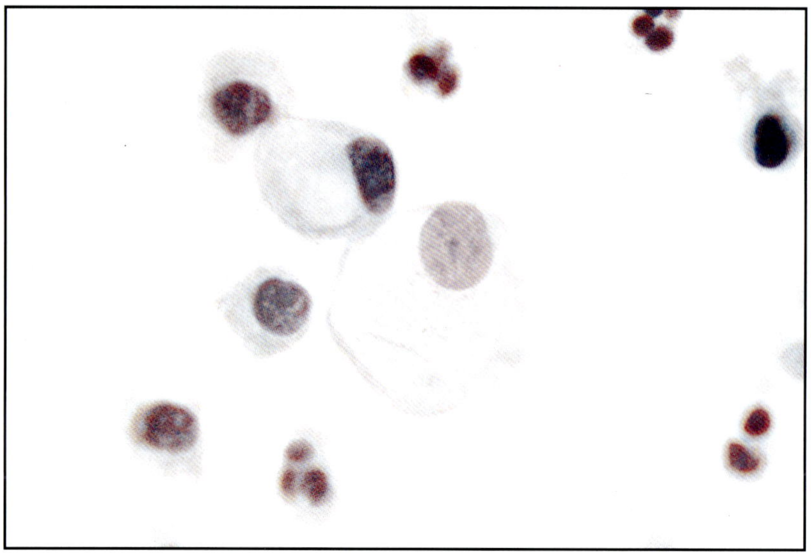

Image 4.7
CSF from a patient with an acute cerebral infarct containing polymorphonuclear leukocytes and foamy macrophages (Papanicolaou, 1,000X).

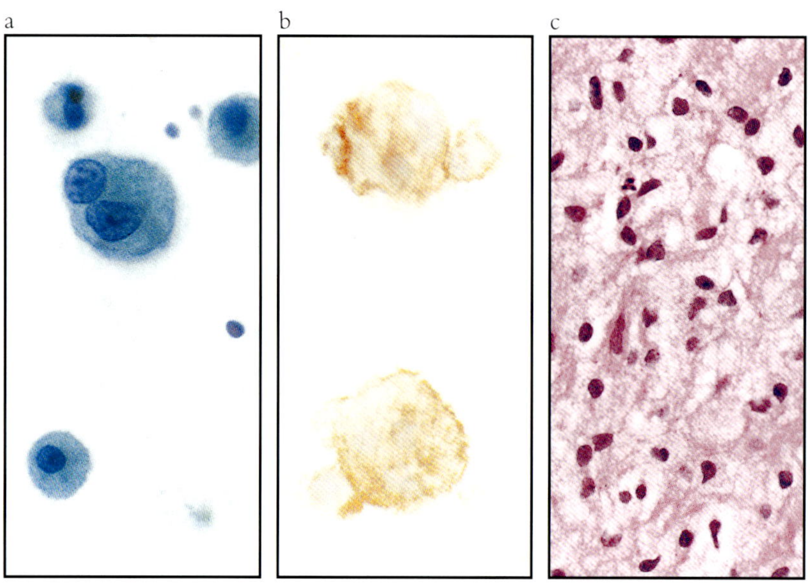

Image 4.8
Needle aspirate of a subacute infarct with numerous foamy macrophages (a) that react with panleukocyte antibody 2D1 (b). Sheets of macrophages in the corresponding biopsy specimen (c) (a, Papanicolaou, 1,000X; b, Panleukocyte antibody 2D1, 1,000X; c, H&E, 400X).

Image 4.9
Erythrophagocytes in CSF from a patient with subarachnoid space (SAS) hemorrhage (a, Papanicolaou; b, Romanowski; both, 1,000X).

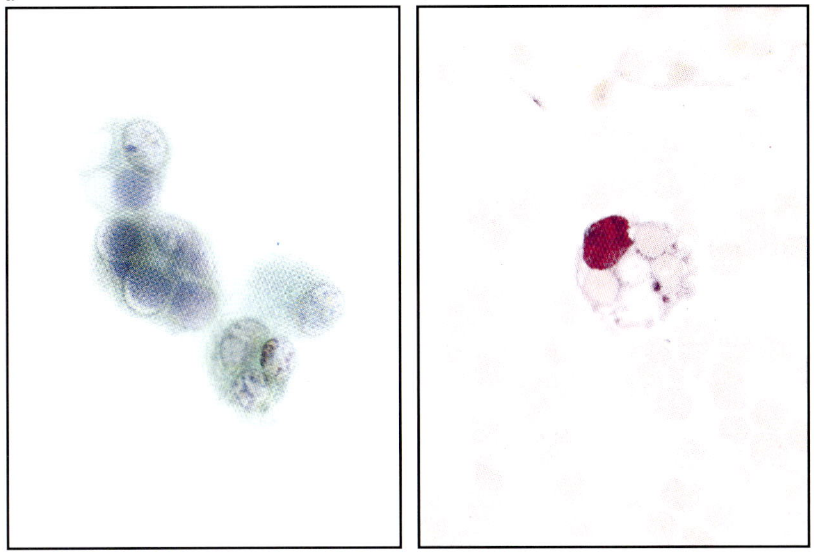

Image 4.10
Hemosiderin-laden macrophage in CSF from a patient with SAS hemorrhage (Papanicolaou, 1,000X).

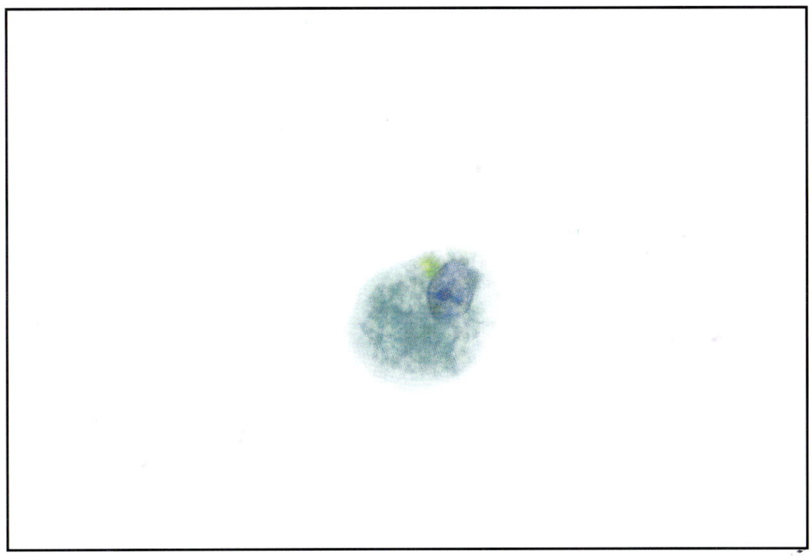

Image 4.11
Multinucleated giant cells (a and b) and macrophages (c) in CSF from a patient with an obstructed shunt. A foreign body reaction occurred on this patient's shunt tip (d) (a through c, Papanicolaou, 400X; d, H&E, 400X).

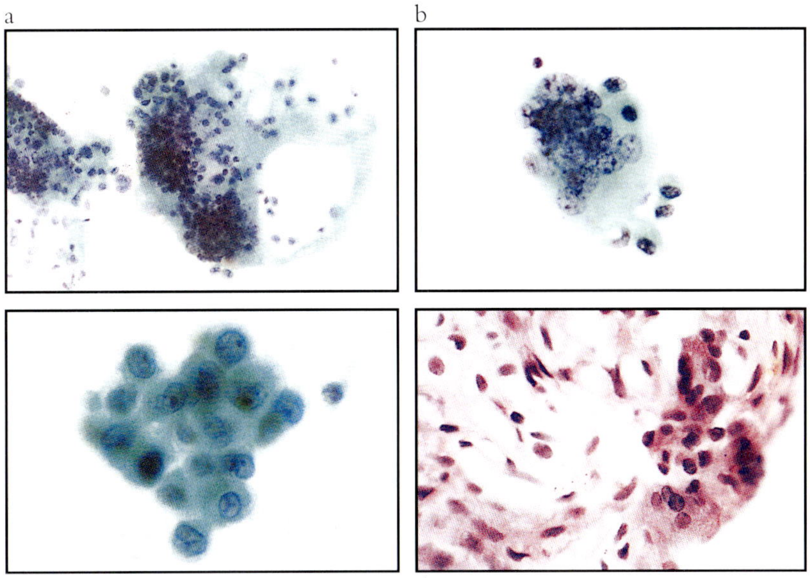

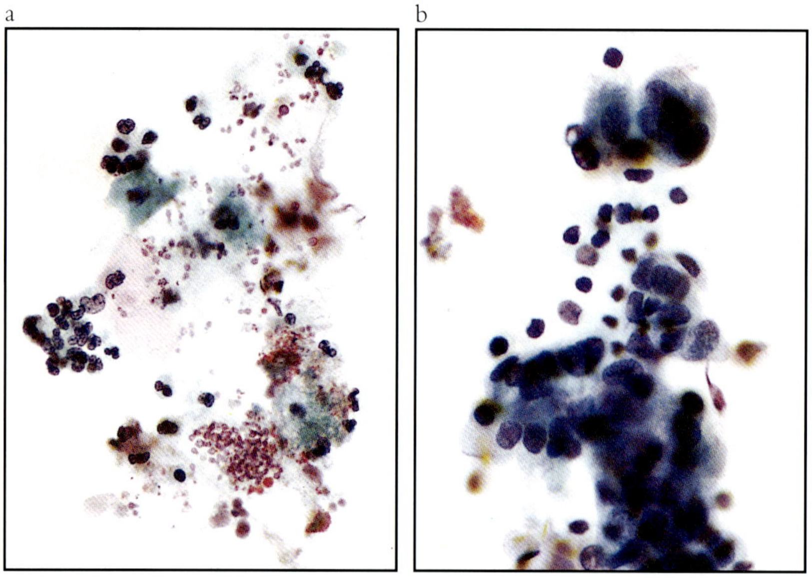

Image 4.12
Mixed bacteria, *Candida*, and ciliated columnar cells in CSF from a patient with a basilar skull fracture (both, Papanicolaou, 1,000X).

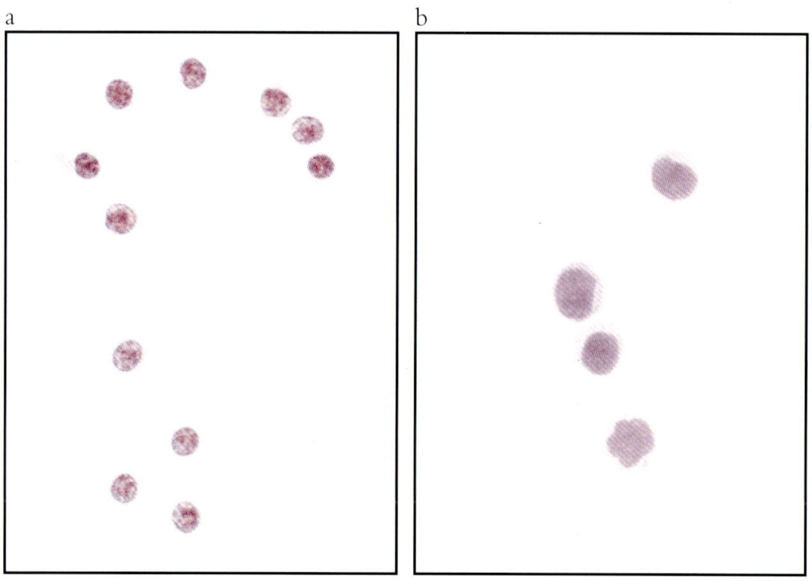

Image 4.13
Reactive lymphocytes in CSF from a 59-year-old woman with granulomatous angiitis (a, Papanicolaou; b, Romanowski; both, 1,000X).

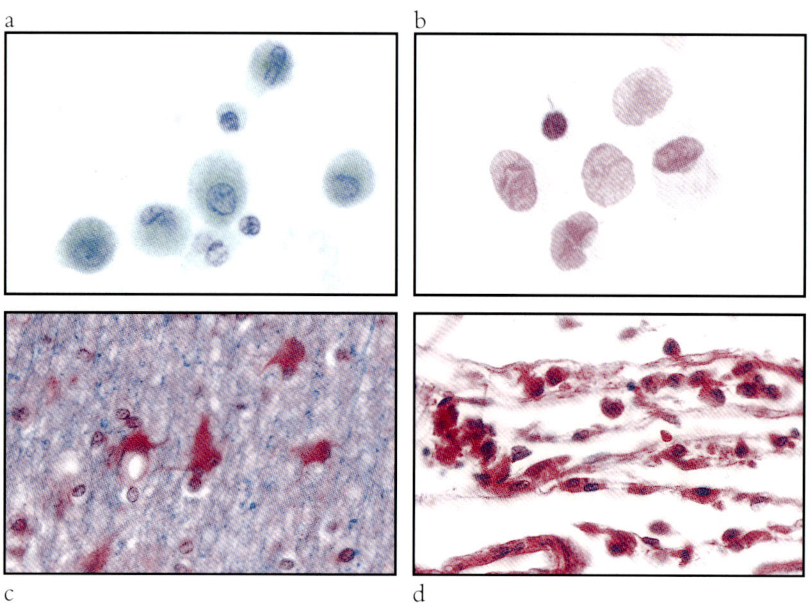

Image 4.14
Foamy macrophages in CSF from a 23-year-old man with necrotizing leukoencephalopathy secondary to therapy for acute leukemia (a and b). Brain at autopsy (c and d). The white matter was infiltrated by reactive astrocytes (c). The SAS contained numerous macrophages similar to these seen in the CSF (d) (a, Papanicolaou, 1,000X; b, Romanowski, 1,000X; c and d, H&E, 400X).

References

1. Bigner SH, Elmore PD, Dee AL, Hoffman M, Johnston WW: Unusual presentations of inflammatory conditions in cerebrospinal fluid. *Acta Cytol* 29:291–296, 1985.
2. Bigner SH, Elmore PD, Dee AL, Johnston WW: The cytopathology of reactions to ventricular shunts. *Acta Cytol* 29:391–396, 1985.
3. Garcia-Riego A, Prats JM, Zarranz JJ: Sanfilippo disease: Buhot cells in the cerebrospinal fluid. *Acta Cytol* 22:282–284, 1978.
4. Gondos B, King EB: Cerebrospinal fluid cytology: diagnostic accuracy and comparison of different techniques. *Acta Cytol* 20:542–547, 1976.
5. Koss LG: *Diagnostic Cytology and Its Histopathologic Bases*, 4th ed, vol 2. Philadelphia, PA, JB Lippincott Co, 1992.
6. McGarry P, Holmquist ND, Carmel SA: A postmortem study of cerebrospinal fluid with histologic correlation. *Acta Cytol* 13:48–52, 1969.
7. Noronha A, Richman DP, Arnason GW: Multiple sclerosis: activated cells in cerebrospinal fluid in acute exacerbations. *Ann Neurol* 18, 6:722–725, 1985.
8. Oehmichen M: *Cerebrospinal Fluid Cytology: An Introduction and Atlas.* Philadelphia, PA, WB Saunders and Co, 1976, p. 148.
9. Polman CH, de Groot CJA, Koestsier JC, Sminia T, Veerman AJP: Cerebrospinal fluid cells in multiple sclerosis and other neurological diseases: an immunocytochemical study. *J Neurol* 234:19–22, 1987.
10. Santoli D, DeFreitas EC, Sandberg-Wollheim M, Koprowski H: Phenotypic and functional characterization of T-cell clones derived from the cerebrospinal fluid of multiple sclerosis patients. *Am Assoc Immunol* 132:2386–2391, 1984.
11. Sornas R: Transformation of mononuclear cells in cerebrospinal fluid. *Acta Cytol* 15:545–552, 1971.
12. Takeda M, King DE, Choi HY, Gomi K, Lang WR: Diagnostic pitfalls in cerebrospinal fluid cytology. *Acta Cytol* 25:245–250, 1981.
13. Tourtellotte WW: A selected review of reactions of the cerebrospinal fluid to disease. In: Fields WS, ed. *Neurological Diagnostic Techniques.* Springfield, IL, Charles C Thomas, 1966, pp. 25–50.
14. Wertlake PT, Markovits BA, Stellar S: Cytologic evaluation of cerebrospinal fluid with clinical and histologic correlation. *Acta Cytol* 16:224–239, 1972.

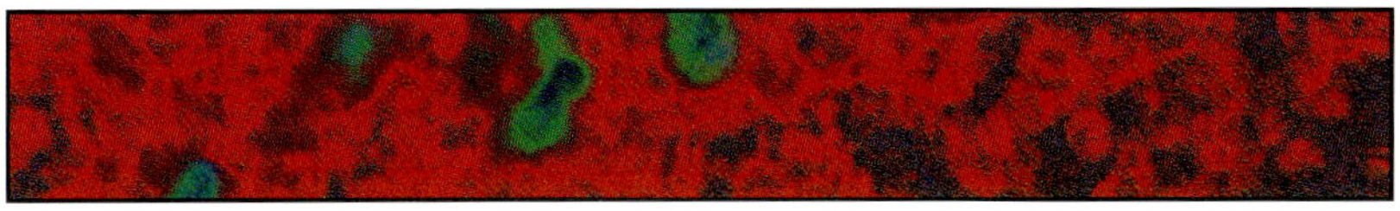

CHAPTER FIVE

Leukemia and Lymphoma

The most common pattern of involvement of the central nervous system (CNS) by lymphoma and leukemia is diffuse seeding of the subarachnoid space (SAS) (Image 5.1). Involvement of the cranial and spinal nerves as they course through this area is common. Parenchymal infiltrates are seen less frequently but are most common in patients with leukemia who have extremely high numbers of circulating blasts ($>100,000/mm^3$). These infiltrates are generally numerous, small, hemorrhagic, perivascular foci composed of both red blood cells (RBCs) and leukemic blasts (Figure 5.1). Patients with lymphoma, particularly those with a heavy systemic tumor burden, may have solid parenchymal infiltrates as well as meningeal disease (Image 5.2). A third pattern of CNS involvement in patients with leukemia and lymphoma is spinal extradural infiltration, which produces symptoms of spinal compression. Because the extradural compartment does not communicate with the SAS, cells are not seen in cerebrospinal fluid (CSF).

Leukemia

Evaluation of CSF from patients with leukemia has become a major task of many cytopathology laboratories. During the last 20 to 30 years, prophylactic CNS radiation and intrathecal chemotherapy have become integral components of the treatment of children with acute lymphocytic leukemia (ALL). In most institutions, these patients undergo cytologic examination of CSF at the time of initial diagnosis and then receive pro-

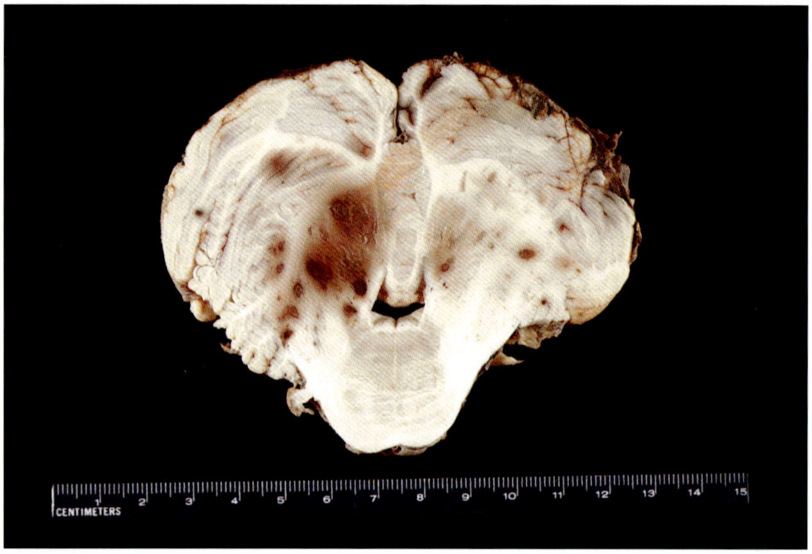

Figure 5.1
Hemorrhagic foci of leukemic infiltrates in a section of cerebellum and brain stem from a patient with acute leukemia.

phylactic CNS therapy. They subsequently have periodic CSF examinations regardless of neurologic condition and CSF cell count. This regimen reduced the overall incidence of CSF involvement to approximately 10% in patients with ALL, whereas those who did not receive such treatment experienced a 60% incidence of CSF involvement.[18]

The blasts of ALL, even when present in small numbers, are generally morphologically distinguishable from normal and reactive inflammatory cells. They are larger than normal lymphocytes with higher nuclear/cytoplasmic ratios, and they usually have visible nucleoli. Nuclei may be round or convoluted (Image 5.3a). Air-dried, Romanowski-stained preparations are particularly helpful in demonstrating the smooth, evenly distributed blastic chromatin pattern (Image 5.3b). This stain also allows direct comparison between cells in CSF and those in the peripheral blood or bone marrow from the same patient. Although reactive lymphocytes may be enlarged and have prominent nucleoli, they have more abundant cytoplasm than leukemic blasts and have the coarsely clumped chromatin pattern typical of mature lymphocytes (Image 5.4). Reactive immunoblasts are greatly enlarged with atypical nuclei, irregular chromatin, and abundant cytoplasm. These differing morphologic features between leukemic blasts and reactive lymphocytes and immunoblasts usually allow their identification using morphologic features alone. In the occasional case where diagnostic problems exist, the application of antileukocyte antibody panels may be useful, particularly if the phenotype of the neoplastic cells has been demonstrated previously in bone marrow or lymph nodes. Image 5.5 demonstrates common acute lymphoblastic leukemia antigen (CALLA)–positive blasts in CSF from a child with CALLA-positive ALL.

Leukemic blasts and reactive lymphocytes and immunoblasts can usually be identified by morphology alone

Cases that present the greatest diagnostic difficulties are generally those in which only a few atypical cells are present for evaluation, and certain determination of whether they are reactive cells or blast forms is impossible. In such cases, antibody studies are of limited value since too few cells are available to be adequately represented on multiple antibody preparations and control slides. Although some observers have used antibodies against CALLA or expression of terminal deoxynucleotidyltransferase in this setting to identify small populations of blast forms, recurrent ALL should probably not be diagnosed using this criterion alone, since rare CALLA-positive cells can be seen in individuals who do not have leukemia.[17,39] Even if a few blast forms can be identified with certainty, these patients present a difficult clinical problem because conflicting evidence exists regarding whether or not these patients should be treated for CNS relapse. Earlier studies suggest that the presence of only rare blast forms in CSF samples of normal cell count should result in aggressive intrathecal therapy. However, recent studies in which these patients have been treated conservatively show spontaneous clearing of the abnormal cells in some patients.[25] The approach suggested by McIntosh and Ritchey[25] for patients with ALL is to treat them for CNS relapse if their CSF contains more than 10 white blood cells (WBCs)/μL with blast forms or less than 10 WBCs/μL if blast forms predominate. For patients with only rare blast forms in CSF samples (<5 WBCs/μL), however, the authors' policy is only to repeat the examination of CSF every few months provided that the patient is in systemic remission and lacks CNS symptoms.

The success of controlling childhood ALL has not been matched in other CNS neoplasms

The dramatic success of controlling childhood ALL has not been matched in any other type of neoplasm that involves the CNS. ALL is unique; not only does chemotherapy effectively control the bone marrow, which is the primary organ of involvement, but prophylactic CNS therapy prevents CNS relapse. In contrast, although prophylactic CNS radiation is effective in patients with acute nonlymphocytic leukemia, the high rate of marrow relapse prevents CNS control from changing survival. In a study of 171 children with acute nonlymphocytic leukemia, a complete remission frequency of 66% was noted, but the median duration of remission was 6 months with a median survival of 10 months.[10]

The nonlymphocytic forms of acute leukemia include acute myelogenous leukemia, acute promyelocytic leukemia, acute myelomonocytic leukemia, acute undifferentiated leukemia, acute monocytic leukemia, and chronic granulocytic leukemia in blast crisis. Myelogenous blasts of the first three types (myelogenous, promyelocytic, and myelomonocytic), and the last (chronic granulocytic) are similar to lymphoblasts on Papanicolaou-stained specimens (Image 5.6). Romanowski stains may show cytoplasmic granules in maturing myeloid cells, which establishes their myelogenous origin (Images 5.7 and 5.8). Monocytic blasts of acute monocytic and acute myelomonocytic leukemias are similar to macrophages with kidney bean–shaped nuclei, prominent nucleoli, and moderate amounts of cytoplasm (Images 5.6b and 5.9). The single-cell presentation, size, and overall morphology of these cells are similar to lobular carcinoma of the breast on Papanicolaou-stained specimens. Romanowski-stained specimens are extremely helpful, because they demonstrate cytoplasmic granules in the monocytes (Image 5.9b).

The possibility of false-positive diagnoses due to contamination from leukemic peripheral blood was recognized by Nies et al,[29] and the possibility of bone marrow from the vertebral bodies contaminating CSF was suggested by Spriggs and Boddington.[38] Rohlfing et al[33] used serial dilutions of leukemic blood in CSF to demonstrate that a single drop of blood, which will not discolor the clear fluid, still contaminates the specimen when prepared by Millipore® filtration. This important pitfall is a result of the extreme efficiency with which membrane filters collect small numbers of blasts combined with the lysis of RBCs by 95% alcohol. This pitfall can be suspected if simultaneous air-dried, Wright-stained preparations are made, because the telltale erythrocytes are preserved by this method. If doubt still persists, the best practice is to repeat the examination several weeks later. Immature hematopoietic elements of bone marrow origin have been described in CSF of both children and adults.[9,21,24] The marrow source can be suspected due to the presence of erythroid precursors in addition to immature myeloid forms.

In marked contrast to the high incidence of CNS involvement in acute leukemia, it is exceedingly rare in patients with chronic lymphocytic leukemia (CLL), a disease that occurs primarily in adults older than 50 years of age. Liepman and Votaw[23] described two patients with symptomatic meningeal involvement of CLL that responded to chemotherapy. Patchy leptomeningeal infiltrates have been described at autopsy in patients with CLL,[32] but only one autopsy-documented case of symptomatic meningeal involvement with CLL has been reported in the literature.[14] Borowitz et al[6] observed that among four patients with CLL with neurologic symptoms, all four showed CSF pleocytosis that was proven to be of infectious, not neoplastic, etiology (Image 5.10).

Cells of CLL are indistinguishable from mature lymphocytes in CSF. When lymphocytes are found in the CSF of these patients, an infectious agent should be sought, since this disorder rarely produces symptomatic CSF involvement. The diagnosis of CLL should be made cautiously by cytologic evaluation of CSF. Detailed clinical information should be obtained, and immunophenotyping should be performed to determine whether the infiltrating cells are indeed monoclonal or represent a mixed population more typical of a reactive process.

Lymphoma

Central nervous system involvement with lymphoma is less common than with leukemia; however, as treatment of lymphoma improves, the incidence of CNS involvement increases. In a series of 1,039 patients with non-Hodgkin's lymphomas, 50 (5%) had CNS disease, 39 (3.7%) had leptomeningeal infiltration, 10 (1%) had cerebral involvement, and two (0.1%) had spinal cord compression.[16] Of the positive cases, 86% had a diffuse, not nodular, histologic pattern. In this series of adult patients with lymphoma, approximately two thirds had either a large-cell or small cleaved cell type. These two cell types comprised 72% of the individuals with lymphomatous involvement of CSF.

As treatment of lymphoma improves, the incidence of CNS involvement increases

When the CSF contains large numbers of bizarre immunoblastic cells, a definitive diagnosis of large-cell lymphoma or immunoblastic sarcoma can be made (Images 5.11 and 5.12). The malignant nature of the infiltrate may be readily apparent, and the diagnostic problem may be to distinguish lymphoma from other large-cell neoplasms such as undifferentiated carcinoma and melanoma. The majority of large-cell lymphomas that involve CSF are B cell in origin (Image 5.12). They may originate systemically (Image 5.11) or may represent meningeal dissemination of a primary CNS lymphoma (Image 5.12). Either of these patterns can be seen in patients with acquired immunodeficiency syndrome (AIDS). Lymphomas of the small cleaved cell variety (termed poorly differentiated lymphocytic lymphoma in the older literature) involve the CNS less commonly than the large-cell varieties. They are characterized by the small size of the cells, which is similar to that of mature lymphocytes; however, in contrast to normal and reactive lymphocytes, these cells have clumped chromatin, visible nucleoli, and convoluted nuclei with bizarre shapes (Image 5.13). Although most lymphomas that involve the CNS are of the B-cell type, T-cell lymphomas of both large- and small-cell morphologies occasionally occur as well. Image 5.14 shows atypical lymphocytic cells in a needle aspirate of a brain mass in a patient with a history of mycosis fungoides. Marker studies confirmed the T-cell origin of this population.

Lymphoma presents in CSF as a monomorphic population of abnormal cells

Lymphoma generally presents in CSF as a monomorphic population of abnormal cells with one of the morphologic patterns just described. The diagnosis of lymphoma, however, is treacherous when dealing with a mixed population containing only small numbers of atypical cells due to morphologic overlap between the malignant cells of immunoblastic sarcoma and reactive immunoblasts and between small-cell lymphomas and reactive lymphocytes. In difficult cases, obtaining an accurate clinical history is imperative, and comparing the cells in CSF with other biopsy material is useful. In addition, the application of lymphoid marker antibody panels to demonstrate the presence or absence of monoclonality often solves the diagnostic dilemma.

CSF involvement is rare in patients with Hodgkin's disease and well-differentiated lymphocytic lymphoma. In these patients, CSF examination is usually done only when neurologic signs and symptoms, particularly those involving the meninges, occur. Since these patients are often immunosuppressed and susceptible to opportunistic infections, the diagnosis of lymphomatous involvement in CSF must be made with caution.

A relatively high incidence of CNS involvement is seen in children with such non-Hodgkin's lymphomas as diffuse lymphoblastic lymphoma and diffuse undifferentiated lymphoma.[28] The cytologic presentations of lymphoblastic lymphoma and undifferentiated lymphoma are similar to that of ALL and are usually easily identified. These lesions are clinically similar to ALL, and prophylactic CNS treatment and periodic CSF examination are part of the normal regimen. CNS involvement is common in Burkitt's lymphoma and was found in 21 of 25 autopsy cases in one series.[19] In a separate study, meningeal involvement was demonstrated either clinically or in CSF in 35 of 77 (46%) patients.[40] These cells are similar to the blast forms of ALL and lymphoblastic lymphoma, but the cytoplasm generally stains a more intense shade of blue on Romanowski-stained preparations (Image 5.15).

Malignant Histiocytosis

Malignant histiocytosis is a rapidly fatal systemic disease characterized by a proliferation of atypical histiocytes. The term is synonymous with histiocytic medullary reticulosis.[31] The most common sites of involvement are lymph nodes, spleen, liver, and bone marrow. CNS involvement is unusual in this disorder, but atypical histiocytes similar to the cells seen in the other involved organs have been reported in the meninges.[22] Similar histiocytic cells have been seen in CSF in eight patients, all of whom had CNS symptoms.[2,3,7,8,15]

Histiocytosis X

The CNS is often involved in histiocytosis X, and the most frequent pattern and location is associated with Hand-Schüller-Christian disease, which involves primarily the hypothalamic region. Histiocytosis X confined to the CNS is rare, but isolated cases have been reported by Den Hartog et al,[11] Bernard and Aguilar,[5] and Kepes and Kepes.[20] Also, cases of Letterer-Siwe disease with a meningoencephalitic character have been described by Batson et al[4] and Rubé et al,[34] who also reviewed the previously reported cases. Hamilton et al[15] have described atypical histiocytes in the CSF of a child with Letterer-Siwe disease and in the CSF of a man with Hand-Schüller-Christian disease.

Multiple Myeloma

Meningeal involvement is unusual in multiple myeloma, but it has occasionally been reported. In 1970, Maldonado et al[27] reported a case with subdural and subarachnoid myeloma at autopsy, but without CSF examination during life. Spriggs[37] described one patient with multiple myeloma in whom myeloma cells were found in the CSF and in the SAS at autopsy. McMenemey and Cumings[26] observed one patient with myeloma cells in CSF. Both of these patients also had spinal extradural myeloma. In 1974, Afifi[1] added two additional cases, and CSF from a patient with multiple myeloma involving the meninges was reported in 1980.[13] Spaar and Argyrakis[36] reported a case with myeloma cells in CSF, confirmed by immunofluorescence, that demonstrated cytoplasmic IgA. Spaar[35] divided cases with CNS myeloma into three categories. The first two groups were patients who presented no diagnostic problems: those with direct CNS invasion from bony lesions and those with widespread myeloma. The third group of patients, however, had primary CNS myeloma without the typical bone marrow or serologic findings. In patients of this latter group, cytologic examination of CSF was particularly useful in establishing a definite diagnosis.

Although plasma cells are not seen in the CSF of normal individuals, they are frequently found in inflammatory CNS diseases, particularly viral infections and neurosyphilis. Intense plasmacytosis with many immature forms has been reported in patients with multiple sclerosis and cerebral cysticercosis.[12,30] The diagnosis of meningeal myeloma, therefore, requires supportive clinical information and should not be made on the presence of atypical plasma cells alone.

Plasma cells are frequently found in inflammatory CNS diseases

Image 5.16a shows plasma cells from the CSF of a patient with multiple myeloma. The well-differentiated morphology of these cells makes the distinction between myeloma and chronic inflammation difficult. Image 5.16b, in contrast, shows atypical plasma cells from the CSF of a patient with multiple plasmacytoma. The undifferentiated nature of this infiltrate makes the distinction between myeloma and other types of neoplasms the diagnostic problem.

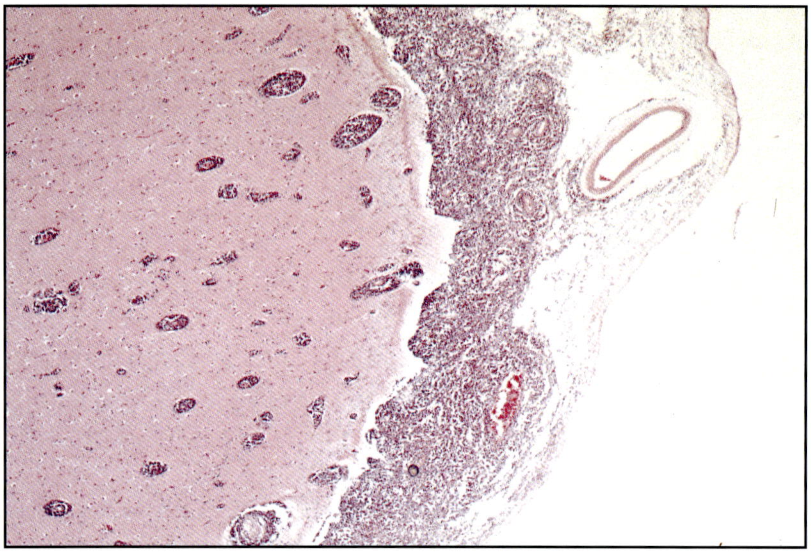

Image 5.1
A dense infiltrate involving the subarachnoid space in a histologic section of the brain of a patient with lymphoma (H&E, 250X).

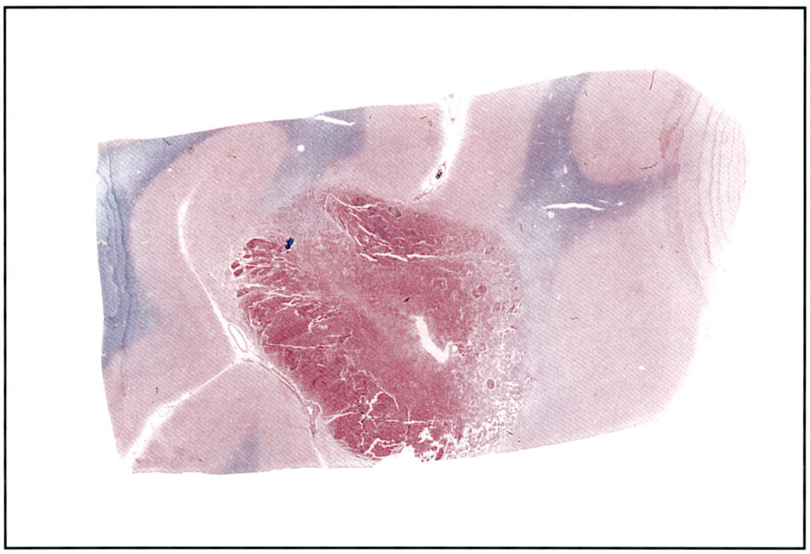

Image 5.2
Grossly evident focal infiltrates of neoplastic cells in a brain section from a patient with lymphoma.

a

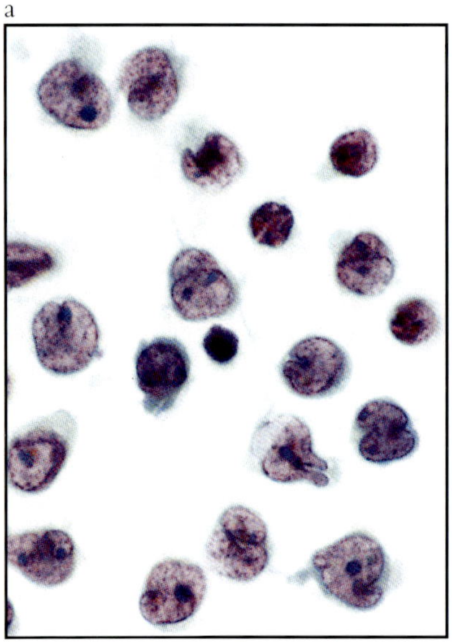

b

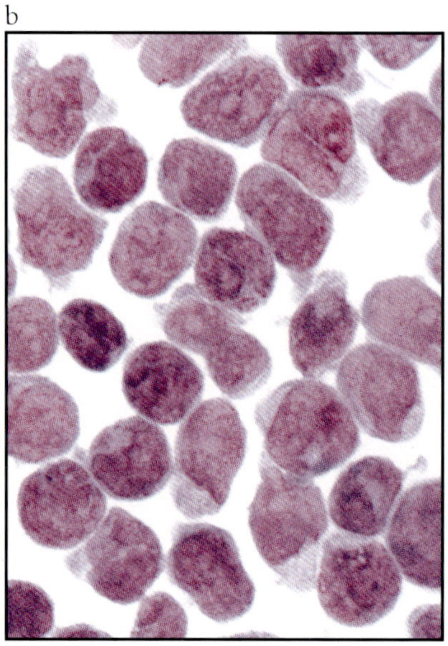

Image 5.3
Lymphoblasts in acute lymphocytic leukemia (ALL). Papanicolaou stain shows the high nuclear/cytoplasmic ratios, bland chromatin, and round or convoluted nuclei with prominent nucleoli (a). On Romanowski-stained preparations, the same general morphology is seen, but the smooth, evenly distributed blastic chromatin pattern is more apparent (b) (a, Papanicolaou, 1,000X; b, Romanowski, 1,000X).

Image 5.4
Reactive lymphocytes in viral meningoencephalitis. The mixed nature of the infiltrate is apparent. Reactive lymphocytes are larger than mature lymphocytes due to an increased amount of cytoplasm, but the characteristic coarse chromatin of lymphocytes is retained. Some of the reactive cells are immunoblasts that are greatly enlarged with abundant cytoplasm. The nuclei contain irregular chromatin and prominent nucleoli, but the chromatin pattern is coarser than that seen in blast forms (a, Papanicolaou, 1,000X; b, Romanowski, 1,000X).

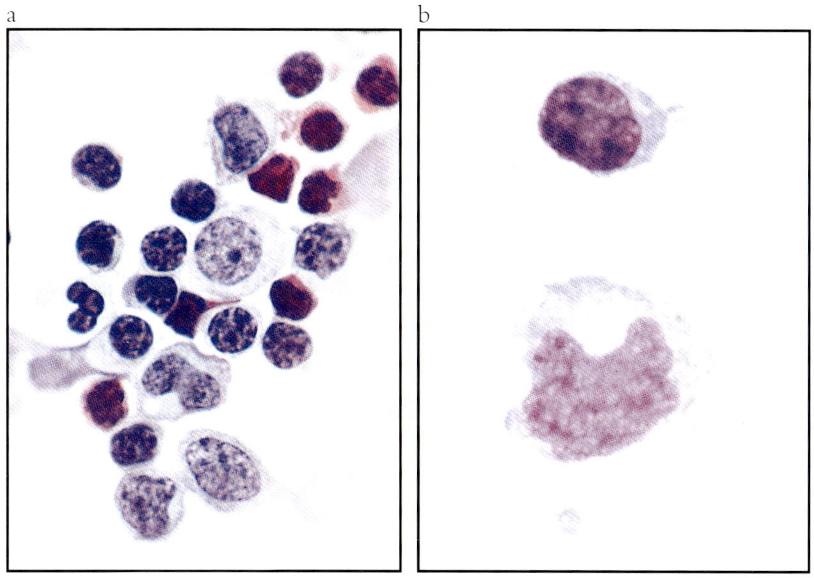

Image 5.5
Blasts in ALL. The morphology of blasts in ALL is generally sufficiently characteristic to allow their identification when enough cells are available for evaluation (a). Reactivity with antibodies against common acute lymphoblastic leukemia antigen (CALLA) is a useful adjunct in problem cases (b) (a, Romanowski, 1,000X; b, Immunoperoxidase, 1,000X).

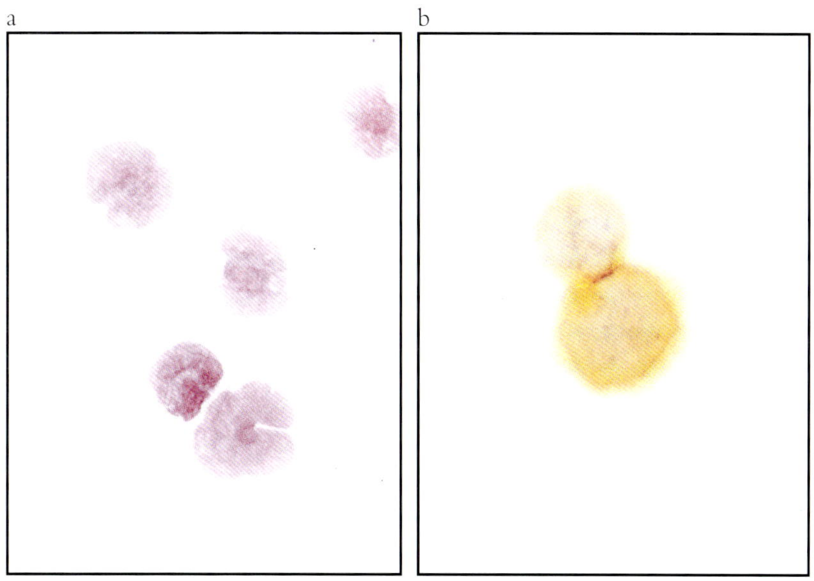

Image 5.6
Blasts in acute myelomonocytic leukemia. Myeloblasts are similar to lymphoblasts in these Papanicolaou-stained preparations (a). The monocytic blasts that are part of this mixed population have more abundant cytoplasm than lymphoblasts or myeloblasts (b) (both, Papanicolaou, 1,000X).

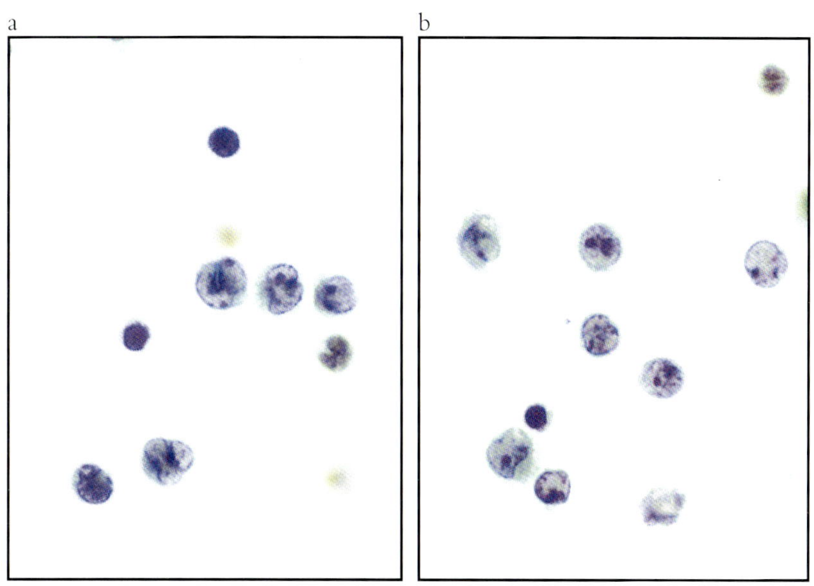

a b

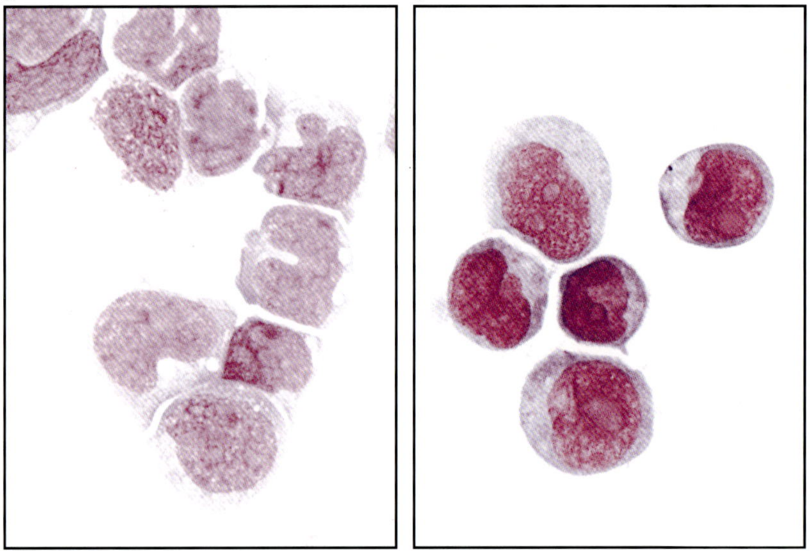

Image 5.7
Early myeloid forms in acute myelogenous leukemia (a) and promyelocytes with cytoplasmic granules in acute promyelocytic leukemia (b) (both, Romanowski, 1,000X).

a b

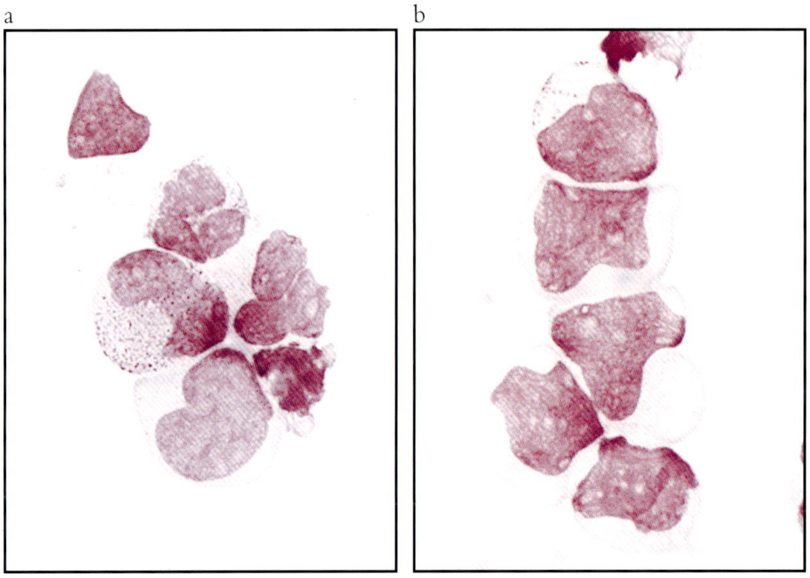

Image 5.8
Chronic granulocytic leukemia in blast crisis showing early myeloid forms similar to those of acute myelogenous leukemia (both, Romanowski, 1,000X).

a b

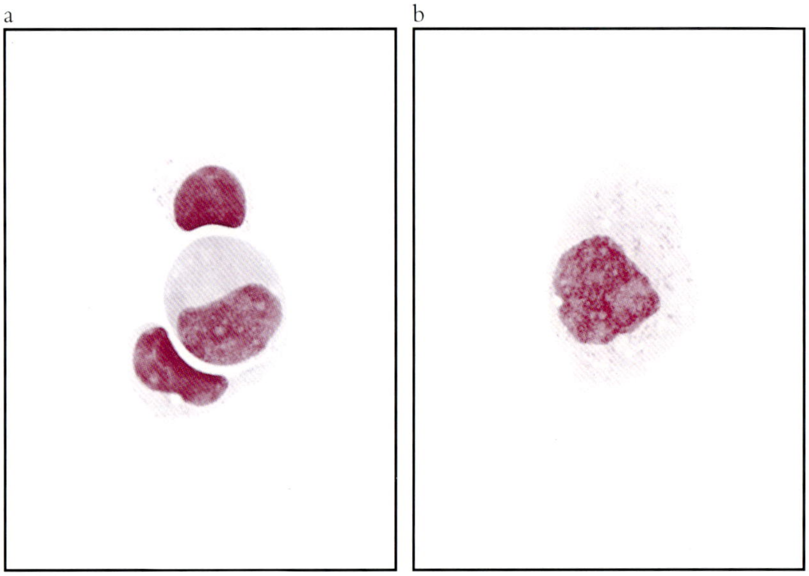

Image 5.9
Romanowski-stained monocytic blasts in acute monocytic leukemia. Blasts have abundant cytoplasm with granules and eccentric nuclei with a smooth, immature chromatin pattern (both, Romanowski, 1,000X).

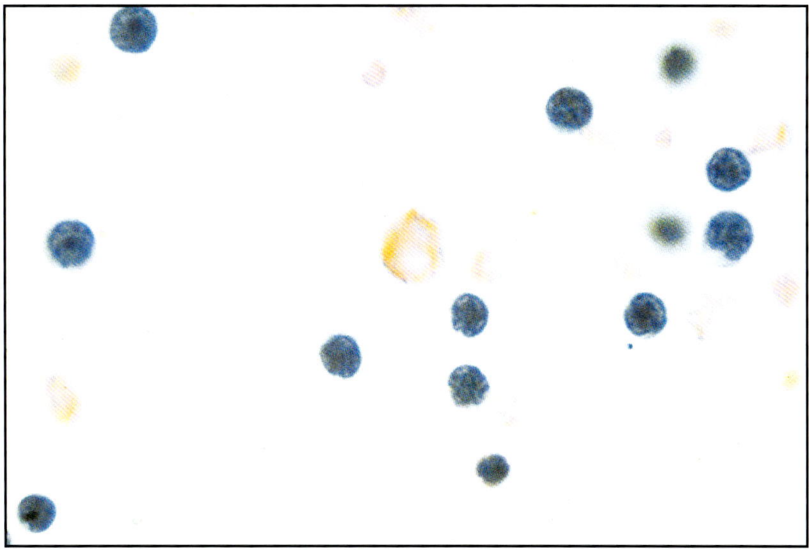

Image 5.10
Reactive lymphocytes in chronic lymphocytic leukemia. These cells are responding to cryptococci and do not represent leukemic involvement (Papanicolaou, 1,000X).

a b

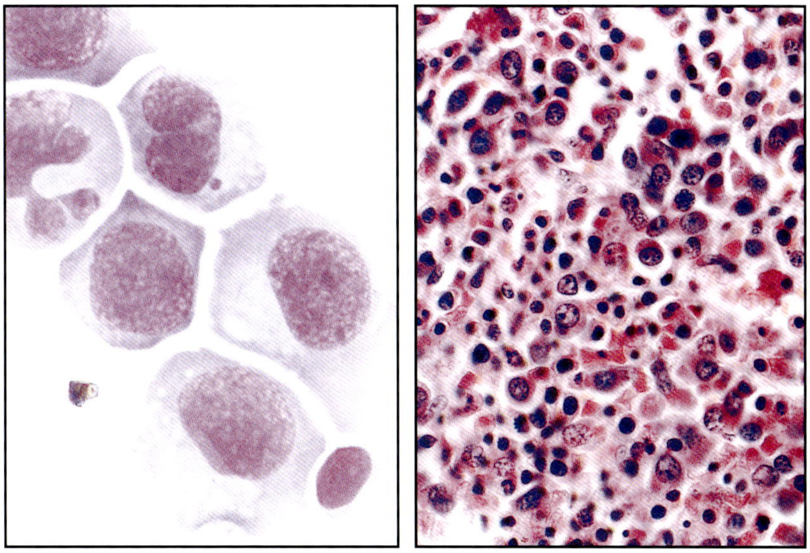

Image 5.11
Large, bizarre immunoblasts with irregular chromatin and prominent nucleoli in systemic lymphoma (a). Marrow biopsy specimen from same patient showing an immunoblastic infiltrate (b) (a, Romanowski, 1,000X; b, H&E, 400X).

a b

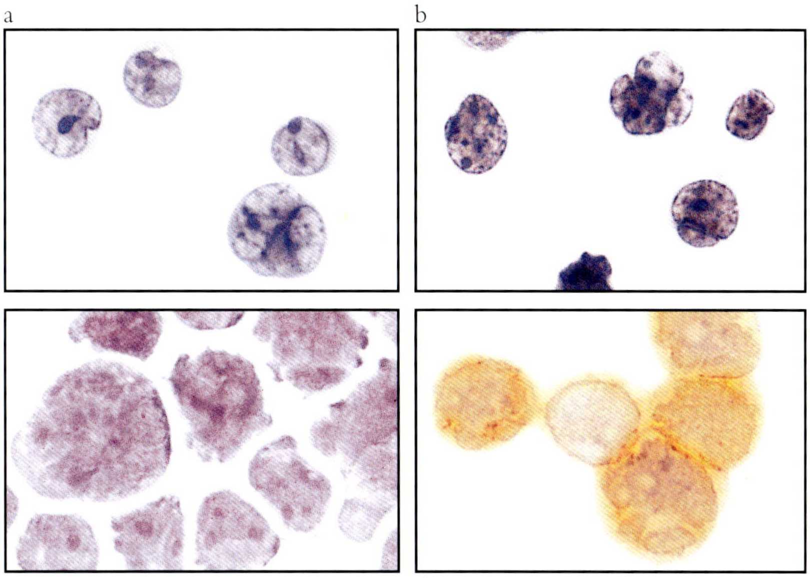

c d

Image 5.12
Large, bizarre immunoblasts in primary cerebral immunoblastic sarcoma. Immunoblasts are readily identifiable on both Papanicolaou- (a and b) and Romanowski- (c) stained preparations. All cells react with an antigamma antibody although they are kappa negative, which confirms the monoclonality of this B-cell lymphoma (d) (a and b, Papanicolaou; c, Romanowski; d, Immunoperoxidase; all, 1,000X).

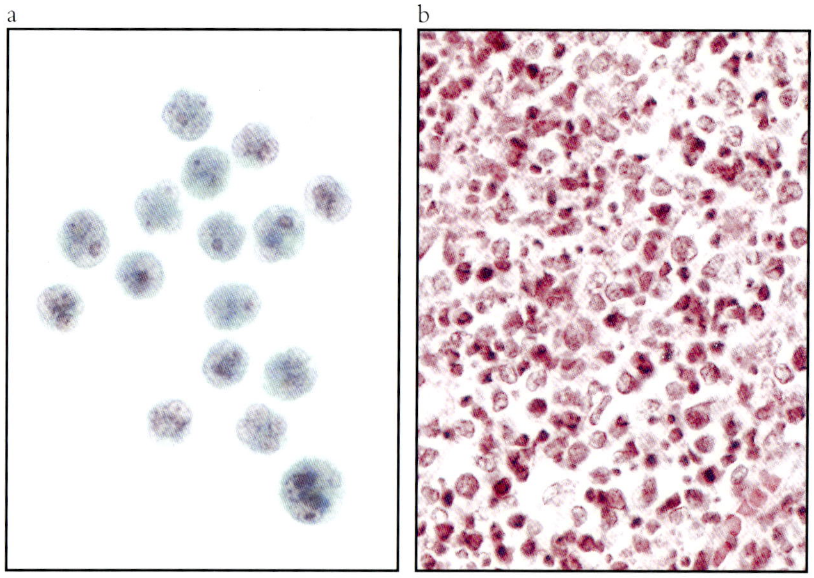

Image 5.13
Malignant lymphocytes of small cleaved cell lymphoma (a). Lymph node biopsy specimen from this same patient displays the diffuse infiltrate of pleomorphic lymphocytes characteristic of this disorder (b) (a, Papanicolaou, 1,000X; b, H&E, 400X).

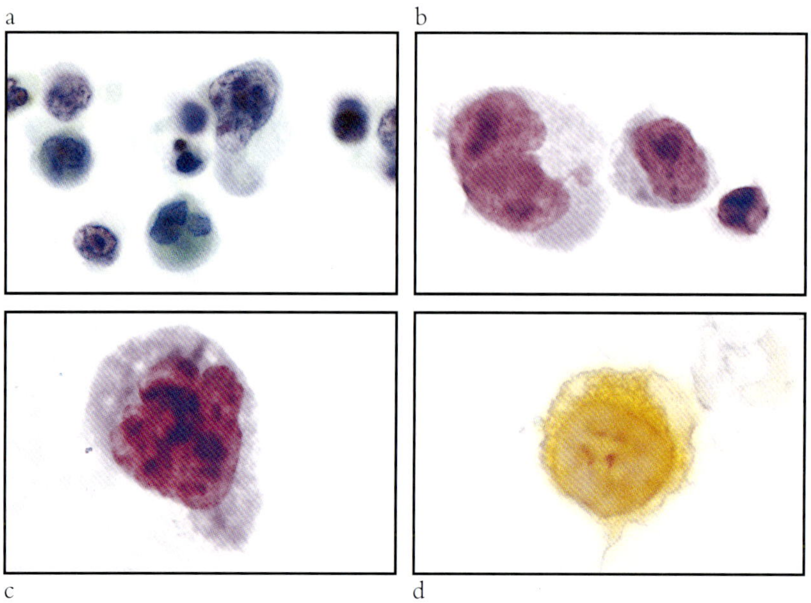

Image 5.14
Atypical lymphocytes with cerebriform nuclei typical of mycosis fungoides (a through c). Reactivity with a pan T antibody confirms their T-cell derivation (d) (a, Papanicolaou; b and c, Romanowski; d, Immunoperoxidase; all, 1,000X).

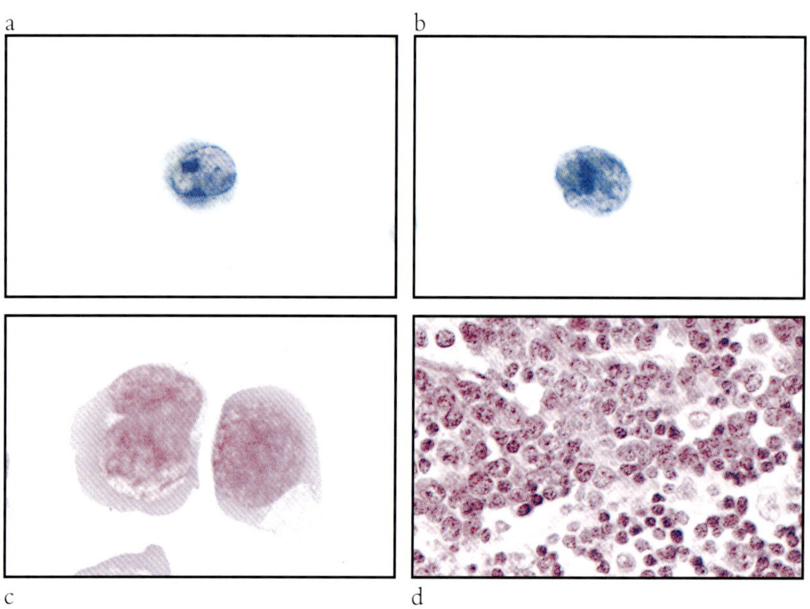

Image 5.15
Papanicolaou-stained blast forms of Burkitt's lymphoma similar to blast forms of other types of acute leukemia and lymphoma (a and b). Romanowski-stained blasts with the intense blue staining of the cytoplasm is characteristic of this tumor type (c). Lymph node biopsy specimen from this patient with typical starry-sky appearance of this type of lymphoma (d) (a and b, Papanicolaou, 1,000X; c, Romanowski, 1,000X; d, 400X).

CHAPTER SIX

Metastatic Tumors and Meningeal Carcinomatosis

Cancer is the second most common cause of death in the United States, killing more than 386,000 Americans annually. As many as 30% of the people who die of systemic cancer are found at autopsy to have had central nervous system (CNS) involvement.[28] When metastatic tumor involves the parenchyma of the brain and spinal cord without disseminating into the ventricular cavities or subarachnoid space (SAS), malignant cells are unlikely to be detected in cerebrospinal fluid (CSF) (Figure 6.1). Similarly, extradural involvement provides no contact between tumor cells and CSF. Meningeal carcinomatosis, however, whether occurring alone or in conjunction with parenchymal lesions, does release tumor cells into the CSF (Figure 6.2 and Image 6.1).

Incidence

Pure meningeal carcinomatosis is considerably less common than parenchymal metastases. In a series of 210 autopsy cases with primary or metastatic CNS tumors reported by Glass et al,[18] 75 had parenchymal metastases alone, 19 had dural metastases alone, and only seven had leptomeningeal metastases alone, although 33 had leptomeningeal disease combined with one of the other patterns. Similarly, of 2,227 autopsy cases with malignant epithelial tumors that had spread to regional lymph nodes and beyond, 306 (18%) had CNS involvement.[19] Only 18 of these 306 had pure meningeal carcinomatosis without parenchymal lesions.

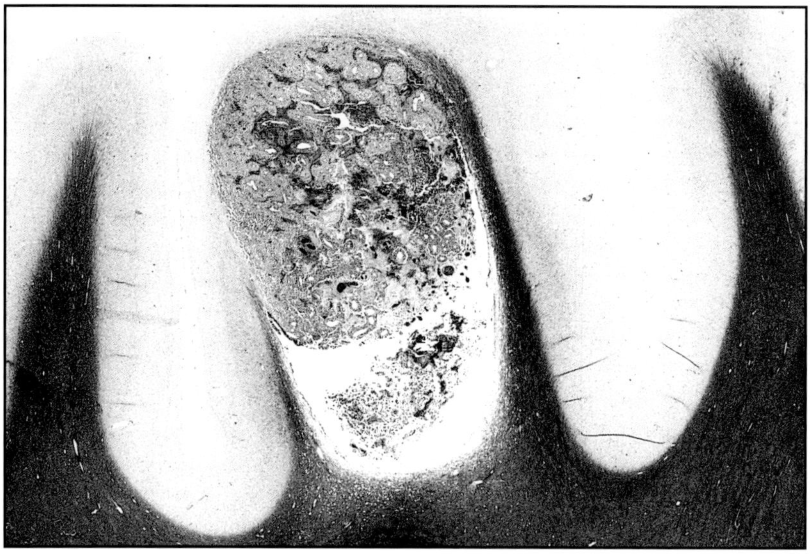

Figure 6.1
A well-circumscribed nodule of metastatic melanoma at the junction of cerebral cortex and white matter.

Whether meningeal carcinomatosis occurs alone or in conjunction with parenchymal lesions, the likelihood of finding malignant cells in CSF depends on the extent of leptomeningeal involvement. Among the 210 patients with CNS tumors described by Glass et al, CSF was examined in 117 cases and malignant cells were found in 31 (26%). Although 65 of 66 cases without leptomeningeal spread at autopsy were negative for malignant cells in the CSF, 30 of 51 (59%) cases with meningeal tumor, either alone or with parenchymal involvement, had such cells. Only five of 13 (38%) patients with focal meningeal disease, as compared with 25 of 38 (66%) patients with multifocal dissemination, showed malignant cells in the CSF.

Pathogenesis

Some observers believe that meningeal carcinomatosis arises when parenchymal metastases discharge cells directly into the subarachnoid space or ventricles. In support of this concept, there are examples of superficial cortical metastases that impinge directly on the SAS (Figure 6.3) and cases with choroidal or subependymal metastases that have direct access to the ventricles (Image 6.2). Cases of pure meningeal carcinomatosis with intravascular and perivascular meningeal deposits of tumor without coexisting parenchymal lesions have also been reported. Such cases support a theory of a purely hematogenous route of dissemination.

Meningeal carcinomatosis likely is initiated by more than one pathway

Malignant tumors may invade the SAS directly. For example, tumors of the eye, such as retinoblastoma, and of the orbit, such as squamous cell carcinoma and embryonal rhabdomyosarcoma, may extend directly along nerve trunks and perivascular spaces through the posterior portion of the orbit into the SAS. Similarly, direct extension has been implicated in cases of other head and neck tumors, such as salivary gland tumors, olfac-

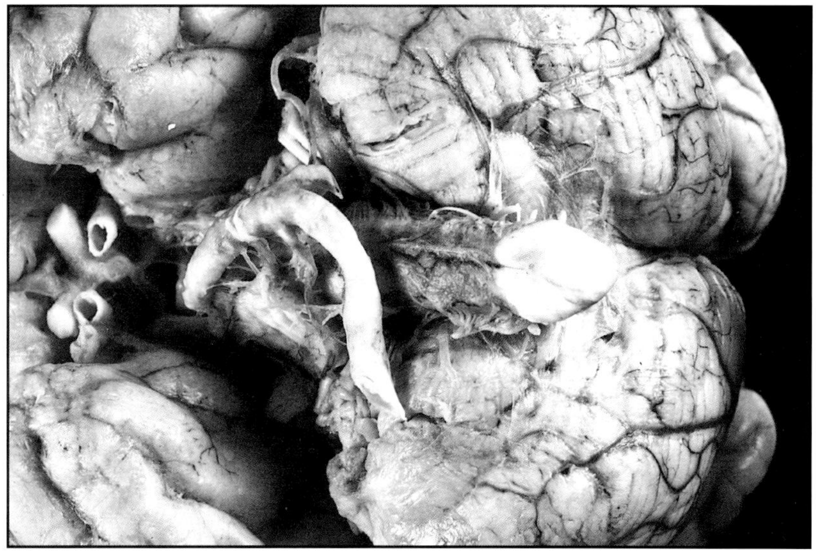

Figure 6.2
Meningeal carcinomatosis manifested grossly by meningeal clouding, which blurs and obscures the underlying cerebellar folia.

tory neuroblastoma,[31] and chordomas. Another pathway for direct extension of tumor into the subarachnoid space is from paravertebral lymph nodes, along perineural lymphatics,[19] or from vertebral, extradural, or subdural deposits of tumor (Figure 6.4).

Since individual cases can be found to support each of these possible routes, it is likely that more than one pathway exists for the initiation of meningeal carcinomatosis. Hematogenous spread, whether meningeal deposits occur directly from meningeal vessels or secondarily from parenchymal lesions, is undoubtedly a common mechanism, especially in tumors such as lung carcinoma that frequently disseminate widely

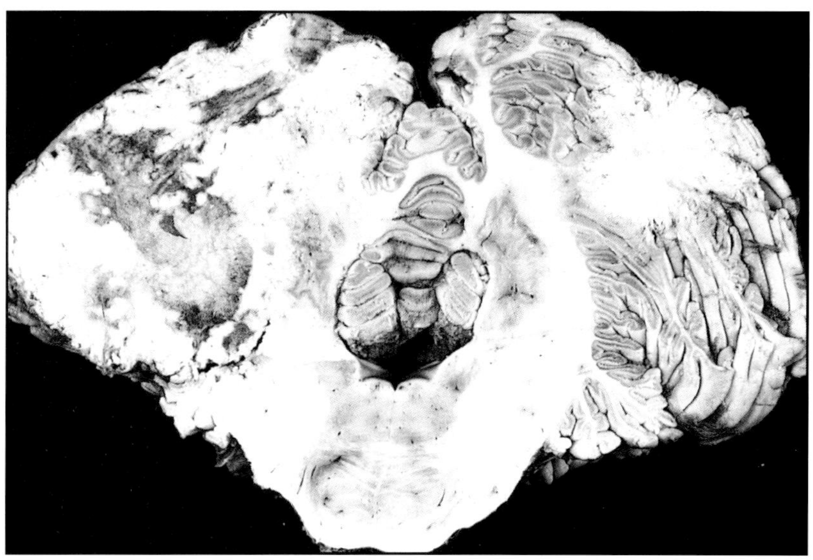

Figure 6.3
Coronal section of the cerebellum and brain stem showing multiple large metastases that impinge directly on the subarachnoid space.

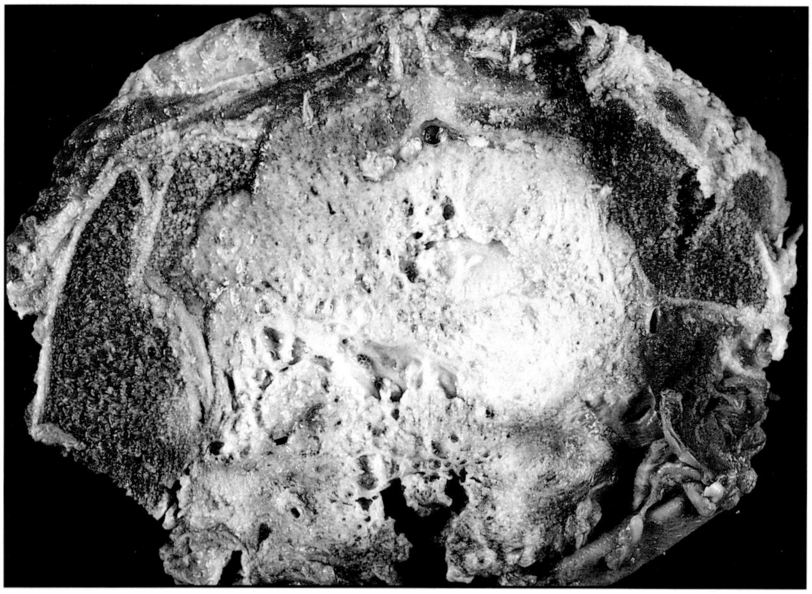

Figure 6.4
Massive replacement of the lumbar vertebrae by carcinoma of the uterine cervix is seen in the brain of a patient with meningeal carcinomatosis.

through the vascular system. The other important pathway is direct extension. The practical implication of this mechanism is that some cases of meningeal carcinomatosis may occur because of the proximity of the primary tumor to the subarachnoid space and may not necessarily reflect widespread dissemination. In such instances, the meninges may be the initial or only site of tumor spread, and treatment of the meningeal infiltrate may increase the survival of the patient.

Prevalence

In 1912 Beerman[5] reported a case of meningeal carcinomatosis in which the primary source of the tumor was never discovered. His review of the previous literature disclosed 11 additional cases. Nine of these were primary in the stomach, while two were primary in the lung. The next large literature review was in 1954 by Spriggs,[33] who found 47 previously reported cases of metastatic lesions diagnosed by cytologic examination of CSF and added two such cases of his own. Although carcinoma of the stomach was the most common primary source in this series, carcinomas of the breast and lung have been most prevalent in all large studies published since then.[7,13,19,24-26,34] Table 6.1 shows the distribution of primary sources of meningeal carcinomatosis diagnosed by CSF examination at Duke University Medical Center from 1971 to 1980.[7] Carcinomas of the lung and breast were the most common primary tumors followed by melanoma. The high number of cases of lung carcinoma is partly explained by the inclusion of all cases from the Durham Veterans Administration Medical Center, with a predominantly male population, in addition to the patients from Duke University Hospital.

Carcinomas of the lung and breast are the most common sources of meningeal carcinomatosis

Table 6.1
Incidence of Meningeal Carcinomatosis Diagnosed by CSF Cytology at Duke University Medical Center 1971 to 1980[7]

Diagnosis	No. of Patients	No. of Patients With Primary Presentation in CSF
Small-cell undifferentiated carcinoma of the lung	16	2
Adenocarcinoma of the lung	15	3
Large-cell undifferentiated carcinoma of the lung	9	0
Undifferentiated carcinoma of the lung (not otherwise specified)	4	3
Carcinoma of the breast	18	0
Melanoma	12	1
Carcinoma of unknown primary	7	5
Adenocarcinoma of the stomach	3	2
Retinoblastoma	2	0
Squamous cell carcinoma of the orbit	2	0
Adenocarcinoma of the bile duct	2	0
Neuroblastoma of the adrenal gland	1	0
Adenocarcinoma of the parotid gland	1	0
Adenocarcinoma of the colon	1	0
Adenocarcinoma of the ovary	1	0
Adenocarcinoma of the endometrium	1	0
Squamous cell carcinoma of the uterine cervix	1	0
Squamous cell carcinoma of the larynx	1	0
Embryonal rhabdomyosarcoma of the orbit	1	0
Total Number of Patients	**98**	**16**

Carcinoma of the Lung

Carcinoma of the lung tends to metastasize to the CNS

Carcinoma of the lung is by far the most common cause of cancer death in men and has recently become the most common cause of cancer death in women.[8] Not only does it have a high incidence in the general population, but it has a pronounced tendency to metastasize to the CNS. From 25% to 41% of patients with lung cancer are shown at autopsy to have CNS metastases.[3,14,15]

The high incidence of lung carcinoma and its predilection for the CNS have made it one of the most common sources of meningeal carcinomatosis. In addition, because of the short time interval between discovery of the primary lung and meningeal involvement, lung carcinoma is one of the most common lesions to manifest early on by CSF spread and even prior to diagnosis of the primary lesion.[7]

All cell types of lung cancer may be seen in CSF fluid. Large- or small-cell undifferentiated carcinoma and adenocarcinoma are the most common; squamous differentiation is rarely identified. Small-cell undifferentiated carcinoma presents in CSF as small cells loosely arranged in clusters or single cells with high nuclear/cytoplasmic (N/C) ratios, nuclear molding, hyperchromatic nuclei, and small nucleoli (Image 6.3a). Occasionally, tightly cohesive tissue fragments with intense nuclear molding are seen (Image 6.3b).

Large-cell undifferentiated carcinoma presents as large isolated cells with irregular nuclei, clumped chromatin, prominent nucleoli, and small-to-moderate amounts of cytoplasm with discrete cell borders (Image 6.4a). Although adenocarcinoma of the lung may rarely present in CSF as well-differentiated, cohesive tissue fragments (Images 6.4c and 6.4d), the usual appearance is that of singly occurring or loosely arranged clusters of large malignant cells (Image 6.4b). Occasionally, cells of adenocarcinoma of the lung display finely granular chromatin and round regular nucleoli and shed in cohesive tissue fragments (Image 6.5). This cytologic picture may be impossible to distinguish from ductal carcinoma of the breast.

Carcinoma of the Breast

Breast carcinoma is currently the second most common cause of cancer death in women in the United States,[8] and 15% to 20% of patients with breast cancer have central nervous system metastases at autopsy.[42] The majority of cases of breast carcinoma are classified histologically as infiltrating ductal carcinoma with a small proportion considered lobular carcinoma. Similarly, ductal carcinoma is the most common type to appear in CSF. Ductal carcinoma presents as large, round cells with centrally placed nuclei, prominent round central nucleoli, and moderate amounts of cytoplasm with discrete cell borders. Cells are usually isolated (Image 6.6a), and they only rarely produce a morula configuration or the in-tandem arrangement with intense molding that is so characteristic in pleural fluid[4] (Images 6.6b–6.6d). Occasionally, ductal carcinoma with anaplastic features metastasizes to CSF (Image 6.7). Similarities in cell shape, nuclear characteristics, and N/C ratio create an illusion of uniformity among cells of infiltrating ductal carcinoma in CSF. In fact, significant variation exists in both nuclear and cytoplasmic diameter from cell to cell within cases and among cases.[40] Lobular carcinoma presents as isolated small cells or loosely cohesive clusters with hyperchromatic nuclei, micronucleoli, and scant cytoplasm. Although overlap in cell size occurs between the smallest cells of ductal carcinoma and the cells of lobular carcinoma, the cells of lobular carcinoma are uniformly small.[40]

Breast carcinoma is the second most common cause of cancer death in women

Malignant Melanoma

Although melanoma is relatively uncommon in the general population as compared to lung and breast carcinoma, it has a much more marked tendency to involve the central nervous system (Figures 6.5 and 6.6). In a series of 122 patients with melanoma, meningeal involvement was found at autopsy in 63 patients (52%) and was confirmed by CSF cytology in nine.[2] Melanoma characteristically presents cytologically as large, single cells with eccentrically placed nuclei, each bearing a single, central macronucleolus.[43] A definite diagnosis, however, requires the demonstration of cytoplasmic melanin (Image 6.8). Since macrophages

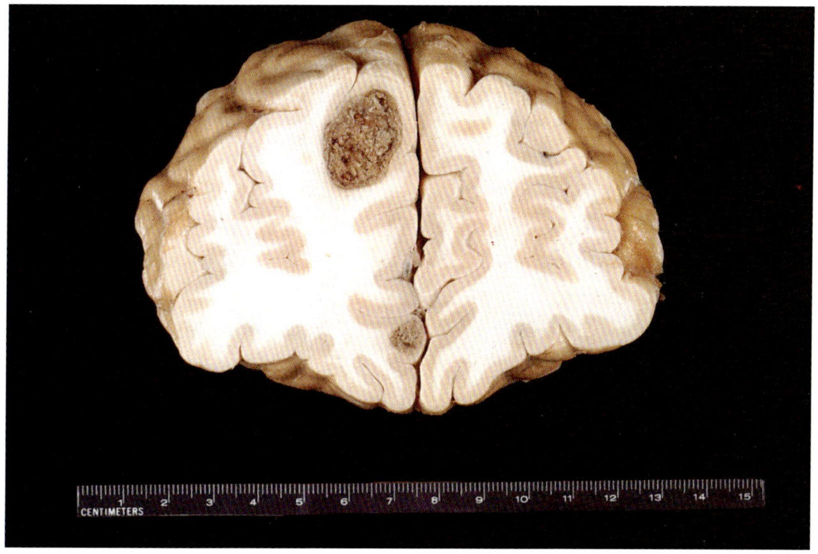

Figure 6.5
The cerebral hemispheres show a pigmented focus of metastatic melanoma.

may phagocytize melanin pigment, care must be taken to verify that the pigment-bearing cells possess malignant features. In some cases, pigment-bearing melanoma cells may be rare and must be carefully sought among amelanotic malignant cells and benign pigment-bearing macrophages.

When malignant melanoma cells are amelanotic, they are difficult to distinguish from other large-cell neoplasms

When the cells of malignant melanoma are amelanotic, it is difficult to distinguish them from other types of large-cell neoplasms such as large-cell undifferentiated carcinoma of the lung and large-cell lymphoma. In such instances, reactivity with antimelanoma monoclonal antibodies such as HMB-45 and Mel-14 and negative reactivity for cytokeratin, anticarcinoma antibodies such as B72.3 and epithelial mem-

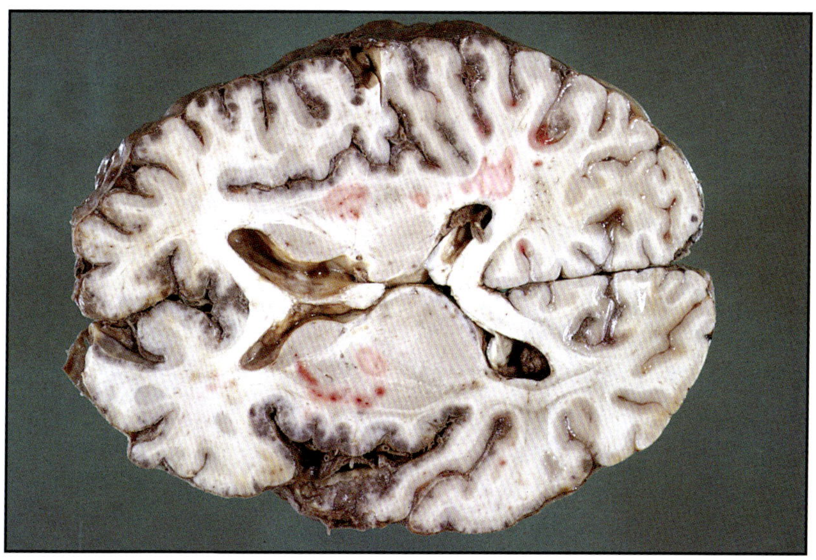

Figure 6.6
The cerebral hemispheres show diffuse meningeal involvement with melanoma.

brane antigen (EMA), and panleukocyte reagents are helpful in making the diagnosis[32,38] (Image 6.9). Although most melanomas express S-100 protein, the antibody cannot be used alone to diagnose melanoma because it also reacts with approximately one third of carcinomas.[12,20,23,35]

Carcinomatosis of Unknown Primary

All series include some cases in which the primary tumor source is not discovered. Sometimes meningeal involvement occurs as a part of widespread carcinomatosis involving multiple organs. The primary source may not be uncovered even with autopsy studies. In other instances, the diagnosis of meningeal carcinomatosis, with its poor prognosis, may precipitate the cessation of further diagnostic procedures. If no autopsy is performed, the primary site will remain unknown.

Adenocarcinoma of the Stomach

Although adenocarcinoma of the stomach was once the most common primary source of meningeal carcinomatosis, it is an uncommon cause of meningeal malignancy in the United States today, probably because of its declining overall incidence.[8] Adenocarcinoma of the stomach typically presents in CSF as isolated cells or clusters of small cells with irregular nuclei bearing prominent characteristics of malignancy. These nuclei are eccentrically placed in small-to-moderate amounts of finely vacuolated cytoplasm (Image 6.10). Occasionally, gastric carcinoma presents in CSF as cohesive tissue fragments (Images 6.10c and 6.10d). The cells shown in Images 6.10a and 6.10b are from a patient whose initial neurologic symptoms prompted the obtaining of this CSF specimen. A diagnosis of adenocarcinoma was rendered. Several days later, a gastric biopsy specimen showed adenocarcinoma. Autopsy confirmed both the primary source and extensive meningeal involvement. This case illustrates the dramatic role that cytopathology can play in solving the puzzling clinical problems that these conditions present.[22]

Uncommon Primary Sources

Many types of cancer occur frequently but rarely involve the SAS

Many types of cancer occur fairly frequently in the general population but seldom involve the subarachnoid space. Squamous cell carcinoma of the cervix rarely metastasizes outside of the pelvis, and, although adenocarcinoma of the colon may produce a solitary cerebral metastasis, it seldom spreads to the meninges. Image 6.11 shows keratinizing squamous cell carcinoma from the uterine cervix[41] (Image 6.11a) and adenocarcinoma from the colon (Image 6.11b) in CSF. Both of these patients had unusual clinical presentations with local recurrence that directly invaded the lumbar vertebrae and gained access to the SAS.[6] Weithman et al[39] reported an additional case of cervical cancer metastatic to CSF.

Renal cell carcinoma, transitional cell carcinoma of the urinary system, and prostatic adenocarcinoma are uncommon etiologies of meningeal carcinomatosis in most series. Ehya et al,[13] however, described five patients with bladder cancer and four patients with prostatic cancer in whom malignant cells were identified in CSF.

When dealing with alleged unusual primary sources of meningeal carcinomatosis, some cases raise doubt as to the true tumor of origin. Image 6.12a shows adenocarcinoma in the CSF from a 42-year-old woman. Her ovaries had been removed three months earlier, and they contained adenocarcinoma (Image 6.12b). Although this case may represent adenocarcinoma of the ovary with meningeal carcinoma, it is also possible that the ovarian lesion is a Krukenberg tumor from an undisclosed primary site. Since the patient died without an autopsy, the question remains unsolved. Similarly, in the case of adenocarcinoma of the parotid in one series, it is impossible to exclude the possibility that this lesion actually represents metastatic carcinoma to a cervical lymph node in the parotid area.

Meningeal Dissemination of Tumors in Childhood

The two major groups of neoplasms involving the CSF of children are small-cell tumors of central and systemic origin and lymphoma/leukemia. The latter group of lesions can be identified based on their single-cell presentation, association with systemic evidence for lymphoma/leukemia, and reactivity of the cells with lymphoid antibodies as described in Chapter Five.

Small-cell neoplasms shed singly in loose clusters or in tight tissue fragments (Images 6.13 and 6.14). Single cells have hyperchromatic nuclei and scant cytoplasm. The similar cytologic presentation of these tumors in CSF often makes the distinction between these systemic and CNS tumors impossible by morphologic criteria alone, but clinical information regarding the body site of origin usually allows the correct interpretation.

Distinction between small-cell neoplasms and CNS tumors is impossible by morphology alone

Small-cell neoplasms of systemic origin that often spread to CSF include embryonal rhabdomyosarcoma, Ewing's sarcoma (peripheral neuroepithelioma), and neuroblastoma.[17] Embryonal rhabdomyosarcoma may arise in the orbit or the ear, and, because of its close proximity to the cranial cavity, it can invade the SAS directly. This tumor presents as single cells with high N/C ratios (Image 6.13a), although Geisinger et al[17] pointed out that these tumors sometimes have more cytoplasm than other small-cell neoplasms. Cross-striations are rarely demonstrated. These authors have also demonstrated that Ewing's sarcoma shows the same small-cell, undifferentiated morphology in CSF as in other body sites. Embryonal rhabdomyosarcomas, Ewing's sarcomas, and extraskeletal Ewing's sarcomas (peripheral neuroepitheliomas) often express neural cell adhesion molecule (N-CAM),[1,27] and thus they cannot be distinguished from neuroectodermal tumors that express this substance, such as neuroblastomas and primary CNS tumors such as retinoblastomas and medulloblastomas.[16] Ewing's sarcomas do, however, express cell surface protein p30/32 MIC2, whereas these other small-cell tumors are negative for this substance.[29] Patients with systemic neuroblastomas usually present with an abdominal mass. These tumors shed small cells with high N/C ratios (Image 6.13b). Rosettes are uncommon in this neoplasm but, when present, are helpful in distinguishing these tumors from rhabdomyosarcomas and Ewing's sarcoma. They do not, however, assist in distinguishing neuroblastomas from retinoblastomas, pineoblastomas, medulloblastomas, and ependymomas, since these tumor types may also form rosettes.

Retinoblastoma is a small-cell tumor of childhood that has a direct line of extension to the meninges by way of the optic nerve. It inevitably manifests in the eye prior to the onset of meningeal involvement. Image 6.14a shows a retinoblastoma in an eye enucleated from a 20-month-old child. Ten months later, the cells shown in Image 6.14b were seen in the CSF. At autopsy, a striking subarachnoid infiltrate was found (Images 6.14c and 6.14d).

Small-cell neoplasms of CNS origin include medulloblastomas, pineoblastomas, and cerebral neuroblastomas. Sometimes anaplastic gliomas may shed in this way. Primary CNS tumors seldom metastasize out of the intracranial and intraspinal cavities. The absence of a systemic lesion at the time of presentation with CNS signs suggests a primary CNS tumor. The differentiation of these primary CNS tumors of small-cell size is difficult but is greatly aided by knowledge of the specific location of the primary lesion within the CNS. Discussion of this problem and cytologic presentation of the individual tumors are included in Chapter Seven.

Meningeal Carcinomatosis as the Initial Manifestation of Cancer

Only rarely is meningeal involvement the primary manifestation of cancer. The majority of patients with malignant cells discovered in CSF already have a prior diagnosis of cancer. Of 98 patients seen at Duke University Hospital from 1971 to 1980, 82 had morphologic documentation of systemic tumor prior to CSF examination (Table 6.1).[7] Of the remaining 16 patients in whom the initial manifestation of carcinoma was found by CSF studies, the most common primary site was the lung. Eight of the 44 patients with lung carcinoma presented in this way. In contrast, although carcinoma of the breast was the second most common primary site, none of the 18 patients with breast carcinoma was among the 16 with initial CSF presentation. The time interval between initial tumor presentation and development of meningeal spread was considerably longer in patients with breast cancer than in patients with lung carcinoma and melanoma. We know of only two cases in the literature of meningeal carcinomatosis from breast carcinoma in which the breast primary was not documented before the finding of meningeal involvement.[11,21]

Most patients with malignant cells in CSF have a prior diagnosis of cancer

One of the 12 patients with melanoma in our series presented initially with CNS involvement. Amer et al[2] described a series of 122 patients with melanoma. Meningeal involvement was confirmed at autopsy in 52%, but only one patient presented initially with meningeal spread.

Although we had only three cases of stomach carcinoma in our series, two presented initially with CNS involvement. In five patients in our series, a primary site was never found. Ringenberg et al[30] described three cases in which the initial manifestation of carcinoma was discovered by CSF examination. In all three cases, autopsy revealed a primary source in the lung.

The distribution of primary sources among patients whose initial manifestation of malignancy is by the shedding of malignant cells into CSF is different than in our overall population of meningeal metastases.[7] Awareness of the tumor types that are likely to present in this way and of their cytomorphology is important when dealing with these patients.

Diagnostic Problems and Immunodiagnosis of Metastatic Tumors

The common diagnostic problems with CSF are distinguishing malignant cells from lymphocytes and macrophages and determining the specific tumor type and organ of origin

In contrast to other body cavity fluids in which reactive mesothelium presents a common problem in differential diagnosis, CSF contains no counterpart of the reactive mesothelial cell to be confused with metastatic carcinoma. Regardless of whether a patient is known to have a malignancy or presents first with meningeal involvement, two common diagnostic problems occur with CSF examination: (1) distinguishing malignant cells, which often occur singly, from lymphocytes and macrophages (Image 6.15), and (2) determining the specific tumor type and organ of origin when cells are clearly malignant.

When tumor cells are present in large numbers in CSF, or when they occur in groups and fragments, the diagnosis of malignancy is straightforward. Frequently, however, the presence of meningeal tumor stimulates a brisk reaction of lymphocytes and macrophages, and the shedding of a small number of tumor cells, particularly in a single-cell presentation, can be difficult to detect. A useful point to remember is that cells of large-cell carcinoma and adenocarcinoma are usually considerably larger than the largest immunoblasts and macrophages and generally exhibit higher N/C ratios than these reactive elements. In addition, several antibodies may be of use. Lymphocytes and macrophages both stain with panleukocytic reagents (Image 6.15d). Lymphocytic subset markers are positive for the former cell type, while monocytic reagents stain the latter. Although these antibodies are positive for the corresponding varieties of lymphoma and leukemia, they are negative for metastatic tumor cells. In contrast, most carcinomas express cytokeratins, and subgroups of these tumors are positive for EMA, carcinoembryonic antigen (CEA), and B72.3.[36] Positive staining for melanoma can be achieved in the majority of cases with S-100, Mel-14,[9,10] and HMB-45 (Images 6.9 and 6.15). These antibodies do not react with lymphoid and hematopoietic elements. Thus, these antibodies, which do react with carcinoma and melanoma, can be useful in highlighting a small population of tumor cells when they are admixed with reactive elements. Thus, using the cytologic features and antibodies described above and in Table 6.2, one can distinguish between lymphohematopoietic cells and malignant cells in the majority of cases.

The second common diagnostic problem with CSF examination (ie, determining the origin of tumor cells that are obviously malignant) can usually be resolved by applying a combination of clinical and morphologic criteria. The primary tumor is already known in the majority of cases of metastases, and meningeal spread in the case of primary brain tumor usually accompanies or follows the discovery of the intracranial tumor. Thus, in the majority of cases, one only needs to determine if the cellular morphology is compatible with the known tumor type. In cases of initial presentation with meningeal disease, it is important to discover whether or not intracranial masses are present or if the neoplastic process is confined to the SAS. Without an obvious intracranial mass, primary brain tumors only rarely present in CSF. Similarly, the location of systemic masses is a critical clue in identifying the primary tumor. Systemic lymphoma inevitably presents with lymphadenopathy, and radiographic lung masses can usually be discerned in cases of lung cancer. The most likely source of a truly occult primary is often the stomach, although melanoma may be present in patients without an identifiable skin lesion either at presentation or by history.

The antibodies described in Table 6.2 and discussed in Chapter Nine are useful in confirming a neoplasm as primary brain tumor, lymphoma, metastatic carcinoma, or melanoma. However, neither these antibodies nor any others available to date will consistently distinguish the primary site of carcinoma. Gastric and lung carcinomas have similar patterns of reactivity with most anticarcinoma antibodies, and the best examples of type-specific antibodies, such as those against prostatic-specific antigen and calcitonin, detect tumor types that are rarely seen in CSF. New antibodies are constantly under development and are being tested in a variety of academic centers and in industry, which will likely result in additional sets of tumor type–specific markers becoming available in the future.

No antibodies can consistently distinguish the primary site of carcinoma

Table 6.2
Antibodies Useful for Diagnosis of Cells in CSF

Antibodies	Antigen Detected	Cell Types Detected
HMB-45*	Unknown	Melanoma, melanocytes
Mel-14[9,10]	Gamma-chondroitin sulfate, proteoglycan	Melanoma, melanocytes
S-100†	S-100 protein	Melanoma, melanocytes, 1/3 of carcinomas
AE1, AE3‡	Cytokeratins	Epithelial cells, carcinoma
B72.3§	TAG-72	Adenocarcinoma
2D1¶	Panleukocyte	Lymphoma, leukemia, inflammatory cells
UJ13A[1,27]	N-CAM	Primary CNS tumors, normal brain and spinal cord elements

* Enzodiagnostics (New York, NY)
† Dakopatts (Glostrump, Denmark)
‡ Boehringer Mannheim Biochemicals (Indianapolis, IN)
§ Biomedical Technologies (Stoughton, MA)
¶ Becton-Dickinson (Mountain View, CA)

Significance and Prognosis of Meningeal Metastases

The demonstration of malignant cells in CSF indicates that they are present in the subarachnoid space or ventricular cavity. Some authors[37] suggest that tumor nodules exposed to these fluid spaces may exfoliate cells into CSF, where they may be identified. Others believe that the presence of tumor cells in CSF virtually always indicates that leptomeningeal seeding has occurred and that therapy directed toward the entire CNS should be instituted.[18]

Patients with metastatic tumor cells in CSF generally have a poor prognosis. In the series reported by Ehya et al,[13] 75% of patients with followup died within 100 days of the first positive CSF result. These findings have grave import, since these patients may receive CNS irradiation or intrathecal chemotherapy. Of equal importance is the fact that many patients are sent home without any further diagnostic or therapeutic procedures.

Immunotherapy

A small number of antibodies may be operationally tumor specific in select situations

In recent years, monoclonal antibodies have been developed that react with a variety of epitopes expressed on tumor cells. Although no truly tumor-specific antibodies have been discovered (and indeed, such a thing may not exist), a small number of antibodies may be operationally tumor specific in select situations, such as when administered directly into the ventricular system (intrathecal administration). Thus, immunotherapy using these antibodies, when they are labelled with isotopes or toxins, holds real promise for some patients. For this purpose, some types of cross-reactivity that would be a drawback for the diagnostic use of a particular antibody might not be important. For example, Images 6.9 and 6.15 show reactivity for monoclonal antibody Mel-14 in cases of meningeal melanoma. Although this antibody also reacts with primary CNS tumors, this cross-reactivity is not important for intrathecal therapy in this patient with melanoma. The critical factor is that this antibody does not react with normal brain, ependyma, peripheral nerve roots, and blood vessels, which are the structures encountered in the ventricles and SAS that could be damaged by this type of treatment.

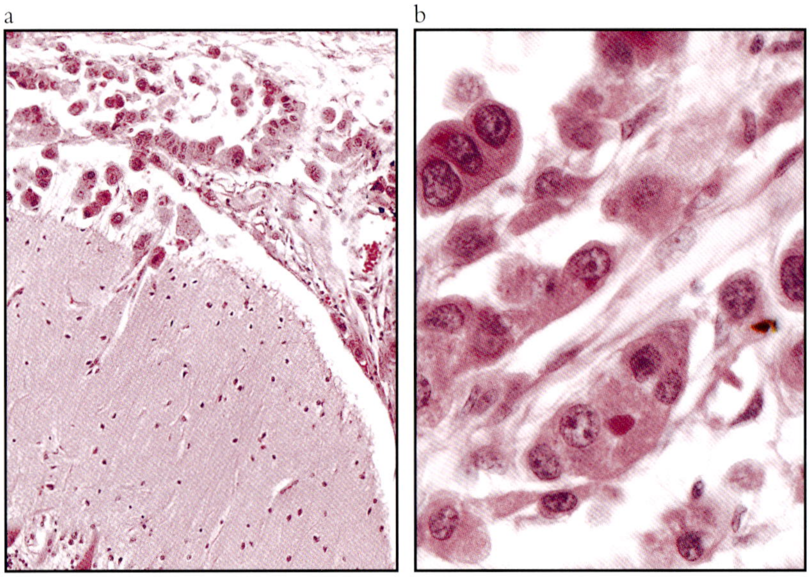

Image 6.1

Meningeal carcinomatosis shows the subarachnoid space (SAS) filled with malignant cells (H&E, Luxol fast blue; a, 200X; b, 400X).

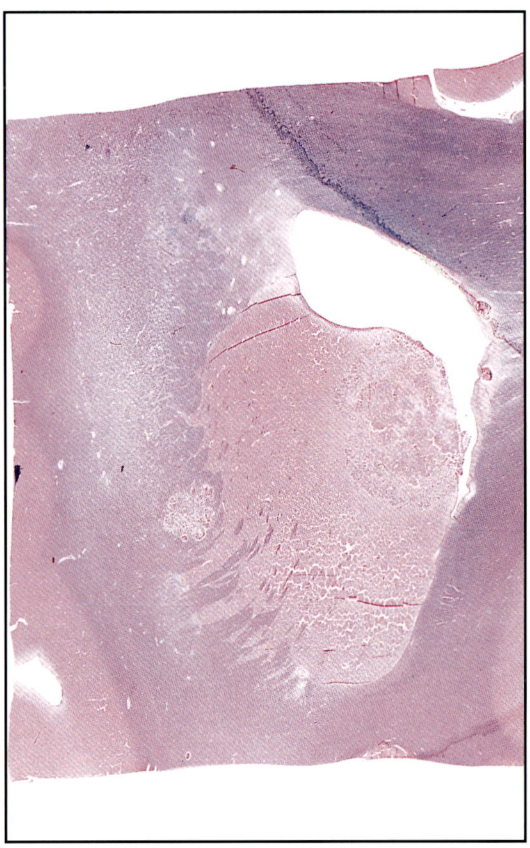

Image 6.2

Section from a patient with meningeal carcinomatosis shows a focus of metastatic breast carcinoma underlying the ependyma and protruding into the lateral ventricle in the brain (H&E, Luxol fast blue, 7X).

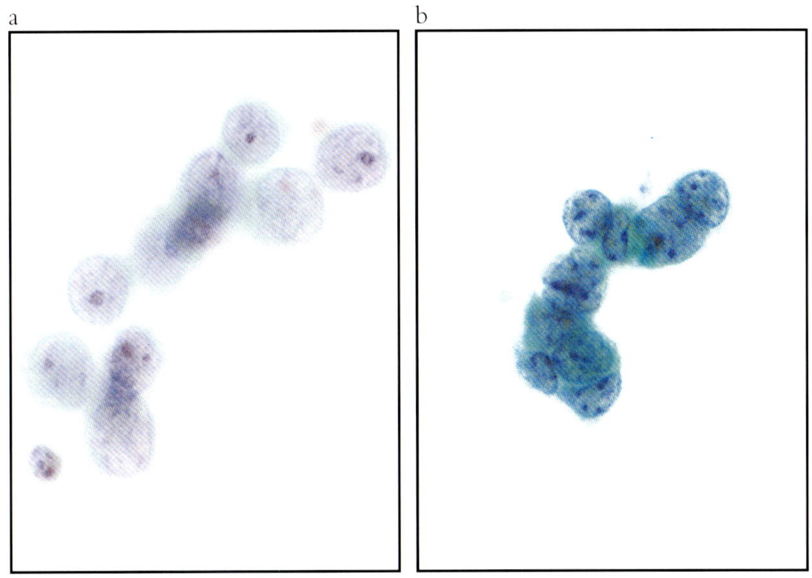

Image 6.3
Metastasis of small-cell anaplastic carcinoma of the lung to the CSF (a). This condition typically presents as loose clusters of cells with high nuclear/cytoplasmic ratios. Cohesive tissue fragments with intense nuclear molding are seen infrequently (b) (both, Papanicolaou, 1,000X).

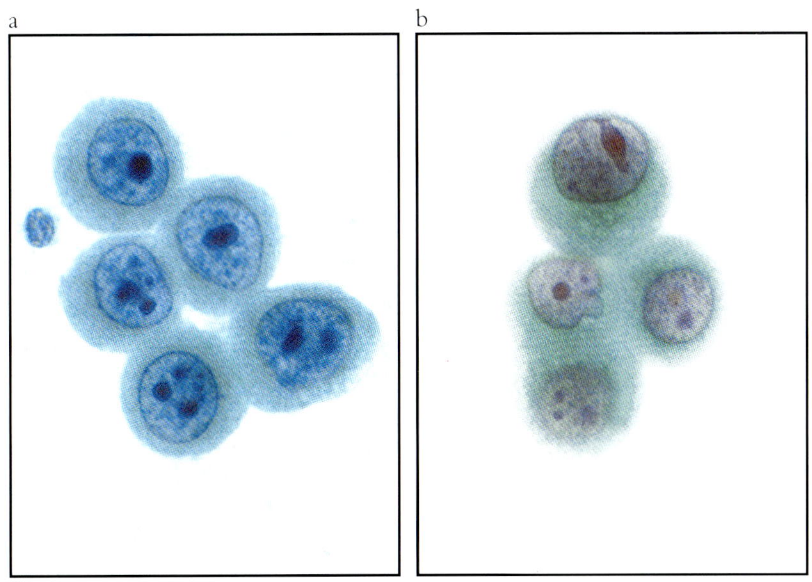

Image 6.4
Large-cell undifferentiated carcinoma of the lung in CSF (a). Adenocarcinoma of the lung commonly sheds as single cells (b) (both, Papanicolaou, 1,000X).

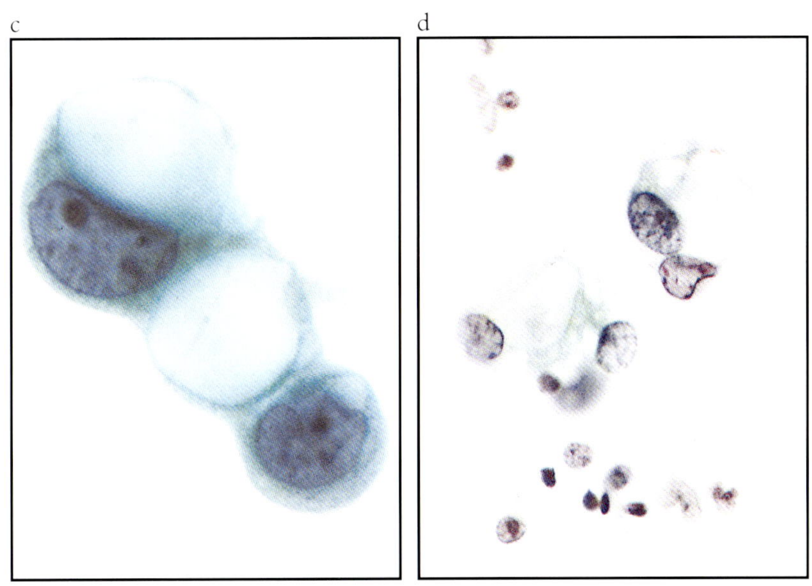

Adenocarcimona of the lung can also shed in small tissue fragments (c). Rarely, well-differentiated adenocarcinoma of the lung metastasizes to CSF as cohesive papillary fragments with hypersecretory vacuoles (d) (both, Papanicolaou, 1,000X).

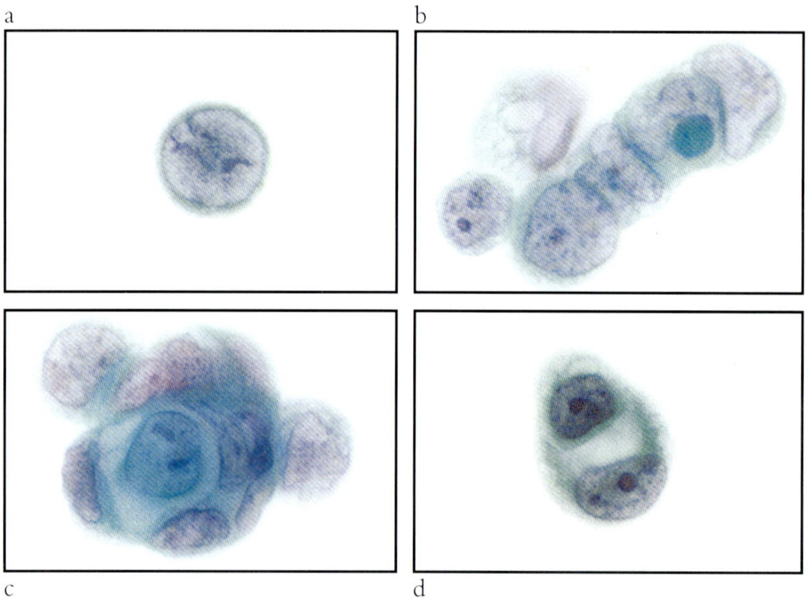

Image 6.5
Bland single cells (a) and cohesive tissue fragments in adenocarcinoma of the lung (b and c). This presentation mimics ductal carcinoma of the breast. A cell-in-cell arrangement is also sometimes seen (d) (all, Papanicolaou, 1,000X).

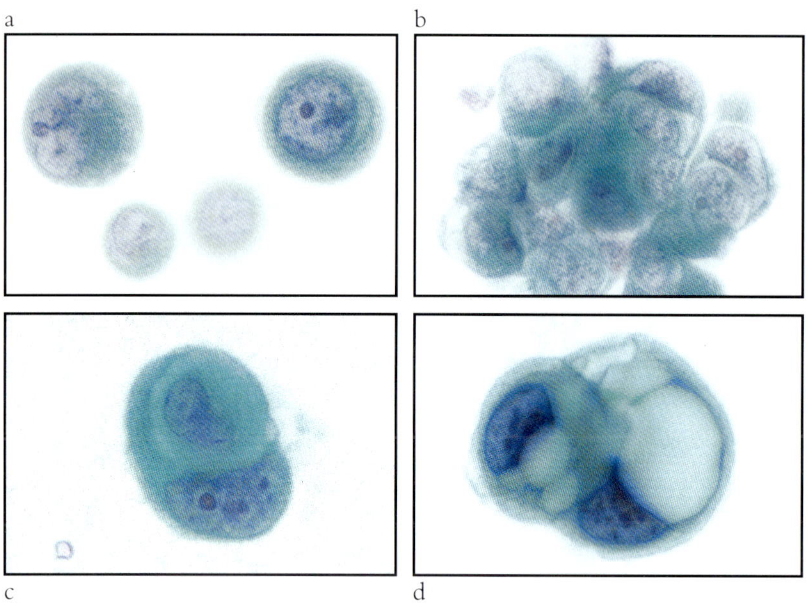

Image 6.6
Ductal carcinoma of the breast typically presents in CSF as single, round cells with moderate amounts of cytoplasm and centrally placed nuclei (a). Cohesive tissue fragments (b) and cell-in-cell arrangements (c) are also produced by ductal carcinoma in CSF, but these formations are not as frequent as in effusions. Breast carcinoma presents occasionally as tissue fragments with hypersecretory vacuoles (d) (all, Papanicolaou, 1,000X).

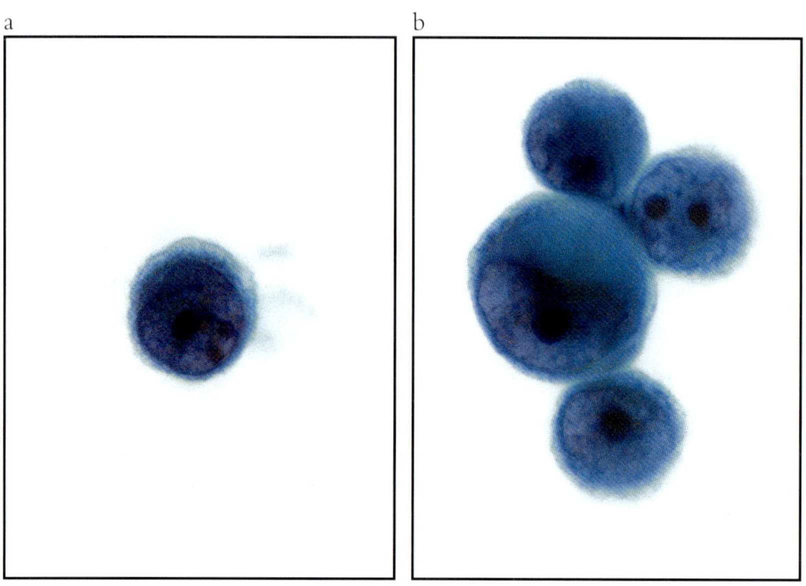

Image 6.7
Ductal carcinoma of the breast with anaplastic features in CSF (both, Papanicolaou, 1,000X).

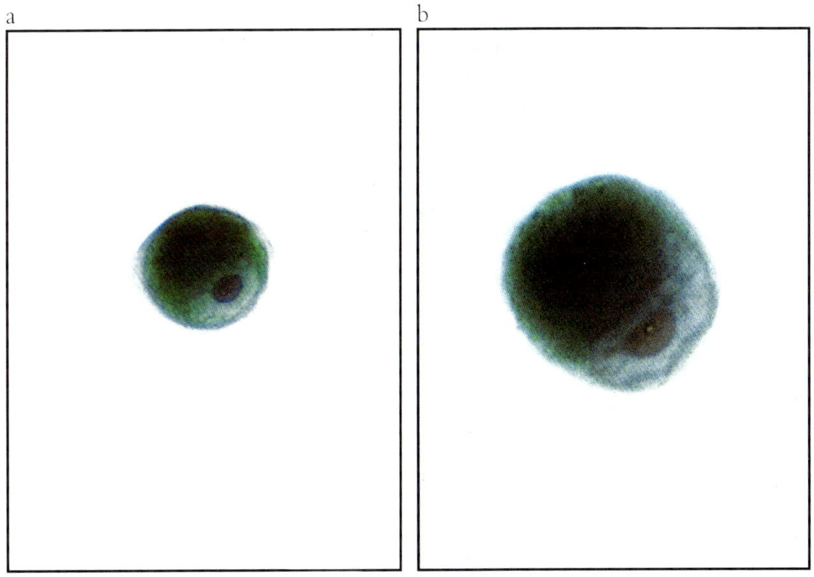

Image 6.8
Large, pigment-bearing cells with coarse chromatin and prominent nucleoli characteristic of malignant melanoma (both, Papanicolaou, 1,000X).

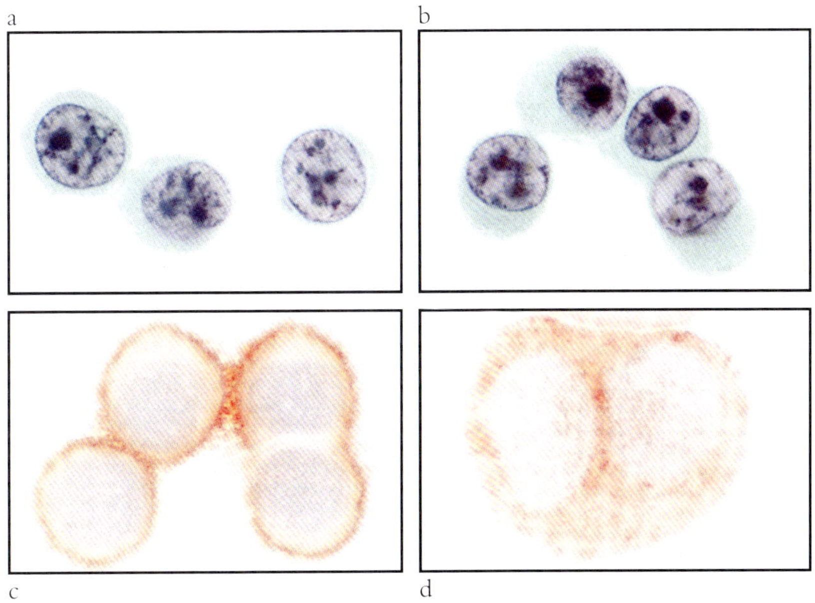

Image 6.9
Amelanotic melanoma presents as undifferentiated malignant single cells (a and b). Reactivity with antimelanoma antibodies Mel-14 (c) and HMB-45,(d) helps to establish this diagnosis (a and b, Papanicolaou; c and d, Immunoperoxidase; all, 1,000X).

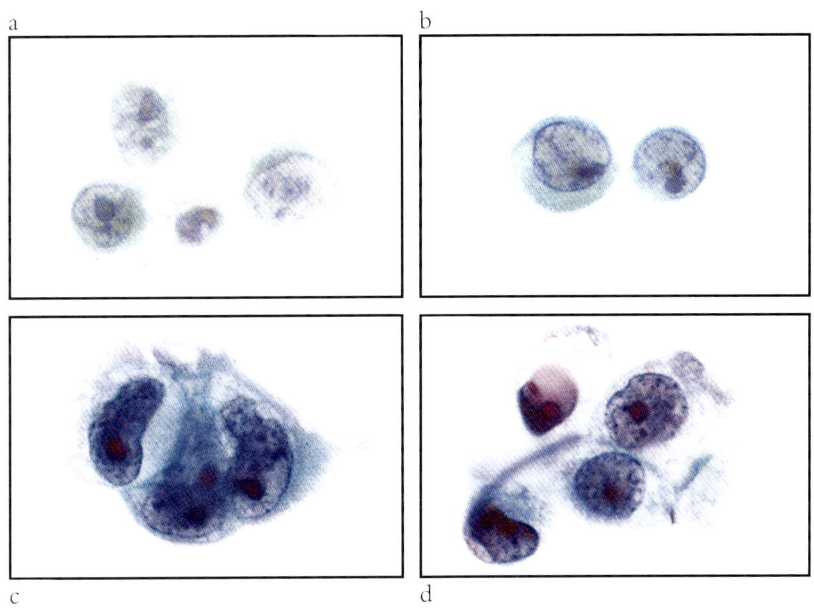

Image 6.10
Adenocarcinoma of the stomach metastatic to CSF. Loosely arranged single cells are noted in some cases (a and b). Tumor cells are shed as cohesive tissue fragments in other patients (c and d) (all, Papanicolaou, 1,000X).

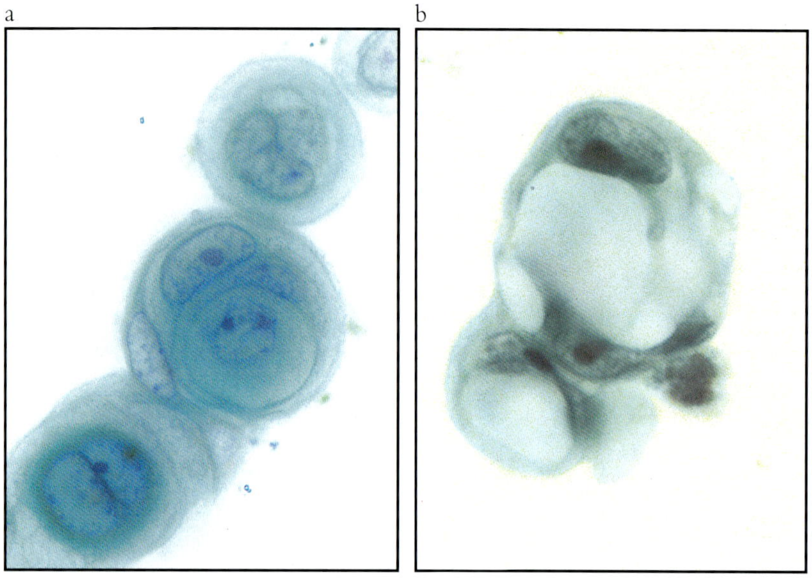

Image 6.11
Squamous cell carcinoma of the uterine cervix producing meningeal carcinomatosis (a) (same patient as Figure 6.4). Well-differentiated adenocarcinoma of the colon metastatic to meninges is seen in another patient (b) (both, Papanicolaou, 1,000X).

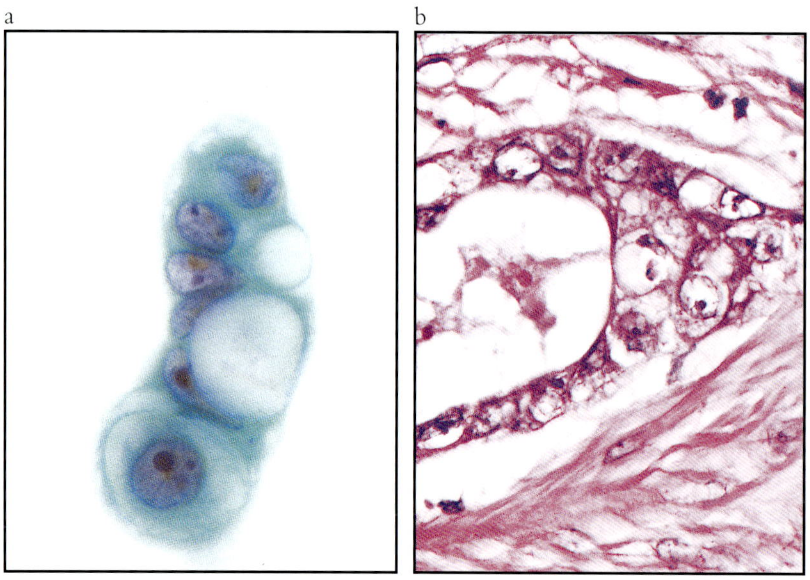

Image 6.12
Metastatic adenocarcinoma in CSF (a). Adenocarcinoma discovered in this patient's ovary several months earlier (b). It is not possible to determine whether this is a primary ovarian neoplasm or a metastatic Krukenberg tumor from an occult primary source (a, Papanicolaou, 1,000X; b, H&E, 400X).

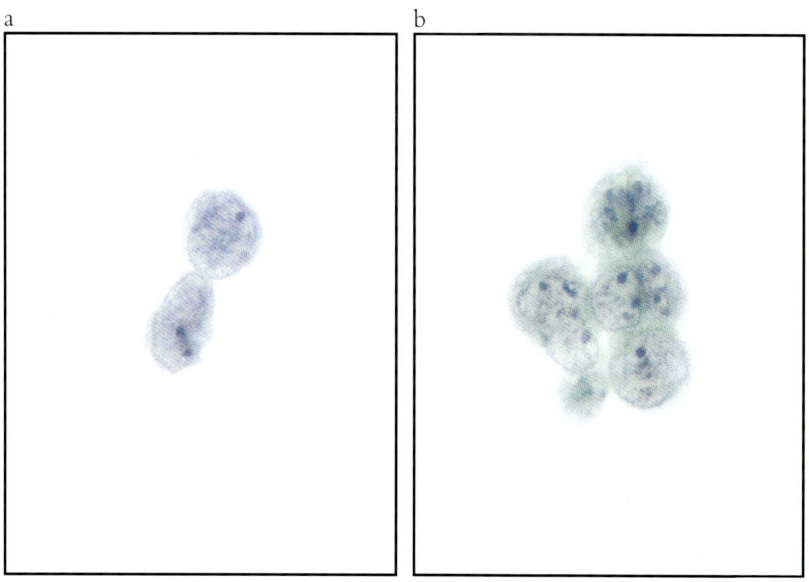

Image 6.13
Pleomorphic, small anaplastic cells with scant cytoplasm characterize embryonal rhabdomyosarcoma of the orbit in this patient (a). Metastatic neuroblastoma originating in the adrenal sheds in CSF as small anaplastic cells with high nuclear/cytoplasmic ratios (b) (both, Papanicolaou, 1,000X).

Image 6.14
Enucleated eye from a 20-month-old child with retinoblastoma (a). Retinoblastoma cells appeared in his CSF 10 months later (b) (a, H&E, 1,000X; b, Papanicolaou, 1,000X).

a b

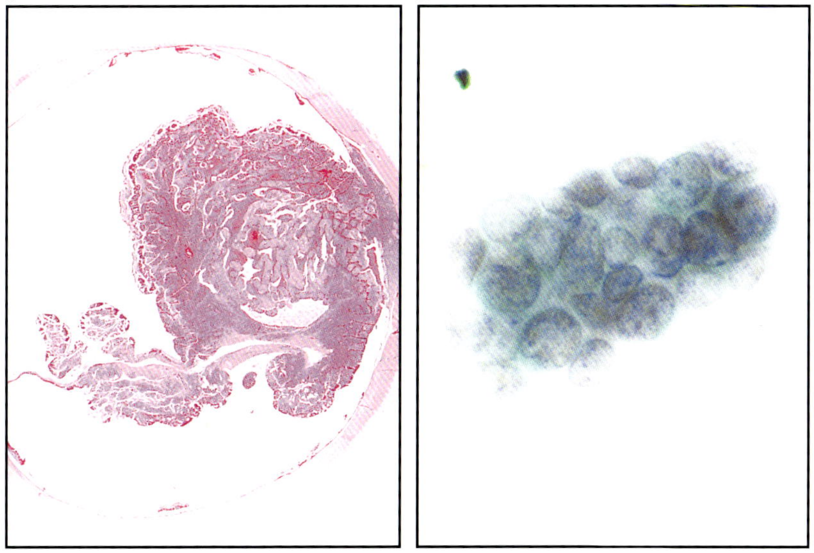

A striking infiltrate filling the spinal SAS at autopsy (c). Histologically, a similar meningeal infiltrate was seen, as had been seen in the cytologic preparation (d) (d, H&E, 400X).

c d

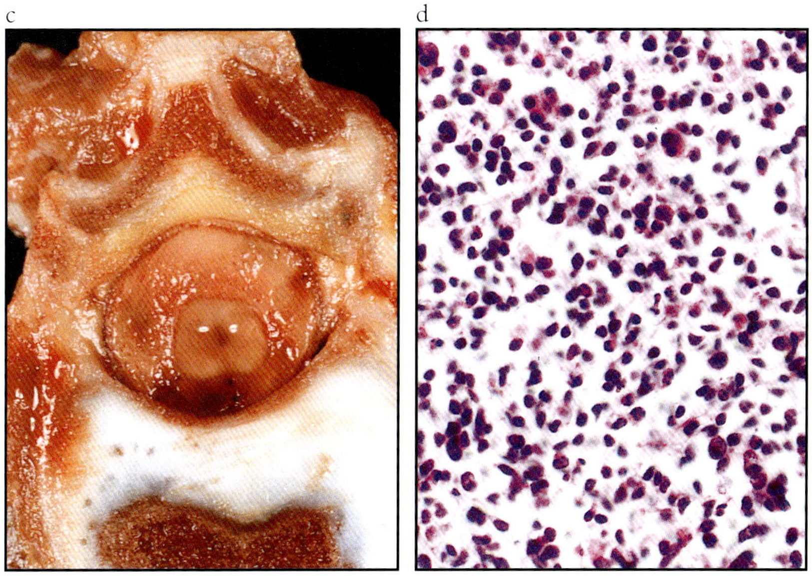

Image 6.15
A mixture of malignant cells and reactive lymphocytes and monocytes (a and b) (a, Papanicolaou; b, Romanowski; both, 1,000X).

a b

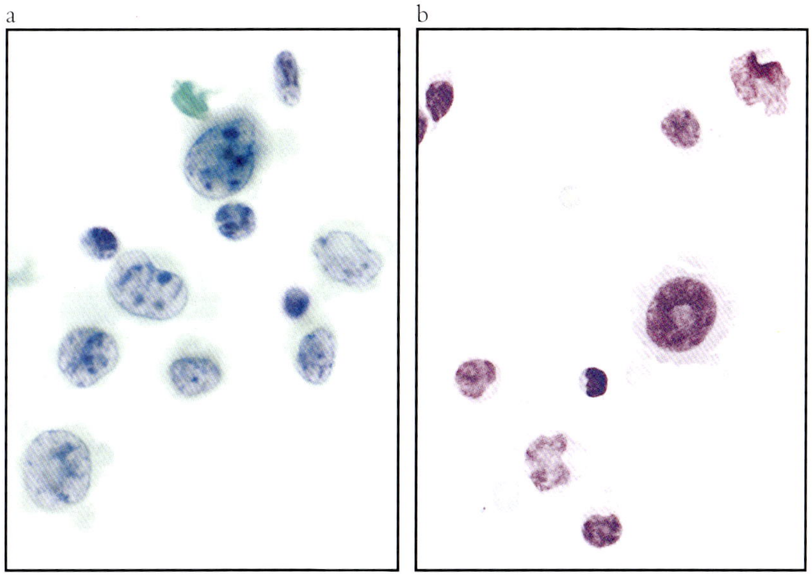

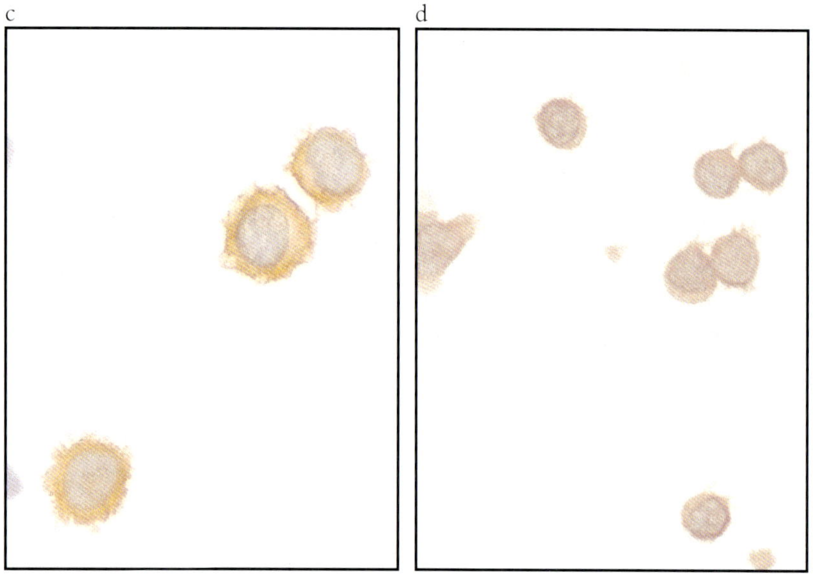

Immunoperoxidase staining with an antimelanoma antibody, Mel-14, distinguishes the cells of malignant melanoma from the background lymphocytes and monocytes (c). Panleukocyte antibody 2D1 stains the inflammatory cells but is negative for the tumor cells (d) (c and d, Immunoperoxidase; both, 1,000X).

References

1. Allan PM, Garson JA, Harper EI, Asser U, Coakham HB, Brownell B, Kemshead JT: Biological characterization and clinical applications of a monoclonal antibody recognizing an antigen restricted to neuroectodermal tissues. *Int J Cancer* 31:591, 1983.
2. Amer MH, Al-Sarraf M, Baker LH, Vaitkevicius VK: Malignant melanoma and central nervous system metastases: incidence, diagnosis, treatment and survival. *Cancer* 42:660–668, 1978.
3. Aronson SM, Garcia JH, Aronson BE: Metastatic neoplasms of the brain: their frequency in relation to age. *Cancer* 17:558–563, 1964.
4. Ashton PR, Hollingsworth AS Jr, Johnston WW: The cytopathology of metastatic breast carcinoma. *Acta Cytol* 19:1–6, 1975.
5. Beerman WF: Meningeal carcinomatosis. *JAMA* 58:1437–1439, 1912.
6. Bigner SH, Johnston WW: The cytopathology of cerebrospinal fluid: a review, part II: metastatic cancer, meningeal carcinomatosis and primary central nervous system neoplasms. *Acta Cytol* 25:461–480, 1981.
7. Bigner SH, Johnston WW: The diagnostic challenge of tumors manifested initially by the shedding of cells into cerebrospinal fluid. *Acta Cytol* 28:29–36, 1984.
8. Boring CC, Squires TS, Tong T: Cancer statistics, 1992. *CA* 42:19–38, 1992.
9. Carrel S, Accolla RS, Carmagnola AL, Mach JP: Common human melanoma-associated antigen(s) detected by monoclonal antibodies. *Cancer Res* 40:2523–2528, 1980.
10. Carrel S, de Tribolet N, Mach JP: Expression of neuroectodermal antigens common to melanomas, gliomas, and neuroblastoma. *Acta Neuropathol* 57:158–164, 1982.
11. Dee AL: Carcinoma of the breast presenting initially in cerebrospinal fluid. *Acta Cytol* 29:909–910, 1985.
12. Drier JK, Swanson PE, Cherwitz DL, Wick MR: S-100 protein immunoreactivity in poorly differentiated carcinomas. *Arch Pathol Lab Med* 111:447–452, 1987.
13. Ehya H, Hajdu SL, Melamed MR: Cytopathology of nonlymphoreticular neoplasms metastatic to the central nervous system. *Acta Cytol* 25:599–610, 1981.
14. Fried BM, Buckley RC: Primary carcinoma of the lungs, IV: intracranial metastases. *Arch Pathol* 9:483–527, 1980.
15. Galluzzi S, Payne PM: Brain metastases from primary bronchial carcinoma: a statistical study of 741 necropsies. *Br J Cancer* 10:408–414, 1956.
16. Garin-Chesa P, Fellinger EJ, Huvos AG, Beresford RH, Melamed MR, Triche TJ, Rettig WJ: Immunohistochemical analysis of neural cell adhesion molecules: differential expression in small round cell tumors of childhood and adolescence. *Am J Pathol* 139:275–286, 1991.

17. Geisinger KR, Hajdu SI, Helson L: Exfoliative cytology of nonlymphoreticular neoplasms in children. *Acta Cytol* 28:16–28, 1984.
18. Glass JP, Melamed MR, Chernik NL, Posner JB: Malignant cells in cerebrospinal fluid (CSF): the meaning of a positive CSF cytology. *Neurology* 29:1369–1375, 1979.
19. Gonzalez-Vitale JC, Garcia-Bunuel R: Meningeal carcinomatosis. *Cancer* 37:2906–2911, 1976.
20. Guillermo HA, Turbat-Herrera EA, Lott RL: S-100 protein expression by primary and metastatic adenocarcinomas. *Am J Clin Pathol* 89:168–176, 1988.
21. Heimann A, Merino MJ: Carcinomatous meningitis as the initial manifestation of breast cancer. *Acta Cytol* 30:25–28, 1986.
22. Johnston WW (moderator), Frable WJ, Naylor B, Patten SF Jr: Diagnostic cytology seminar. *Acta Cytol* 20:410–445, 1976.
23. Lee AK, Dwarkanath S, DeLellis RA, Rosen PP, Silverman ML, Bator L, Wolfe HJ: S-100 protein positivity in breast carcinoma. *Lab Invest* 54:35A, 1986.
24. Little JR, Dale ADJ, Okazaki H: Meningeal carcinomatosis: clinical manifestations. *Arch Neurol* 30:138–143, 1974.
25. Naylor B: The cytologic diagnosis of cerebrospinal fluid. *Acta Cytol* 8:141–149, 1964.
26. Olson ME, Chernik NL, Posner JB: Infiltration of the leptomeninges by systemic cancer: a clinical and pathologic study. *Arch Neurol* 30:122–137, 1974.
27. Patel K, Rossell RJ, Bourne S, Moore SE, Walsh FS, Kemshead JT: Monoclonal antibody UJ13A recognizes the neural cell adhesion molecule (NCAM). *Int J Cancer* 44:1062, 1989.
28. Posner J (chair), Bigner DD, D'Angio GJ, Shapiro W, Walker MD: Subpanel on neoplasms in report of the panel on stroke, trauma, regeneration, and neoplasms to the National Advisory Neurological and Communicative Disorders and Stroke Council. United States Department of Health Education and Welfare. Public Health Service, National Institutes of Health. September 15, 1978, pp. 152–153.
29. Rettig WJ, Garin-Chesa P, Huvos AG: Ewing's sarcoma: new approaches to histogenesis and molecular plasticity. *Lab Invest* 66:133–137, 1992.
30. Ringenberg SQ, Francis R, Doll DC: Meningeal carcinomatosis as the presenting manifestation of tumors of unknown origin. *Acta Cytol* 34:590–592, 1990.
31. Russell DS, Rubinstein LJ: *Pathology of Tumours of the Nervous System*, 5th ed. Baltimore, MD, Williams and Wilkins Co, 1989, p. 919.
32. Shoup SA, Johnston WW, Siegler HF, Tello JW, Schlom F, Bigner DD, Bigner SH: A panel of antibodies useful in the cytologic diagnosis of metastatic melanoma. *Acta Cytol* 34:385–392, 1990.
33. Spriggs AI: Malignant cells in cerebrospinal fluid. *J Clin Pathol* 7:122–130, 1954.
34. Twijnstra A, Ongerboer der Visser BW, van Anten AP: Diagnosis of leptomeningeal metastasis. *Clin Neurol Neurosurg* 89:79–85, 1987.

35. Vanstapel MJ, Gatter KC, Wolf-Peeters C, Mason DY, Desmet VD: New sites of human S-100 immunoreactivity detected with monoclonal antibodies. *Am J Clin Pathol* 85:160–168, 1986.

36. Vick WW, Wikstrand CJ, Bullard DE, Kemshead J, Coakham HB, Schlom J, Johnston WW, Bigner DD, Bigner SH: The use of a panel of monoclonal antibodies in the evaluation of cytologic specimens from the central nervous system. *Acta Cytol* 31:815–824, 1987.

37. Wagner JA, Frost JK, Wisotzkey H Jr: Subarachnoid neoplasia: incidence and problems of diagnosis. *South Med J* 53:1503–1508, 1960.

38. Walts AE, Said JW, Shintaku IP: Cytodiagnosis of malignant melanoma: immunoperoxidase staining with HMB-45 antibody as an aid to diagnosis. *Am J Clin Pathol* 90:77–80, 1988.

39. Weithman AM, Morrison G, Ingram EA: Meningeal metastasis of squamous cell carcinoma of the uterine cervix: case report and review of the literature. *Diagn Cytopathol* 3:170–172, 1987.

40. Wallace RM, Bigner SH, Johnston WW: Metastatic breast carcinoma in cerebrospinal fluid: a cytomorphometric study. *Acta Cytol* 26:787–792, 1982.

41. Weed JC Jr, Creasman WT: Meningeal carcinomatosis secondary to advanced squamous cell carcinoma of the cervix: a case report. *Gynecol Oncol* 3:201–204, 1975.

42. Willis RA: 163 Secondary tumors. In: Minckler J, ed. *Pathology of the Nervous System*, vol. 2, part XIII. New York, NY, McGraw-Hill Book Co, 1971, pp. 2178–2196.

43. Woodward BH, Ideker RE, Johnston WW: Cytologic detection of malignant melanoma in urine. *Acta Cytol* 22:350–352, 1978.

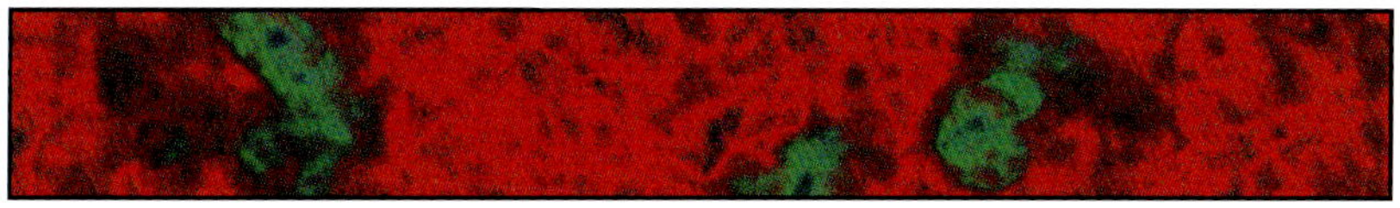

CHAPTER SEVEN

Primary Central Nervous System Neoplasms

The presentation of leukemia, lymphoma, and metastatic tumors in cerebrospinal fluid (CSF) is sufficiently similar to that in other body cavity fluids to present little problem for the cytopathologist and cytotechnologist. By contrast, primary central nervous system (CNS) tumors, with their confusing nomenclature and vast array of individual tumor types each having its own characteristic clinical and cytologic presentation, pose more of a diagnostic challenge.

Cytologic Techniques

Examination of CSF is appropriate in some cases to make the initial diagnosis of a primary brain tumor. For this approach to work, four prerequisites must be met: (1) the tumor type must have a high incidence of CSF involvement; (2) CSF must be obtained without unnecessary risk to the patient; (3) the neoplastic cells must be morphologically identifiable; and (4) an advantage to obtaining a preoperative diagnosis must be present.

For tumor types with a low incidence of CSF involvement, direct sampling techniques are most appropriate. Cyst fluid aspirates and fine needle aspiration biopsy can be accomplished through a burr hole with computed tomography (CT)–guided stereotactic techniques. The low morbidity and mortality rate and the short hospitalization time, as compared to open craniotomy, make these procedures advantageous when dealing with lesions for which direct surgical approach is impossible or unnecessary. During craniotomy and open biopsy, imprint and touch preparations provide an important adjunct to frozen section and permanent section evaluation.

A more widely used application of CSF examination is to document CSF spread in patients known to have primary CNS tumors. In an individual patient, this may precipitate whole neuraxis therapy. This procedure is particularly useful to document recurrence in patients whose posttreatment CT scans and arteriograms are difficult to interpret. In addition, documentation of a high rate of CSF dissemination for a specific tumor type may lead to prophylactic whole neuraxis treatment for future patients.

Nomenclature

In 1926, Bailey and Cushing[2] provided the first widely accepted nomenclature for brain tumors. In 1949, Kernohan et al[26] presented an alternate scheme based on histologic grade of individual tumor types. In 1965, Zulch[49,50] provided a third set of terms. More recently, the terminology presented by Russell and Rubinstein[38,39] has become widely used in the United States and Britain. This confusing situation of overlapping classification schemes for primary brain tumors was alleviated in 1979 with the publication of the World Health Organization's brain tumor classification,[47] which represents a reconciliation of the conflicting terminology previously used. The World Health Organization classification was updated at a conference in 1988, and the revised version was published in 1989.[10]

The WHO brain tumor classification reconciles previous conflicting terminology

Tumors of Neuroectodermal Origin

The two major cell types that comprise the brain and spinal cord are the neurons or ganglion cells and the supporting cells or glia. The glia consist of macroglia, which include astrocytes, oligodendroglia, and ependymal cells, and microglia. The choroid plexus lining cell is considered to be a specialized form of ependymal cell. These cell types can all give rise to neoplasms, each of which generally derives its name from its presumptive cell of origin (see Table 7.1).

Astrocytoma

One of the most common gliomas is the slow-growing astrocytoma. This tumor occurs throughout the brain and spinal cord in patients of all ages. Grossly, these neoplasms appear as ill-defined diffuse expansions of the white matter, which may be predominantly cystic (Figure 7.1). Histologically, they are composed of stellate or bipolar astrocytes with bland nuclei embedded in a fibrillary background (Image 7.1). In smears and imprints, the cells of astrocytomas have round to slightly ovoid regular nuclei with fine chromatin and small nucleoli. The cytoplasm of individual cells is often indistinct; the nuclei appear embedded in a fibrillar matrix. In both histologic and cytologic preparations, the astrocytoma

Table 7.1
Tumors of Neuroepithelial Origin

I. Astrocytic Tumors
   A. Astrocytoma
   B. Pilocytic astrocytoma
   C. Subependymal giant cell astrocytoma (tuberous sclerosis)
   D. Astroblastoma
   E. Anaplastic (malignant) astrocytoma
   F. Glioblastoma multiforme
   G. Gliomatosis cerebri

II. Oligodendroglial Tumors
   A. Oligodendroglioma
   B. Mixed oligoastrocytoma
   C. Anaplastic oligodendroglioma

III. Ependymal and Choroid Plexus Tumors
   A. Ependymoma
   B. Anaplastic ependymoma
   C. Choroid plexus papilloma
   D. Anaplastic (malignant) choroid plexus papilloma

IV. Neuronal Tumors
   A. Gangliocytoma
   B. Ganglioglioma
   C. Ganglioneuroblastoma
   D. Anaplastic gangliocytoma and ganglioglioma
   E. Neuroblastoma

V. Poorly Differentiated and Embryonal Tumors
   A. Medulloblastoma
   B. Medulloepithelioma
   C. Primitive polar spongioblastoma

when compared to normal white matter shows increased cellularity, nuclear hyperchromasia, and variability in nuclear size and shape (Image 7.1). These neoplastic astrocytes retain expression of glial fibrillary acidic protein (GFAP) and other neuroectodermal antigens, such as neural cell adhesion molecule (N-CAM), but no immunohistochemical methods are currently available to distinguish these tumors from reactive gliosis (Image 7.2). A common variant of this tumor is the piloid astrocytoma, which is composed of bipolar astrocytes with elongated processes. This tumor frequently contains waxy, amorphous bodies called Rosenthal fibers (Image 7.3). Low-grade astrocytomas are uncommonly identified in cerebrospinal fluid, probably because even when these cells have access to CSF, their benign cytologic characteristics render them indistinguishable from normal and reactive cells.

Anaplastic astrocytomas are morphologically and biologically aggressive

Anaplastic Astrocytoma

The morphologically and biologically more aggressive variant of the astrocytoma is the anaplastic astrocytoma, according to the World Health Organization classification.[47] Anaplastic astrocytomas are hypercellular infiltrative neoplasms composed of sheets of cells that retain

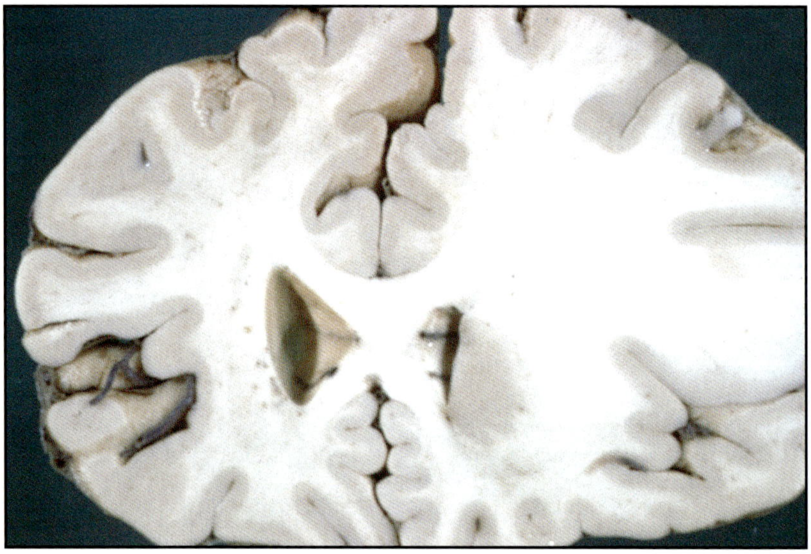

Figure 7.1
This coronal section through the frontal lobes shows a diffuse astrocytoma expanding one hemisphere.

astrocytic morphology but have irregularly shaped, convoluted, hyperchromatic nuclei (Image 7.4). In CSF, they show these same nuclear features and generally have only small amounts of wispy cytoplasm.

Glioblastoma Multiforme

Glioblastoma is the most common malignant primary brain tumor of adults. It is frequently seen in the deep white matter or in the basal ganglia of middle-aged adults and also occurs in the brain stem and spinal cord. This tumor presents occasionally in childhood, but its presentation in the cerebellum of patients of all ages is extremely rare.

Glioblastoma is the most common malignant primary brain tumor of adults

Grossly, this neoplasm is an ill-defined area typically containing regions of necrosis and hemorrhage (Figure 7.2). Although surgical excision is usually performed, the infiltrative nature of the cells makes total resection impossible, so adjunctive radiation and chemotherapy are used. Even with this aggressive regimen, the tumor is inevitably fatal.

Glioblastomas contain the same cellular populations as are seen in anaplastic astrocytomas, including fibrillary and protoplasmic astrocytes and gemistocytes (Images 7.5 and 7.6). These tumors often show more cellular pleomorphism than do anaplastic astrocytomas, and they frequently contain bizarre multinucleated tumor giant cells and/or small anaplastic cells. The two most characteristic features in histologic sections are necrosis with surrounding pseudopalisading of cells and exuberant endothelial proliferation (Image 7.5). The presence of necrosis is the most useful feature in distinguishing between anaplastic astrocytoma and glioblastoma, because its presence correlates with the more malignant clinical course that characterizes glioblastoma.[7]

The incidence of spinal fluid dissemination of glioblastoma ranges from 30% to 40% in most series[6,17,28,33] (Table 7.2). The incidence of positive cytologic findings at the time of initial presentation, however, is probably considerably lower.[43] The cytologic presentation of glioblas-

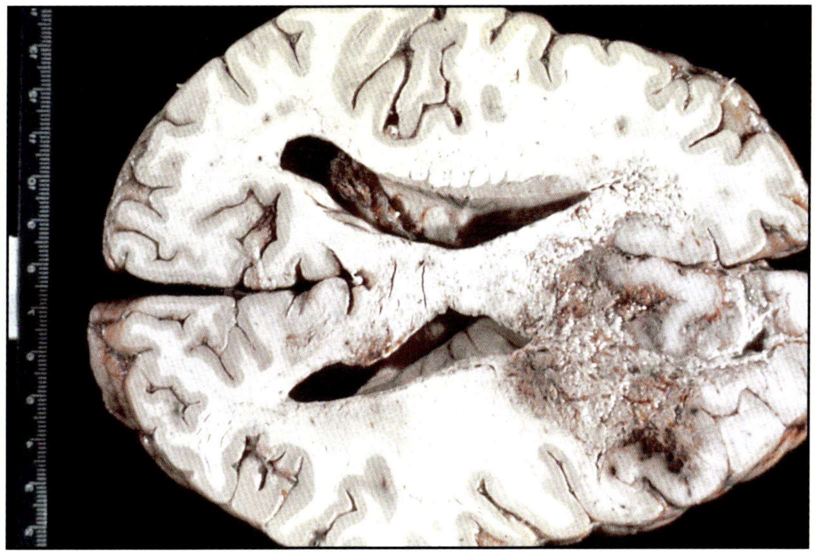

Figure 7.2
Glioblastoma multiforme produces a mass and contains areas of hemorrhage and necrosis. This frontal lobe tumor has spread across the midline and back into the corpus callosum.

toma is variable and depends on which components reach the subarachnoid space (SAS) (Image 7.7). Sometimes exfoliated cells are large and pleomorphic, with multiple overlapping nuclei and cytoplasm that has a tendency to trail off. Other common cell types are multinucleated cells and round cells with discrete cell borders, dense cytoplasm, and hyperchromatic nuclei. Frequently undifferentiated cells of large or small size are seen.

Glioblastomas are especially problematic when they exfoliate only one cell type

Glioblastomas are especially problematic when they exfoliate only one cell type. Image 7.8 shows small anaplastic cells in CSF from a 5-year-old girl with a pontine mass. At surgery, she had a pontine glioblastoma multiforme, but only the small anaplastic component was seen in the CSF (Image 7.8a). With the development of anti-GFAP antibodies, immunohistochemical approaches have aided greatly in this problem, since expression of this marker can identify malignant cells as glial in origin, as was done in this case (Image 7.8b).

Gliomatosis Cerebri

Gliomatosis cerebri is an unusual astrocytic proliferation that diffusely involves large portions of the brain. Histologically, the proliferating cell varies from a well-differentiated stellate astrocyte to a more elongated spindle form. Although one would predict exfoliation of bland cells with indistinct cytoplasm, the only report of this lesion in CSF describes small, anaplastic cells.[31]

Primary Meningeal Gliomatosis

Gliomas sometimes spread in the subarachnoid space, producing meningeal gliomatosis. Rarely, however, the tumor cells are seen in the meninges alone without a primary parenchymal source.[23] Image 7.9 shows anaplastic cells in the CSF of an 18-year-old woman with ascend-

Table 7.2
Frequency of Detection of Primary Central Nervous System Tumors by CSF Cytology

	Bischoff[6]	Kline[28]	Naylor[33]	Gondos & King[17]	Balhuizen et al[3,4]
		(Number detected by CSF cytology/Total number)			
Neuroectodermal Tumors					
Medulloblastoma	3/4	2/2	3/17	16/26	12/17
Astrocytoma grades I and II	4/16	4/13	2/17	7/28	5/27
Astrocytoma grades III and IV	6/20	11/26	3/7	6/21	14/38
Ependymoma	—	0/2	5/15	3/13	5/28
Oligodendroglioma	2/5	0/1	1/1	—	4/17
Choroid plexus carcinoma	—	1/1	—	—	—
Olfactory neuroblastoma	—	—	1/1	—	—
Tumors of the Pineal Gland					
Pineal germinoma	—	—	1/4	3/8	—
Malignant teratoma	—	1/1	—	—	1/1
Pineal choriocarcinoma	—	—	—	—	1/1
Tumors of the Pituitary Region					
Craniopharyngioma	2/2	1/2	0/6	—	2/17
Pituitary adenoma	2/7	—	3/12	0/6	2/63
Tumors Originating in the Meninges and Supporting Structures					
Meningiosarcoma	1/1	—	—	—	1/3
Meningioma	1/15	3/6	0/6	0/7	—
Neurinoma	—	0/5	0/4	—	—
Tumors of Uncertain Origin					
Hemangioblastoma	2/2	—	0/4	—	—
Other	2/6	—	—	5/15	—

ing paralysis and no demonstrable brain or spinal cord tumor by radiographic studies.[5] At autopsy, no lesions were within the brain or spinal cord, but a striking meningeal infiltrate covered the spinal cord (Figure 7.3 and Image 7.10). A glial heterotopia was found outside the thoracic spinal cord, which is presumably the source of this neoplastic process. Most cases of primary meningeal gliomatosis can be traced to glial heterotopias, and the cells that disseminate can be well differentiated or anaplastic and may be of astrocytic, ependymal, or oligodendroglial origin.[23]

Oligodendroglioma

Oligodendrogliomas comprise from 5% to 12.4% of intracranial gliomas, and they occur most frequently in the cerebral hemispheres of adults.[39] Grossly, they are more discrete than astrocytic tumors and typically contain calcifications that are occasionally of sufficient density to be seen on skull films (Figure 7.4). Histologically, they contain sheets of uniform polygonal cells with round nuclei (Image 7.11a). Perinuclear clearing in the cytoplasm is a frequent artifact that produces a "fried egg" appearance. A delicate fibrovascular stroma and microcalcification are other typical features (Image 7.11b). Although cases of oligodendrogliomas have been reported in CSF by Bischoff,[6] Naylor,[33] and Balhuizen,[4] none mentioned specific features of these neoplasms. Smears

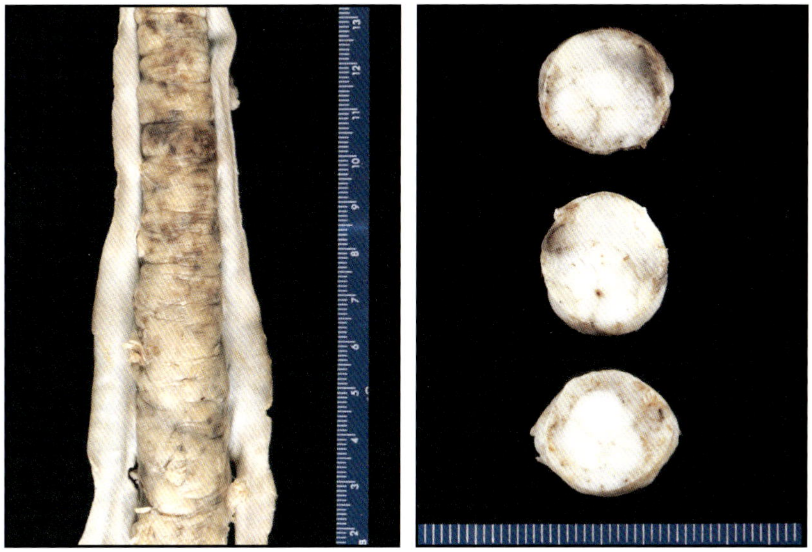

Figure 7.3
At autopsy, the spinal subarachnoid space of an 18-year-old woman with ascending paralysis was filled with tumor representing primary meningeal gliomatosis (see Image 7.9).

GFAP studies confirm the glial nature of oligodendrogliomas

and needle washings reveal distinctive round regular nuclei with powdery chromatin, small nucleoli, and indistinct wispy cytoplasm (Image 7.12a). These features are important clues in correctly identifying this tumor, which may be confused with high-grade gliomas, metastases, or lymphomas due to its high cellularity. GFAP studies confirm the glial nature of these tumors and are useful in distinguishing them from lymphoma and metastases. Although generally classified as a benign neoplasm, the oligodendroglioma is prone to recurrence. Even a pure oligodendroglioma generally becomes more highly cellular and anaplastic when it recurs repeatedly. Image 7.12b shows cells from a tumor washing of an

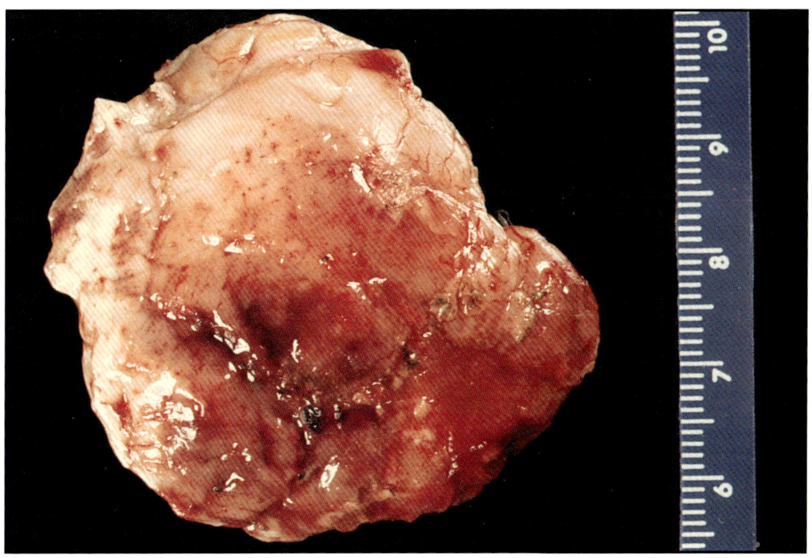

Figure 7.4
Grossly, the oligodendroglioma is usually a solid, well-circumscribed mass.

anaplastic oligodendroglioma. These preparations reveal no distinctive characteristics, and this lesion could easily have been confused with a metastasis without the history of multiple prior excisions of an oligodendroglioma from this same site. Many of these lesions are, in fact, mixed oligoastrogliomas (Image 7.13). When these mixed tumors recur, the astrocytic component tends to become progressively more malignant, finally resulting in a glioblastoma.

Ependymoma

Ependymomas may occur anywhere throughout the brain and spinal cord of an individual of any age, but they are most frequent in the fourth ventricles of children (Figure 7.5). Although anaplastic variants occur, many ependymomas are slow growing and discrete, lending themselves to successful surgical excision.

Many ependymomas lend themselves to successful surgical excision

Histologically, this tumor consists of sheets of cells with bland, oval nuclei, and a tendency for unipolar cytoplasmic processes to surround blood vessels forming pseudorosettes (Image 7.14a). Less frequently, true rosettes may be seen (Image 7.14b). Cytologically, these cells contain bland, round-to-oval nuclei with small nucleoli, and they may display a columnar orientation (Images 7.15 and 7.16).

Anaplastic Ependymoma

The anaplastic ependymoma contains sheets of closely packed cells with high nuclear/cytoplasmic (N/C) ratios. Its ependymal derivation is suggested by a perivascular pseudorosette pattern (Image 7.17a). This tumor exfoliates as clusters of anaplastic cells that resemble cells from medulloblastomas (Images 7.17b and 7.17c). When the cells retain a

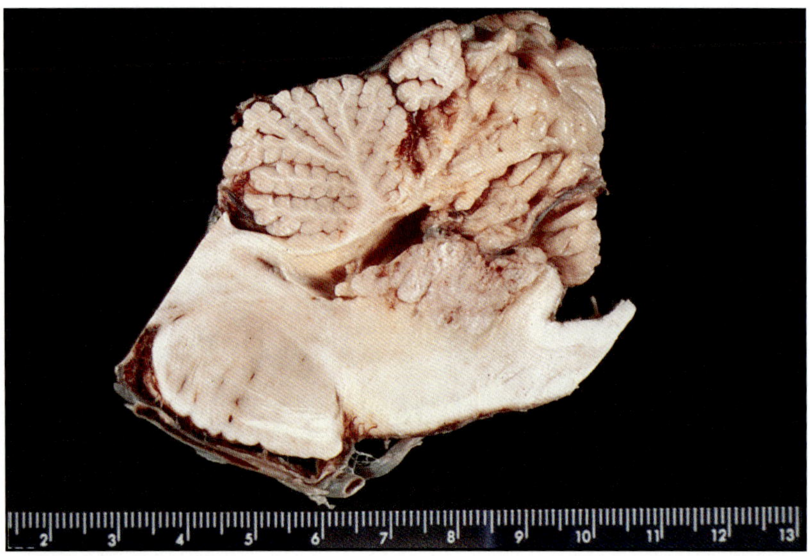

Figure 7.5
Midsagittal section through the cerebellum and brain stem reveals a granular friable mass in the floor of the fourth ventricle. This is a common site and gross appearance for an ependymoma.

columnar configuration they may be difficult to distinguish from metastatic adenocarcinoma (Image 7.17d).

Choroid Plexus Papilloma

The choroid plexus papilloma is a rare benign tumor found most commonly in the ventricles of small children (Figure 7.6). This lesion often produces hydrocephalus, because of both mechanical obstruction and an overproduction of CSF. Due to its location in the ventricular cavity and the friable nature of the tissue, it commonly exfoliates into CSF.

Choroid plexus papilloma commonly exfoliates into CSF

Histologically, this lesion resembles the papillary structures of normal choroid plexus. The chief distinguishing feature is abundance of tissue in excess of normal choroid plexus (Images 7.18a and 7.18b). Papillomas exfoliate as cohesive tissue fragments composed of regular cuboidal cells with round nuclei, often occurring in papillary fronds (Images 7.18c and 7.18d). These benign tissue fragments are indistinguishable from normal ependymal/choroidal cells. Since numerous fragments of normal choroid plexus may be seen in ventricular fluids from hydrocephalic children who do not have papillomas, final interpretation of these specimens may depend on the radiographic demonstration of the presence or absence of an intraventricular mass.

Malignant Choroid Plexus Papilloma

The malignant counterpart of the choroid plexus papilloma also occurs in the ventricles of children. It may be well differentiated and recognized only by its aggressive invasion of surrounding brain in histologic sections, or it may be anaplastic, as shown in Image 7.19. In an adult, this lesion could be confused with metastatic papillary adenocarcinoma. In a young child, adenocarcinoma is rare in CSF, and this cytologic presenta-

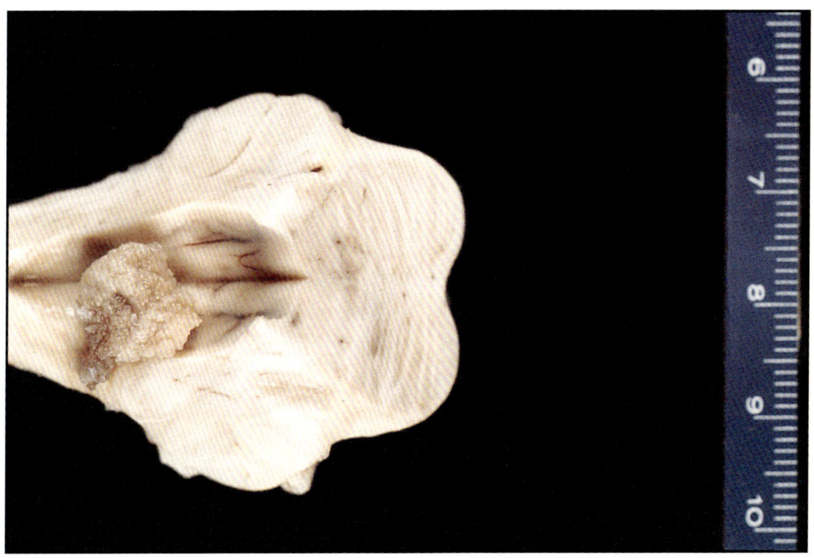

Figure 7.6
Grossly, this choroid plexus papilloma presents as a friable intraventricular mass and is often associated with hydrocephalus.

tion (Images 7.19d–7.19f), especially if a large ventricular lesion is present, is virtually diagnostic of malignant choroid plexus papilloma.

Tumors of Neuronal Origin

This group of tumors includes neuroblastomas, which are presumably derived from neuronal precursors, and neoplasms containing mature ganglion cells.

Neuroblastoma

Neuroblastoma is a primitive, small-cell, childhood tumor that may arise in the adrenal medulla or peripheral ganglia and involve the CNS secondarily with metastases. Less commonly, it may arise in the brain.[13] Histologically, it contains sheets of small anaplastic cells that may form rosettes (Image 7.20). By electron microscopy, neurosecretory granules and synaptic vesicles are seen, and these tumors express synaptophysin, neurofilament protein, and N-CAM immunohistochemically.[14,25] Cytologically, this tumor resembles other small-cell tumors of childhood (Image 7.20a). If rosettes or neurosecretory granules are demonstrated or if neuroectodermal antigens are expressed, leukemia, Ewing's sarcoma, and embryonal rhabdomyosarcoma can be excluded. Since retinoblastoma, medulloblastoma, and pineoblastoma can also exhibit these signs of neuronal differentiation, however, it is necessary to know the location of the primary tumor to distinguish among these tumors. If extra-CNS involvement is present, the lesion is probably a systemic neuroblastoma. Alternatively, a retinal lesion implies a retinoblastoma, a pineal lesion a pineoblastoma, and a cerebellar lesion a medulloblastoma. Primary CNS neuroblastomas generally arise in the cerebral hemispheres.

Ganglion Cell Tumors

The major type of primary CNS tumor that contains ganglion cells is the ganglioglioma. Since mature ganglion cells are incapable of division and are therefore benign, the biologic behavior of the lesion is dependent on the degree of malignancy of the glial component. Histologically, ganglion cells can be identified by their large size, round nuclei, and round macronucleoli. The most characteristic feature is basophilic cytoplasmic clumps known as Nissl substance, which is best demonstrated with cresyl fast violet stains. The most reliable evidence of their identity, however, is the demonstration of synapses by electron microscopy. Firpo and Watson[11] have demonstrated the cytologic appearance of two gangliogliomas in imprint preparations. Although abnormal cells were seen in the CSF from one of these patients, the presentation was nonspecific. Peripheral nervous system tumors that contain ganglion cells (ganglioneuromas) are usually benign. If a neuroblastic component is identified, however, the lesion will behave like a neuroblastoma and is called a ganglioneuroblastoma. It is important to recognize a ganglion cell component when evaluating cytologic and histologic preparations of central and peripheral nervous system tumors. Despite their alarming appearance, these cells

The biologic behavior of a ganglioglioma depends on the degree of malignancy of the glial component

behave in a benign fashion. Misinterpretation of the ganglion cells can lead to erroneous diagnoses of sarcoma in systemic ganglioneuromas and glioblastoma in gangliogliomas.

Medulloblastoma

Medulloblastoma is a highly malignant small-cell tumor that occurs in the cerebellum of children and young adults (Figure 7.7).[12] Lesions arising in the midline vermis have access to the fourth ventricle, whereas those occurring laterally in the cerebellar hemispheres may invade the SAS. This tumor commonly spreads in CSF.

Medulloblastoma commonly spreads in CSF

The prevailing concept concerning the histogenesis of medulloblastoma is that it arises from nests of primitive cells located in the posterior medullary velum or the external granular cell layer of the cerebellum. Whether this primitive cell is indeed a medulloblast (ie, capable of glial as well as neuronal differentiation) is a matter still being discussed and debated. Regardless of the histogenesis of this tumor, the term "medulloblastoma" is widely utilized for this small-cell anaplastic cerebellar tumor of childhood.

Histologically, this tumor presents as sheets of small anaplastic cells (Image 7.21a). Rosette formation may occur (Image 7.21b), and lesions that invade the meninges may stimulate a brisk fibroblastic response. Medulloblastoma presents in CSF as small, undifferentiated tumor cells shedding singly or in tissue fragments (Image 7.22). Although the nuclei are usually hyperchromatic with small nucleoli (Image 7.22), in occasional cases the chromatin is coarsely clumped and nucleoli are prominent (Image 7.23). When seen in histologic sections, these features may be associated with a poorer prognosis.[15] Immunohistochemically, these cells express markers of neuroectodermal derivation such as synaptophysin and N-CAM[18] (Image 7.24). Many of these tumors display evidence for neu-

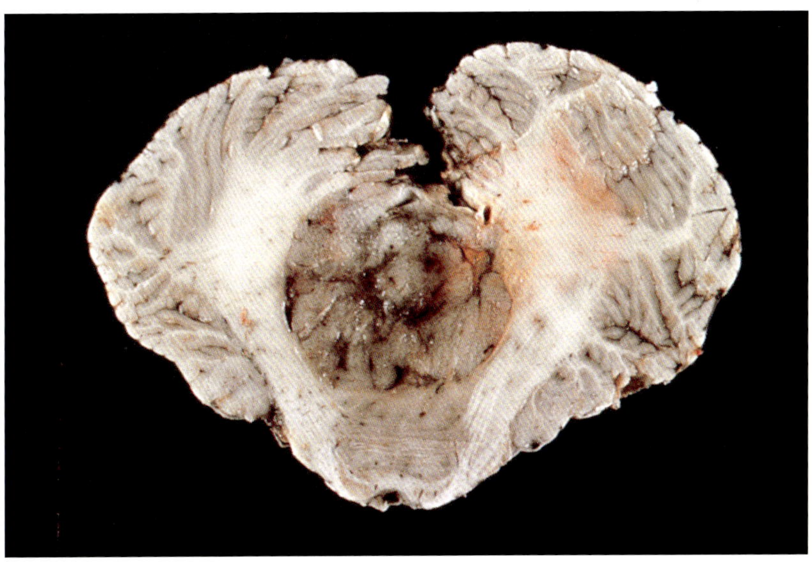

Figure 7.7
Grossly, the medulloblastoma is a solid mass arising in the cerebellum (Courtesy of Paul Kleihues, MD).

ronal differentiation with the expression of one or more of the neurofilament proteins. Although astrocytic differentiation has been described occasionally, these cases are difficult to evaluate due to the problem of distinguishing GFAP positivity in tumor cells from antigen expression in residual astrocytic elements in the underlying brain.

Medulloblastoma may spread early in cerebrospinal fluid, and an occasional patient presents initially with signs of meningeal irritation.[44] This clinical presentation mimics bacterial meningitis, but the correct interpretation can be made by cytologic examination of CSF. The majority of patients with medulloblastoma present initially with signs and symptoms of a cerebellar mass. Since the usual regimen of diagnostic procedures utilized for cerebellar masses includes ventriculography, CSF samples can easily be obtained without additional risk to the patient. Although medulloblastoma is cytologically and immunohistochemically indistinguishable from the other neurogenic small-cell tumors of childhood, a cerebellar mass distinguishes this lesion from retinoblastoma, pineoblastoma, and neuroblastoma. Childhood glioblastoma may exfoliate as small undifferentiated cells, but these tumors virtually never arise in the cerebellum. Fourth ventricular anaplastic ependymomas may, however, be clinically, cytologically, and histologically impossible to distinguish from medulloblastomas. Antibodies against GFAP are helpful in distinguishing medulloblastomas from glioblastomas and malignant ependymomas, since medulloblastoma does not express the large amounts of GFAP that are usually demonstrable in tumors of glial origin.

Medulloblastoma has a high incidence of CSF involvement in all reported series, ranging from 25% to 100%[4,6,17,28,33] (Table 7.2). The tendency for this tumor to disseminate in the subarachnoid space was appreciated in autopsy studies as early as 1925 by Bailey and Cushing,[1] and prophylactic whole neuraxis irradiation has been a part of the therapy for medulloblastoma since the early 1930s.[34] Medulloblastoma is also known to metastasize outside the central nervous system, although this phenomenon is uncommon. The most frequent sites for metastasis are lymph nodes and bones. Image 7.25 shows metastatic medulloblastoma in a fine needle aspirate from the iliacus muscle of a 2-year-old girl with a cerebellar medulloblastoma.

CSF can be used to document the primary diagnosis of medulloblastoma, and such examination is useful in the initial staging. For example, Harisiadis and Chang[20] showed that radiation therapy is generally effective in preventing subarachnoid seeding, but patients who present initially with CSF spread generally do not do as well. Furthermore, CSF cytology is useful in confirming recurrence, although most deaths are due to relapse in the posterior fossa, rather than meningeal spread.

Primitive Neuroectodermal Tumor and Peripheral Neuroepithelioma

Many primary brain tumors in children are composed of primitive embryonal cells

Although many anaplastic childhood brain tumors can readily be classified as medulloblastomas, cerebral neuroblastomas, or glioblastomas based on their location and histologic pattern, a significant proportion of primary brain tumors in children are composed of primitive embryonal cells with minimal evidence for differentiation or with differentiation along multiple histogenetic lines. In 1983, Rorke[37] introduced the term "primitive neuroectodermal tumor (PNET)" to deal with this confusing group of tumors, which can be qualified as showing neuronal or glial differentiation, or both. Although this term is useful when applied to embryonal neoplasms of uncertain or mixed differentiation occurring within the CNS, the designation PNET has been widely and inappropriately applied to virtually any type of anaplastic neuroectodermal tumor both within and outside the CNS. This terminology is particularly confusing when it is used to designate tumors for which more specific names already exist, such as medulloblastoma, neuroblastoma, and glioblastoma.

Primitive small-cell neoplasms showing variable levels of neuronal differentiation arising in the adrenal gland and in sympathetic ganglia are generally termed neuroblastomas. Small-cell childhood neoplasms of bone and soft tissue that lack neuronal differentiation have generally been referred to as Ewing's sarcoma and extraskeletal Ewing's sarcoma, respectively. Indeed, recent studies have shown cytogenetic and molecular genetic differences in these two groups of tumors. Neuroblastomas frequently show chromosome 1p deletions and double-minute chromosomes associated with amplification of the N-*myc* gene. Ewing's sarcomas, in contrast, lack these features and contain translocations between chromosomes 11 and 22. In addition, immunohistochemical studies have shown that Ewing's tumors express a surface protein, p30/32 MIC2, which is generally lacking in neuroblastomas.[14] Although the cell of origin of Ewing's sarcoma remains an enigma, these tumors seldom express neuronal markers or N-CAM, which makes the terms "peripheral neuroepithelioma" and PNET (which are sometimes applied to these tumors) confusing and of dubious value. It is even more inappropriate to apply the term PNET to neuroendocrine tumors arising in various organs in the adult.

With regard to systemic tumors, we prefer the terms neuroblastoma, Ewing's sarcoma, and neuroendocrine tumors in reference to the tumor types described above, and we avoid the terms PNET and peripheral neuroepithelioma. Within the CNS, we reserve the designation PNET for those rare primitive neoplasms of uncertain or mixed differentiation that usually arise in the supratentorial region of young infants, and we avoid applying the term to other well-defined intracranial neoplasms, such as medulloblastoma and glioblastoma.

Tumors Originating in the Pineal Gland

Cytologic techniques are useful for diagnosing tumors of the pineal area

The pineal gland is a small, midline body located just posterior to the third ventricle, overlying the brain stem (Figure 7.8). Lesions involving this structure often compress the cerebral aqueduct leading to enlargement of the lateral and third ventricles with midbrain compromise and resultant aberrations in eye movements. This set of clinical findings is specific for a pineal lesion. A variety of different neoplastic and non-neoplastic lesions can involve the pineal gland. Although they all produce similar symptoms, the histogenesis, prognosis, and treatment of these different lesions are variable. This variation in biologic behavior and the difficulty in approaching this region surgically make cytologic techniques particularly important for diagnosing tumors of the pineal area.

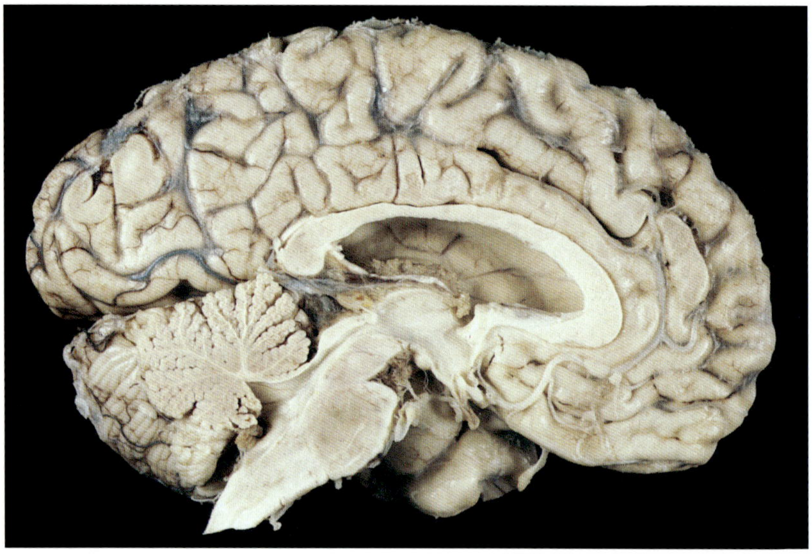

Figure 7.8
Midsagittal section of a brain shows the pineal gland located in the midline, posterior to the third ventricle.

Germ Cell Tumors

The entire spectrum of gonadal germ cell tumors that occur in other midline structures, such as the mediastinum and retroperitoneum, may also originate in the pineal gland. The pineal germinoma, which has been called atypical teratoma or pinealoma, comprises only 0.4% to 1% of all intracranial neoplasms but is the most common tumor to arise in the pineal gland, accounting for over 50% of neoplasms of the region.[9,40] In this location, it is usually restricted to adolescent males, but ectopic pinealomas occurring elsewhere in the midline, particularly around the third ventricle, may be seen in females as well. Grossly, it is usually solid and may be hemorrhagic (Figure 7.9). Microscopically, it contains the same monotonous population of polygonal cells with round nuclei and accompanying lymphocytes that are seen in germinomas arising elsewhere in the body (Image 7.26a). The cytologic presentation is a population of large cells with round nuclei and prominent nucleoli occurring singly or in loose clusters (Image 7.26b).[16,48] The accompanying lymphocytic population is nonspecific.

All histologic types of germ cell tumors may originate in the pineal gland

The other types of germ cell tumors (teratoma, choriocarcinoma, embryonal carcinoma, and endodermal sinus tumor) may also arise in the pineal gland. They occur alone or as mixtures of the different germ cell tumor types. Teratomas are frequently cystic, whereas necrosis and hemorrhage often occur in the more malignant varieties (Figure 7.10). Histologically and cytologically, these lesions are the same as when seen in the gonads.

Pineal Cell Origin

Two varieties of primary pineal cell tumors occur: the mature variant, a pineocytoma (pinealocytoma), and the more primitive type, a pineoblastoma (pinealoblastoma). Both are uncommon and together account for less than one fifth of the pineal region tumors. The pinealoblastoma usu-

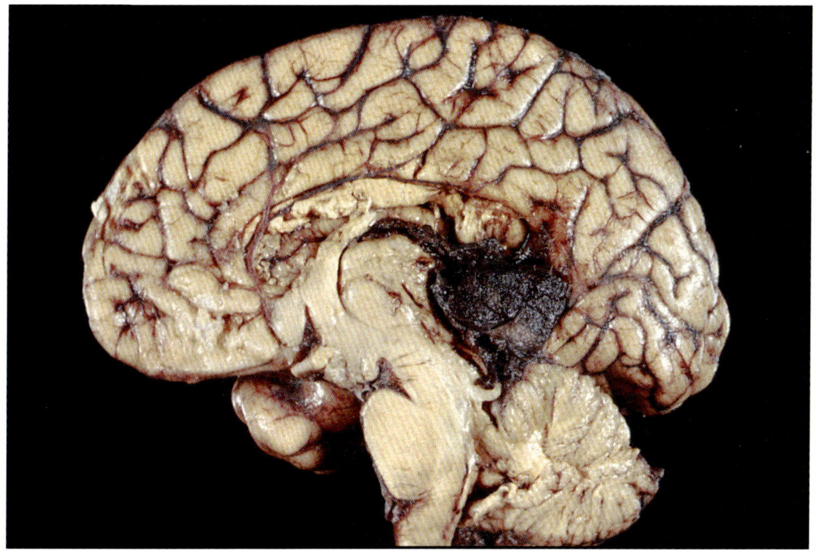

Figure 7.9
Grossly, the pineal germinoma forms a mass that is often hemorrhagic.

ally occurs during the first decade of life, while the pineocytoma has been seen in patients of various ages.

The pineocytoma retains the architecture of the normal pineal gland

The pineocytoma is a well-differentiated tumor that retains the architecture of the normal pineal gland. Rosette formation is common (Image 7.27a). The pineoblastoma is an anaplastic small-cell tumor similar to the medulloblastoma and neuroblastoma (Image 7.27b). It generally occurs in young children and frequently exfoliates into CSF as loose clusters (Image 7.28) or cohesive tissue fragments (Image 7.29) of small anaplastic cells.

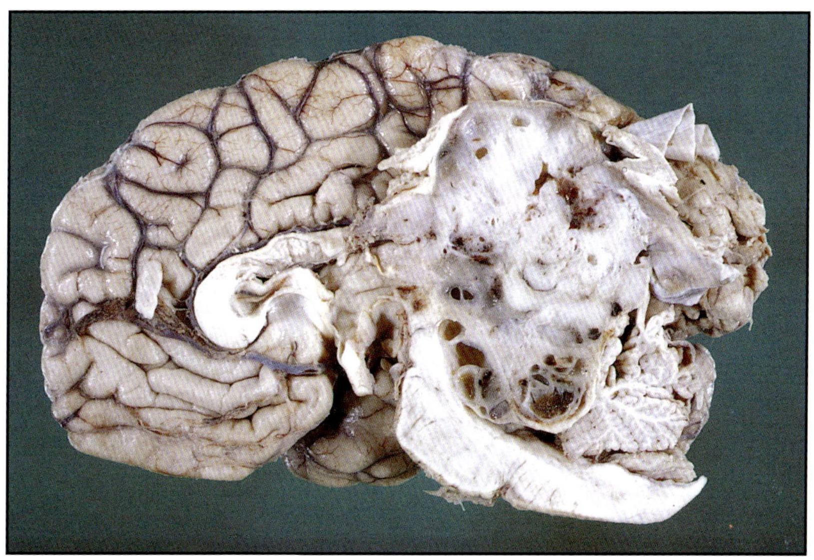

Figure 7.10
Midsagittal section of a large pineal mass in a boy. The mass proved to be a malignant teratoma with rhabdomyosarcomatous elements.

Glial Tumors

The astrocyte is a component of the normal pineal gland. Astrocytic tumors may involve this structure. Their morphology, both histologically and cytologically, is the same as when seen elsewhere in the central nervous system.

Non-neoplastic Lesions

A variety of non-neoplastic and cystic lesions may involve the pineal gland. Among these are arachnoid cysts, dermoid and epidermoid cysts, and vascular malformations. These are all relatively rare in this location, and reports of their morphology in cytologic preparations are incomplete.[48] Presumably, their presentation would be the same as that seen in other locations.

Tumors of the Pituitary Gland and Suprasellar Region

The suprasellar area of the brain may contain primary brain tumors such as astrocytic tumors, ependymomas, and oligodendrogliomas. Tumors arising from the meninges, such as meningioma and non-neoplastic berry aneurysms of the cerebral vessels, may also present as mass lesions in this area. In addition, the area above the sella, surrounding the third ventricle, is a favored site for the same spectrum of germ cell tumors as is seen in the pineal region.

Tumors arising in the meninges may also present as mass lesions in the suprasellar area

In children, one of the most common neoplasms of the suprasellar region is the craniopharyngioma (Figure 7.11). This is a frequently cystic, calcified lesion, presumably derived from Rathke's pouch. The lining

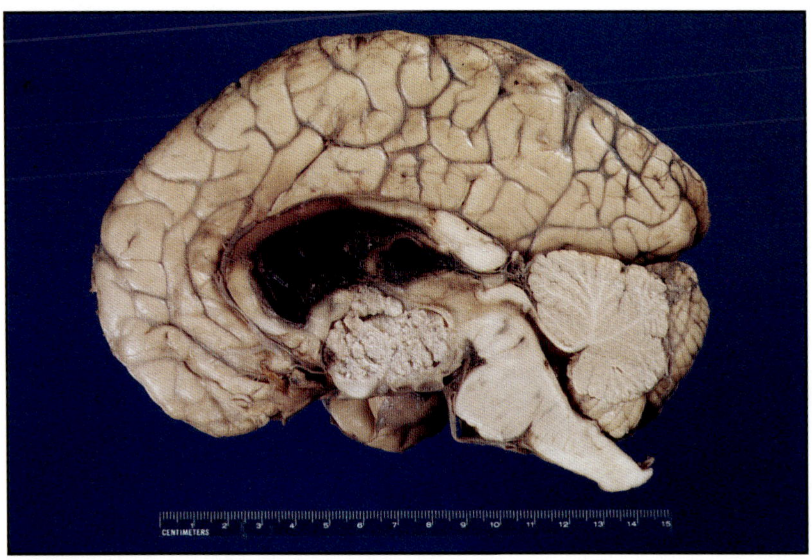

Figure 7.11
This brain section contains a friable granular mass in the suprasellar region that is a craniopharyngioma. Marked intraventricular hemorrhage is also noted.

may be predominantly benign squamous epithelium or sheets of basaloid adamantinomatous cells (Image 7.30). Cyst fluid aspirates contain cholesterol crystals, keratin debris, and benign squamous cells, but the basaloid epithelial component is necessary for a definite diagnosis, since the former features may also be seen in non-neoplastic epidermoid cysts.[48]

The specific identification of pituitary tumors depends on the hormone produced

Tumors arising in a pituitary fossa may expand upward to involve the suprasellar region. The most common of these lesions in adults is the pituitary adenoma (Figure 7.12). Any of the cell types of the adenohypophysis may become neoplastic, but their specific identification depends on the hormone(s) produced. This determination may be made by radioimmunoassay or immunohistochemistry. The different types are usually indistinguishable by light microscopy and cytology, and they are best lumped together as pituitary adenomas. They contain sheets of cuboidal or columnar cells that may form glandlike structures or a papillarylike pattern (Images 7.31 and 7.32). In imprints and needle aspirates, they appear as benign cuboidal or columnar cells (Image 7.31). The regular appearance and bland chromatin are useful in distinguishing them from metastatic well-differentiated adenocarcinoma, which may also involve the sellar area. These tumors are usually benign, but they occasionally spread in CSF. Image 7.32 shows cells from recurrent pituitary adenoma that spread in CSF.

Tumors of the Meninges, Nerve Sheath, and Other Surrounding Structures

The two most common tumors to present as extracerebral masses are meningioma and schwannomas. Rarely, metastatic tumors to the dura grow as discrete masses. Tumors involving the meninges less commonly are hemangioblastomas and hemangiopericytomas, which are discussed in the section on "Vascular Tumors and Malformations."

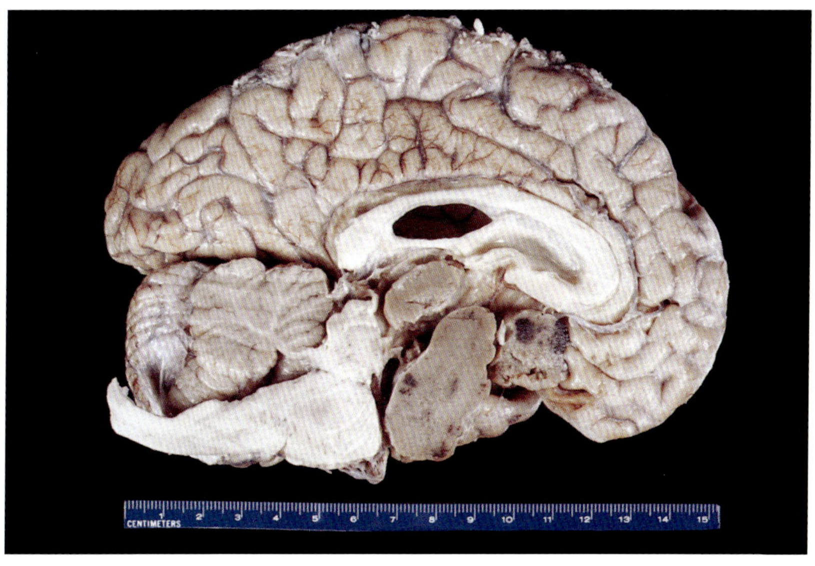

Figure 7.12
This brain section shows a large, brown, solid pituitary adenoma in the suprasellar region.

Meningiomas

Meningiomas are slowly growing, benign neoplasms, presumably derived from the arachnoid lining cell. They are most common in the parasagittal region, near the sylvian fissure, or at the base of the brain, particularly along the sphenoid ridge, the olfactory groove, or near the sella. Meningiomas also occur in the spinal canal, predominantly in the cervical region. They are more common in women than in men and usually occur in adults.

Grossly, meningiomas are round, firm, well-defined masses that are located outside the parenchyma of the brain and spinal cord (Figure 7.13). Histologically, they are composed of sheets and whorls of cells with bland, oval nuclei, and indistinct cytoplasmic borders (Image 7.33). Psammoma bodies are calcifications in the centers of these whorls. Meningiomas are common, comprising about 14% of all intracranial neoplasms. Few reports, however, have detected meningioma cells in CSF. The cohesive nature of these benign cells and their usual location outside of the SAS presumably prevent their shedding into CSF.

Few reports have detected meningioma cells in CSF

The cytologic morphology of meningiomas in imprint preparation is characterized by oval nuclei with delicate chromatin, which are seen within indistinct masses of cytoplasm. Cellular whorls and psammoma bodies are helpful diagnostic features (Image 7.34).

Although most all meningiomas are benign, occasional malignant variants occur, as manifested by aggressive invasion of underlying brain tissue or dissemination within the SAS. Ludwin and Conley[29] reviewed the literature in 1975 and found eight acceptable cases of meningeal spread of meningiomas.

Schwannoma

The schwannoma (neurinoma, neurolemmoma acoustic neuroma) is a benign tumor arising from the Schwann cell of cranial and peripheral

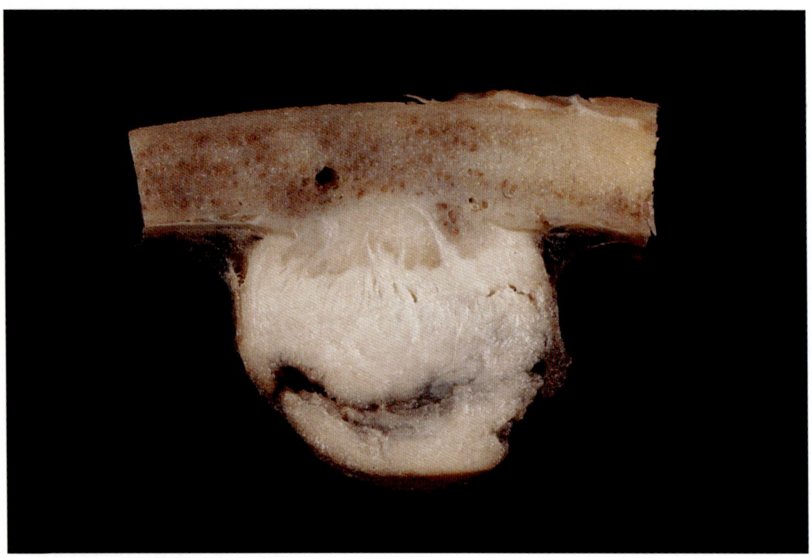

Figure 7.13
This meningioma is a discrete, firm, lobulated mass.

nerves. This tumor is commonly located where the nerve penetrates the pia of the brain and spinal cord. This tumor occurs most frequently in adults and has a marked predilection for sensory nerves, particularly the eighth or acoustic nerve. The next most frequent intracranial site is along the trigeminal or fifth nerve. This tumor is also found frequently in the spinal canal around the lumbar and sacral cord.

Histologically, schwannoma is composed of sheets and interlacing bundles of spindle-shaped cells with bland, elongated nuclei (Image 7.35a). Although these tumors may be cellular with nuclear pleomorphism and hyperchromasia, they lack frank malignant features and seldom, if ever, spread in CSF. Imprints are sparsely cellular, containing only a few spindle cells with nuclei that are more thin and elongated than the plump nuclei of meningiomas (Image 7.35b). Schwannomas lack whorls and psammoma bodies.

Neurocutaneous Melanosis

Neurocutaneous melanosis is a syndrome that usually presents in childhood and is characterized by multiple cutaneous nevi that may include giant hairy nevi and melanocytic proliferations in the meninges.[21,36,41] The meningeal component ranges from a pigmented meningeal infiltrate differing minimally from the melanocytic elements that normally populate the leptomeninges to aggressive proliferations of pigmented melanocytes that infiltrate the brain and fill the SAS and ventricular foramina producing hydrocephalus. Image 7.36 illustrates cells in the CSF from a patient who displayed the classic elements of neurocutaneous melanosis—cutaneous nevi and a melanocytic meningeal proliferation. In keeping with other examples of this syndrome, the cells are cytologically bland, resembling nevus cells more than anaplastic cells of melanoma. Diffuse filling of the SAS, however, leads to hydrocephalus and increased intracranial pressure. The differential diagnosis of this disorder includes metastatic malignant melanoma arising cutaneously or intracranially. Neurocutaneous melanosis generally presents in childhood, while melanoma is rare before puberty. Both the cutaneous and meningeal lesions often show benign cytologic features in the former disorder, while melanomas show more cellular anaplasia.

Melanin does not necessarily mean that a cell is melanocytic in origin

A number of other primary CNS neoplasms often contain melanin pigment, and many of them occur in childhood.[39] An unusual variant of medulloblastoma with papillary features and intracytoplasmic pigment has been reported in young children. The rare melanotic neuroectodermal tumor of infancy (also termed retinal anlage tumor or melanotic progonoma), which usually arises in bones of the jaw and head, may occasionally originate intracranially. These tumors can spread widely in the SAS but, unlike melanocytic proliferations, are composed of small anaplastic cells with scant cytoplasm. Rarely, more common tumors such as meningiomas, neurofibromas, ependymomas, and choroid plexus tumors may contain pigment.[39] Thus, the presence of melanin does not necessarily mean that a cell is melanocytic in origin, and overall cellular morphology, clinical presentation, and location of the tumor should always be considered.

Lesions of Non-neuroectodermal and Unknown Origin

Vascular Tumors and Malformations

Vascular malformations are common in the central nervous system. They include berry aneurysms that form a protrusion from the walls of the large cerebral vessels and arteriovenous malformations that usually occur within the brain or spinal cord parenchyma. Either type of lesion can give rise to sudden, severe, intracerebral or subarachnoid hemorrhage that may manifest in CSF as described in Chapter Four. Venous and capillary malformations are more likely to remain asymptomatic.

True vascular neoplasms are uncommon in CNS

True vascular neoplasms are uncommon in the CNS. The hemangiopericytoma may occur intracranially, most commonly attached to the dura. Grossly, it resembles a meningioma, although it is slightly softer to palpation. Histologically, this tumor is indistinguishable from hemangiopericytomas seen elsewhere in the body. It is composed of sheets of oval cells with intervening slitlike spaces (Image 7.37a). This tumor has not been described in CSF, but imprint preparations show sheets of cells with oval nuclei, delicate chromatin, small nucleoli, and indistinct cytoplasm (Image 7.37b).

Hemangioblastoma

The hemangioblastoma is a highly vascular tumor, occurring most commonly in the cerebellar hemispheres of adults. The second and third most frequent locations are the spinal cord and the meninges. It is generally considered a benign tumor, since total excision is curative. Grossly, it may be well defined, hemorrhagic, and partly cystic, or it may constitute only a small mural nodule in a large cystic space (Figure 7.14). Histologically, the cyst wall is composed of densely gliotic brain tissue that may contain Rosenthal fibers. The hemorrhagic nodule itself contains numerous blood vessels with intervening foamy stromal cells (Image 7.38a). It is undecided whether these stromal cells, the accompanying vascular cells, or the surrounding astrocytes are the active neoplastic elements. The cytologic presentation of this neoplasm has not been fully described. No reports have given specific features in CSF from these patients. Cyst fluid aspirates are also nonspecific. In imprint preparations, the stromal cells are polygonal with round regular nuclei and prominent nucleoli (Image 7.38b). Histologically and cytologically, this tumor may be indistinguishable from metastatic renal cell carcinoma. This problem is compounded because renal cell carcinoma may be associated with hemangioblastoma in the von Hippel-Lindau syndrome.

Primary Cerebral Lymphoma

Historically, considerable confusion has existed over the name and derivation of the primary brain lymphoma. This tumor has been variously called a microglioma or has been considered to represent a form of lymphoma, either primary reticulum cell sarcoma, primary histiocytic lymphoma, or immunoblastic sarcoma, according to the lymphoma nomenclature in vogue. The demonstration of surface immunoglobulin in most primary brain lymphomas[42] and the ready classification of these

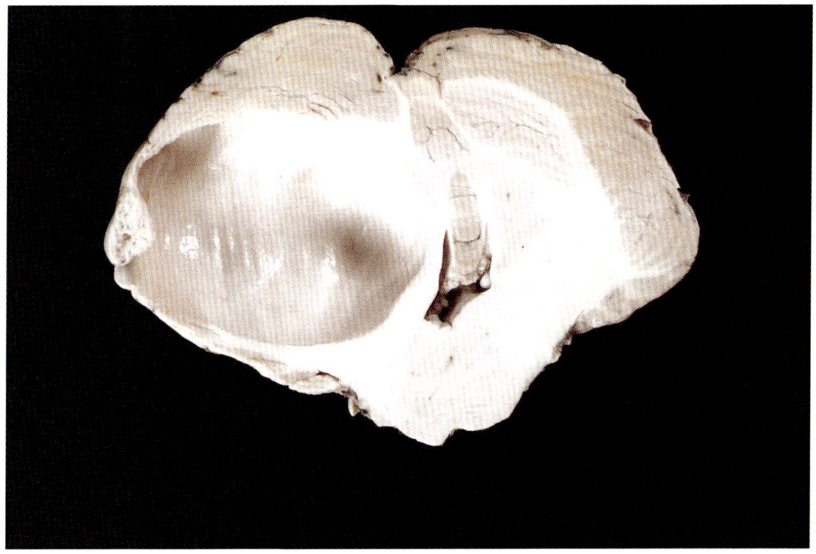

Figure 7.14
This cerebellar hemangioblastoma appears as a well-defined hemorrhagic nodule in the wall of a cyst in the cerebellum.

tumors by both the Rappaport[35] and Lukes/Collins[30] systems support the concept that these lesions are true lymphomas, analogous to those beginning elsewhere in the body.

Primary cerebral lymphoma occurs in the brain or spinal cord in the absence of systemic involvement with lymphoma

Regardless of the genesis and specific name, the primary lymphoma occurs in the brain or spinal cord of adults in the absence of systemic involvement with lymphoma.[22,24,32] Grossly, it is a poorly defined, somewhat granular lesion that may be multifocal. Histologically, it is composed of sheets of anaplastic cells similar to lymphomas seen elsewhere in the body (Image 7.39a). Many are bizarre with convoluted nuclei and are considered histiocytic lymphomas (Rappaport[35]) or large-cell lymphomas or immunoblastic sarcomas (Lukes and Collins[30]). Other types of follicular center cell lymphomas, including those with plasmacytoid features, have been seen as well. Most of these lesions are of B-cell derivation, but some of these lesions prove to be of T-cell origin. Histologically, the neoplastic cells characteristically encircle and invade blood vessel walls (Image 7.39b). In imprints and aspirates, this lesion shows single cells with scant cytoplasm similar to cells from systemic lymphoma (Images 7.39c and 7.39d). This tumor can be easily confused with anaplastic gliomas or metastases, and it should be considered in the differential diagnosis in all cases of anaplastic CNS lesions in adults. The correct classification of this tumor can easily be demonstrated by its reactivity with antileukocyte antibodies and its failure to express GFAP or carcinoma-related antigens. Image 7.40 shows cells of large-cell lymphoma in CSF from a 49-year-old woman with a primary cerebral lymphoma. Demonstration of a monoclonal B-cell population confirms that these cells represent meningeal dissemination of lymphoma.

Primary Cerebral Histiocytosis

In 1979, Wolfson[46] reported the CSF and autopsy findings in a 13-year-old girl with a diffuse proliferation of abnormal histiocytes that was restricted to the central nervous system. He termed this condition "cerebral histiocytosis." We have seen two cases bearing some resemblance to this patient. The first was a 50-year-old woman who presented with cranial and spinal nerve palsies. Atypical histiocytes with moderate amounts of cytoplasm were seen in her CSF specimen (Images 7.41a and 7.41b). At autopsy, her brain and subarachnoid space were infiltrated by massive numbers of similar cells (Images 7.41c and 7.41d), but no tumor was found outside the CNS. Whereas in the older terminology this would be considered a case of "microgliomatosis," the abundant cytoplasm of this population with malignant nuclei suggests that these cells may be "true histiocytes" or macrophages of reticuloendothelial, not lymphoid, origin. Perhaps this case would more properly be considered one of primary cerebral histiocytosis.

The second case was that of a 7-year-old girl who presented with symptoms of chronic meningitis. Her CSF contained numerous atypical histiocytes (Images 7.42a–7.42c). Arachnoid biopsy showed accumulations of similar cells (Image 7.42d) that were positive for lysozyme but contained no immunoglobulins. No organisms have been identified morphologically or by CSF culture, and she has no extra-CNS findings. She was considered to have a malignant histiocytic proliferation and was treated with intrathecal methotrexate and a ventriculoperitoneal shunt. She has continued to have atypical histiocytes in her CSF as of her most recent examination. Although the final diagnosis is not clearly established in this patient, the morphologic characteristics of her lesion and the histochemical aspects of her case suggest that this too is an instance of cerebral histiocytosis. Although these histiocytoses are uncommon, it is important to include this unusual category of lesions in the differential diagnosis when a CSF infiltrate contains atypical histiocytic cells.

Sarcomas

Historically, the term "sarcoma" has been applied to a variety of primary CNS tumors. In the early part of the 20th century, meningeal sarcomatosis was a term generally applied when any tumor spread in the subarachnoid space. In retrospect, most of these tumors were metastatic carcinomas, glioblastomas, or medulloblastomas.[2,8] In the 1940s, Kernohan and Uihlein[27] introduced the term "circumscribed arachnoidal sarcoma" to describe a desmoplastic lesion in the cerebellum of young adults. This term has produced widespread confusion because others, such as Willis,[45] considered the lesion a variant of medulloblastoma.

Primary CNS sarcomas include meningeal sarcomas, mixed tumors, and those occurring within the brain parenchyma

If these categories of "sarcoma" are excluded, true primary CNS sarcomas fall into three groups. The first consists of the meningeal sarcomas, which include malignant meningiomas as well as dural fibrosarcomas and are discussed in the section on "Tumors of the Meninges, Nerve Sheath, and Other Surrounding Structures." Due to their location and aggressive biologic nature, these tumors may spread in the SAS. The second group includes mixed tumors containing both a component of glioblastoma and sarcoma (Image 7.43). The sarcomatous component of these gliosarcomas is usually a fibrosarcoma. These tumors frequently invade the meninges directly and, therefore, have access to the SAS. In imprint preparations, a gliosarcoma can be suspected if clusters of anaplastic spindle cells are seen with more typical anaplastic glia. A definite cytologic

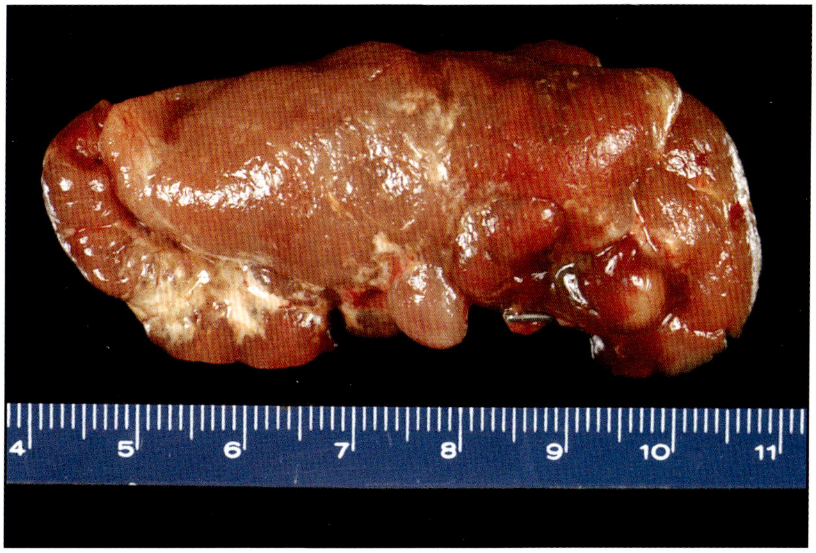

Figure 7.15
This well-circumscribed, fleshy, intracerebral neoplasm is the typical presentation of a primary sarcoma.

diagnosis of this lesion should be made cautiously, however, as any anaplastic glioma that reaches the subarachnoid space generally elicits a proliferation of benign fibroblasts. In addition, anaplastic glia may assume a bipolar configuration and mimic sarcoma. The third group of CNS sarcomas occurs within the brain parenchyma. They are most frequently primary cerebral fibrosarcomas, although primary cerebral and cerebellar rhabdomyosarcomas have been reported as well. These tumors are relatively discrete fleshy lesions (Figure 7.15), which are histologically and cytologically the same as when seen elsewhere in the body (Image 7.44). Although relatively rare, primary sarcomas are actually more common than sarcomas metastatic to the CNS.

Most cases of primary meningeal sarcomatosis probably represent meningeal spread of medulloblastomas as suggested by Willis.[45] Hajdu[19] presented a case with similar morphologic and clinical presentation in which glial differentiation was proven immunohistochemically by demonstrating intracellular GFAP. These findings suggest that cases termed "primary meningeal sarcomatosis" may actually represent a heterogeneous group of tumors of diverse origin, including primitive embryonal neoplasms discussed previously as "PNETs" as well as more typical medulloblastomas.

a b

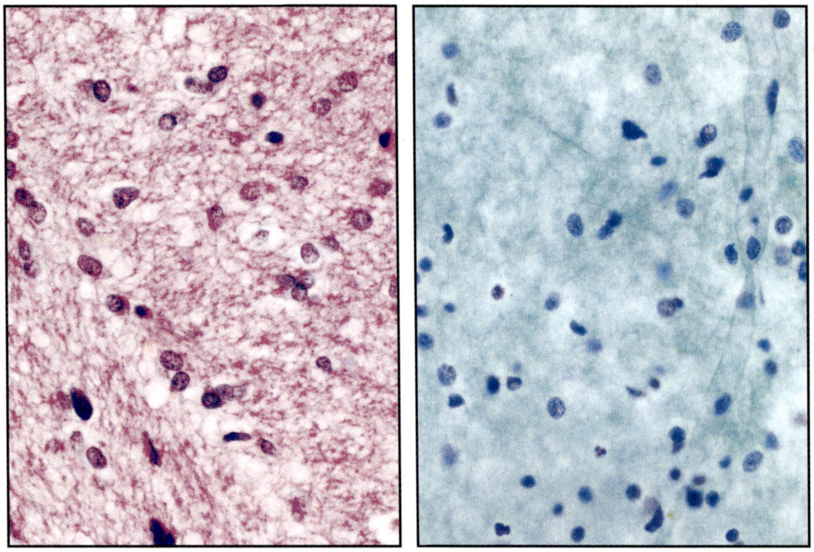

Image 7.1
Hypercellularity is the main feature of this low-grade astrocytoma (a, H&E, 400X; b, Papanicolaou, 400X).

a b

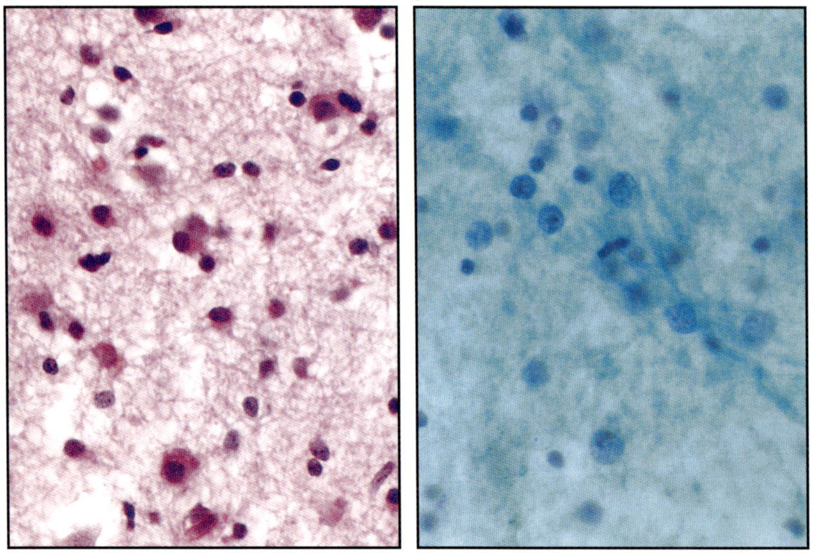

Image 7.2
Histologically, gliotic brain tissue contains an increased number of astrocytes, many of which have abundant cytoplasm (a). Imprint preparations reveal the same features (b) (a, H&E, 400X; b, Papanicolaou, 400X).

a b

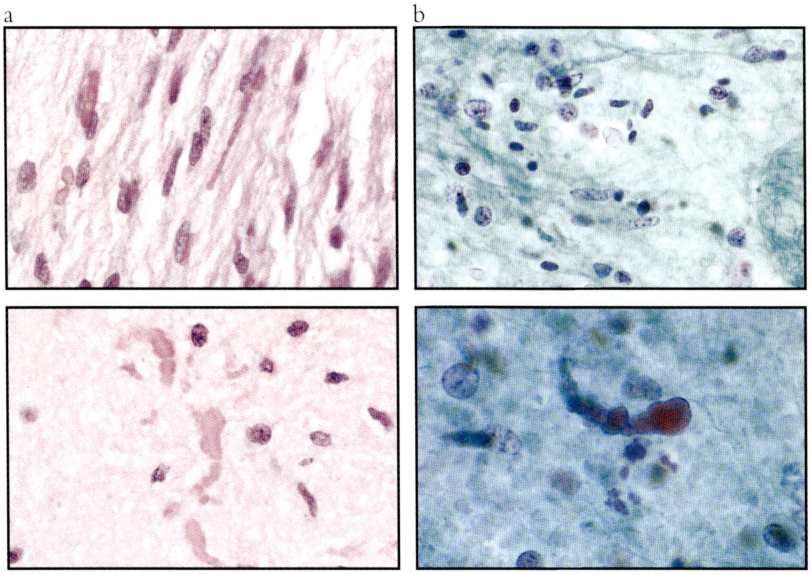

c d

Image 7.3
Bipolar astrocytes of the piloid astrocytoma (a and b). Amorphous, waxy elongated bodies called Rosenthal fibers are characteristic of this tumor (c and d) (a, H&E, 400X; b, Papanicolaou, 400X; c, H&E, 1,000X; d, Papanicolaou, 600X).

a b

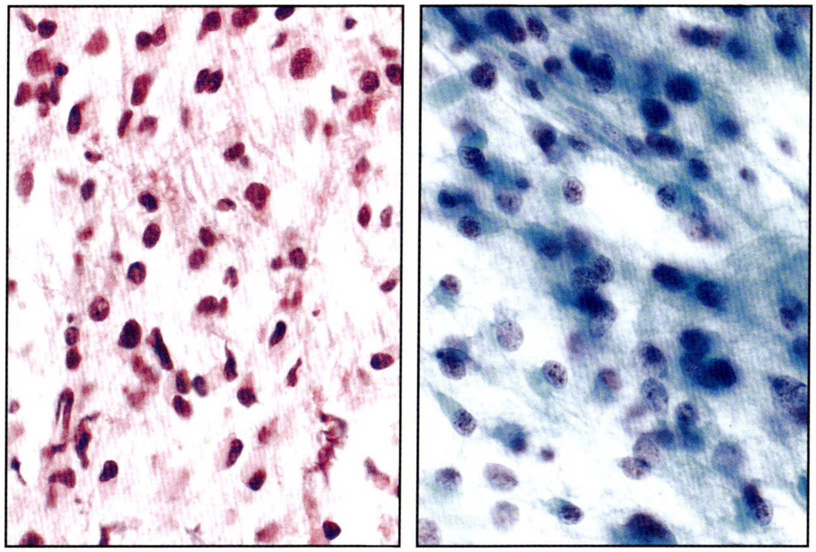

Image 7.4
Histologically, the anaplastic astrocytoma shows intense hypercellularity, nuclear hyperchromasia and irregularity, and a fibrillary background (a). The same features are apparent in imprint preparations (b) (a, H&E, 400X; b, Papanicolaou, 400X).

a b

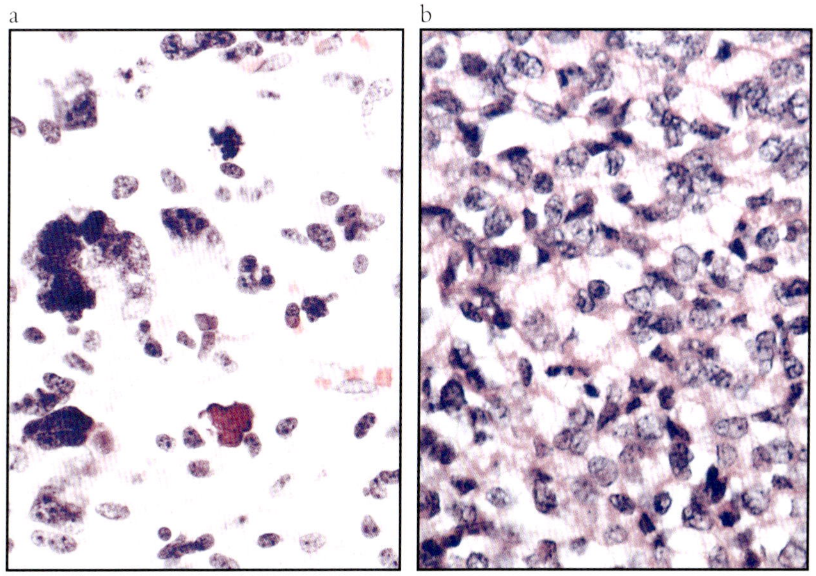

Image 7.5
The cells of this highly cellular neoplasm of glioblastoma multiforme may be pleomorphic with multinucleated giant cells (a). Sheets of anaplastic cells are also often present (b) (both, H&E, 400X).

c d

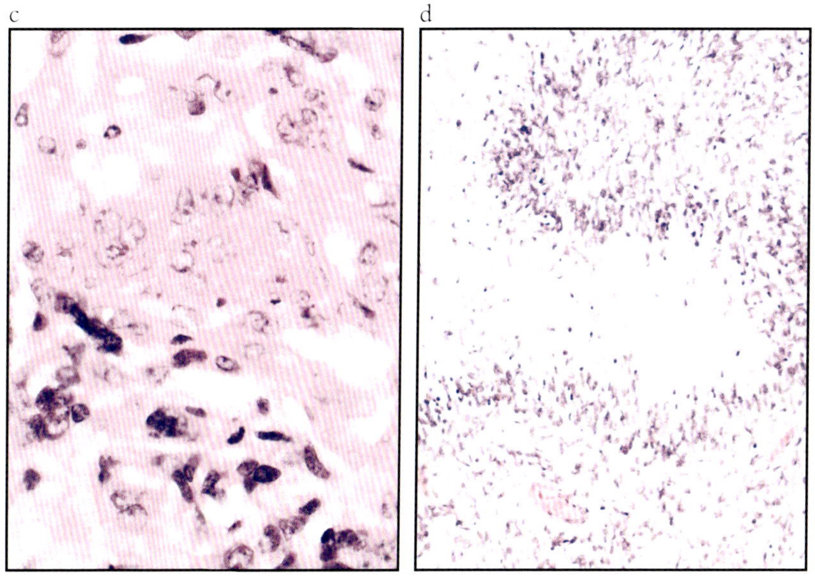

Plump endothelial cells form glomeruloid structures called endothelial proliferations (c). This neoplasm typically contains serpentine areas of necrosis lined by pseudopalisading (d) (both, H&E; c, 400X; d, 200X).

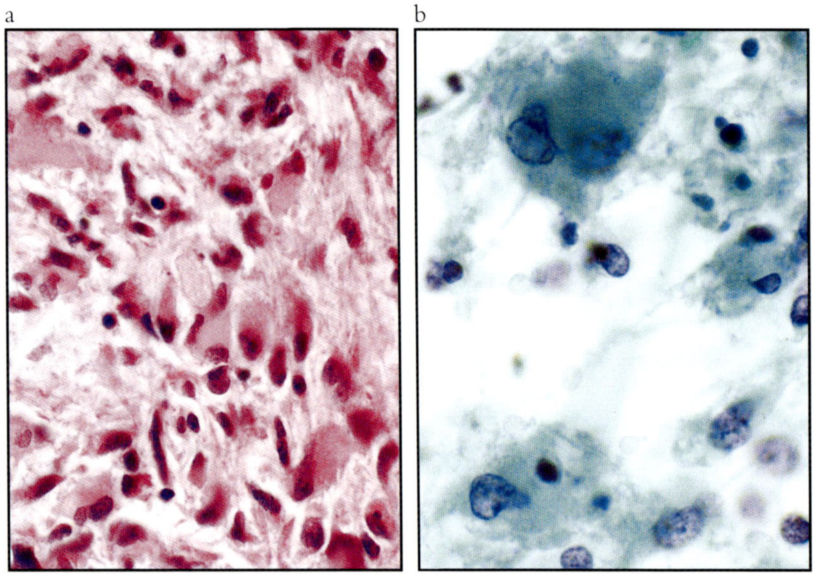

Image 7.6
This glioblastoma contains a mixed population of fibrillary, protoplasmic, and gemistocytic astrocytes (a and b) (a, H&E, 400X; b, Papanicolaou, 600X).

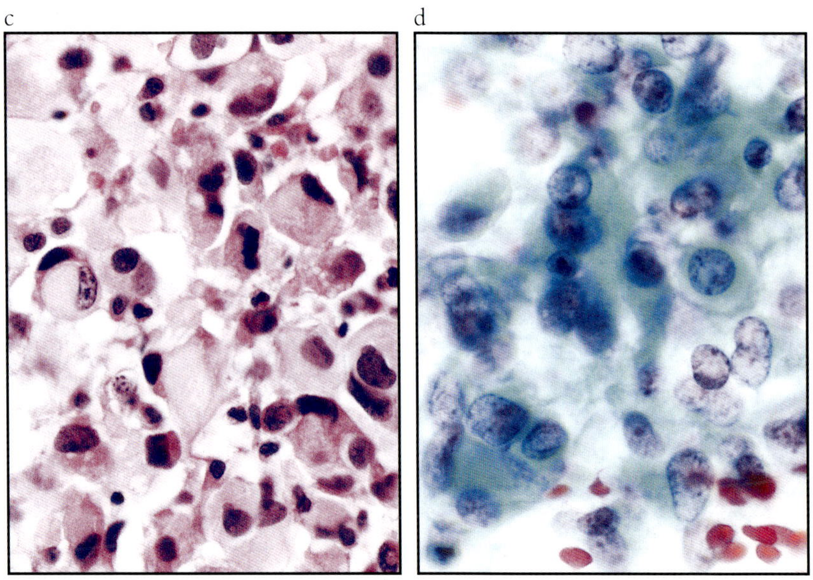

This glioblastoma consists mainly of pleomorphic gemistocytic astrocytes (c and d) (c, H&E, 400X; d, Papanicolaou, 600X).

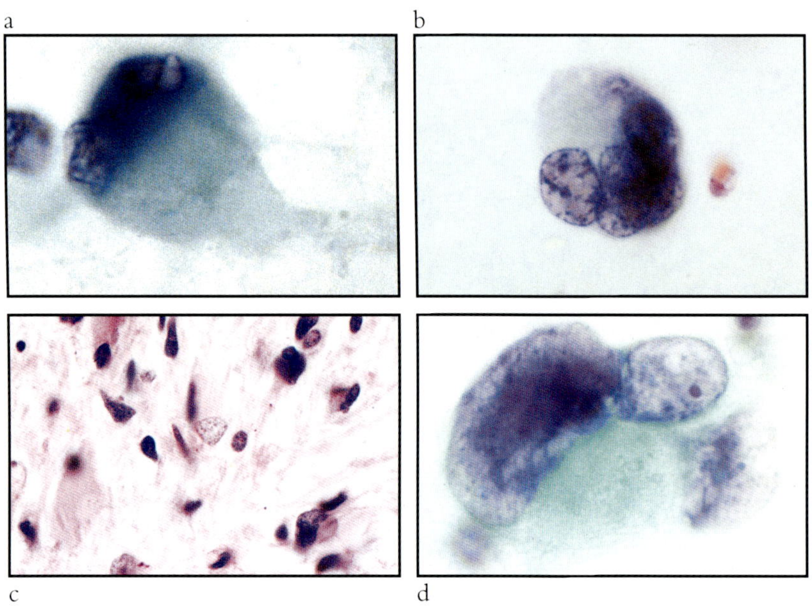

Image 7.7
The cytologic presentation of glioblastoma in CSF is dependent on which cells reach the subarachnoid space. Tumor cells in the CSF of a patient with a pontine glioblastoma represent a variety of cell types ranging from gemistocytes with distinct cell borders (a) to multinucleated giant cells (b and d). Tumor cells are shown in histologic sections from this patient's glioblastoma (c) (a, b, and d, Papanicolaou, 1,000X; c, H&E, 400X).

In addition to the pleomorphic cell types seen in CSF in the histologic section, a population of small undifferentiated cells are represented both histologically (e) and cytologically (f) (e, H&E, 400X; f, Papanicolaou, 1,000X).

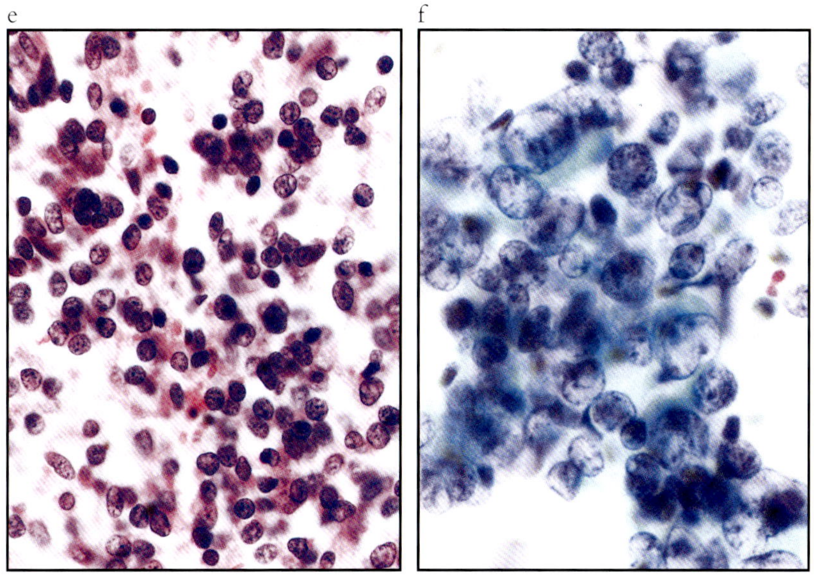

Image 7.8
Small anaplastic cells in the CSF of a 5-year-old girl with a pontine glioblastoma (a). Strong glial fibrillary acid protein (GFAP) positivity confirms the glial origin of these cells (b) (a, Papanicolaou, 1,000X; b, Immunoperoxidase, 1,000X).

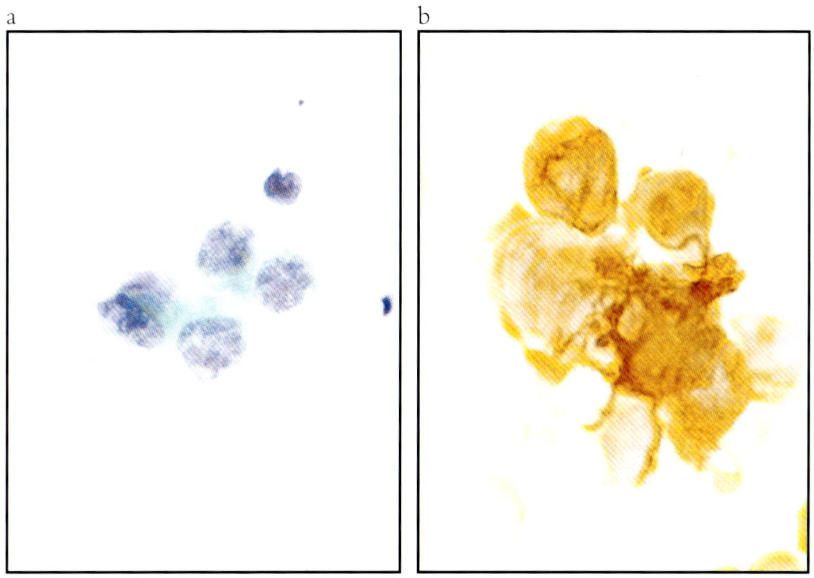

Image 7.9
Anaplastic cells in CSF of an 18-year-old woman with ascending paralysis show primary meningeal gliomatosis (Papanicolaou, 1,000X).

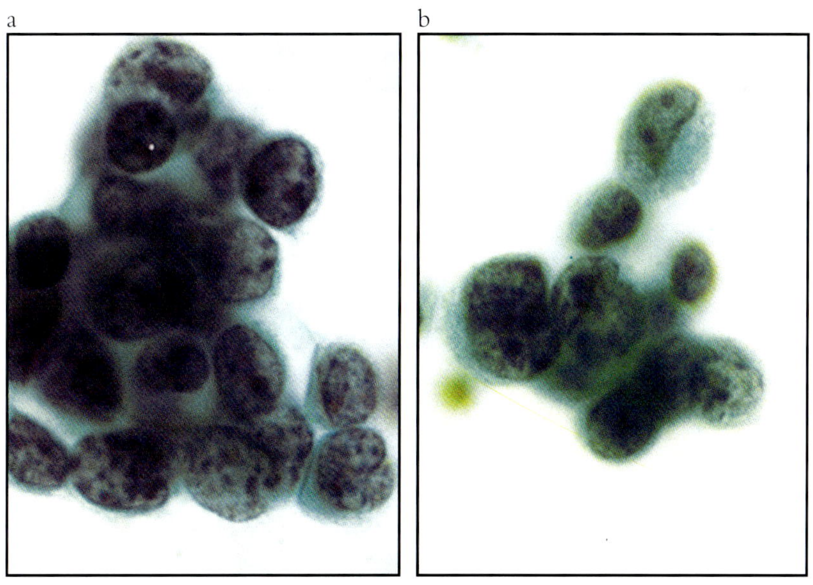

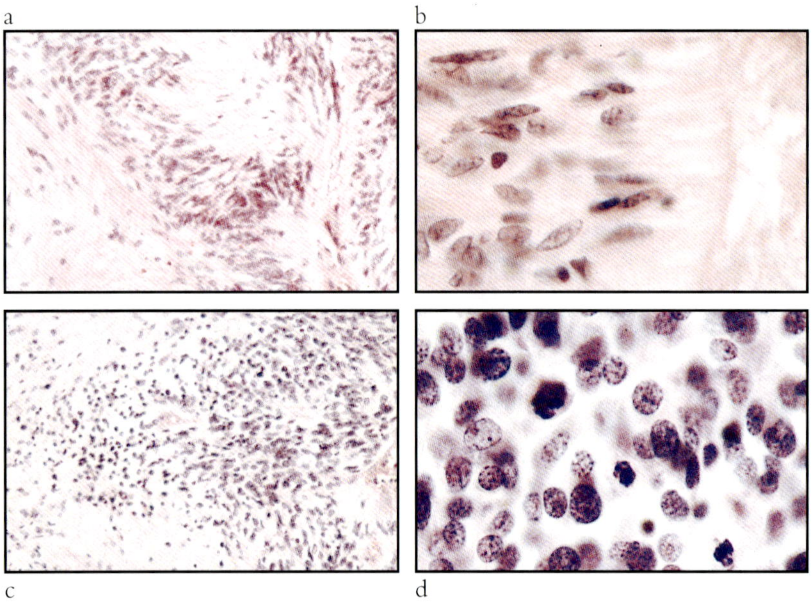

Image 7.10
The neoplastic process of the patient described in Image 7.9 and Figure 7.3 probably began in this glial heterotopia (a and b). In these regions (c and d), undifferentiated elements similar to those seen in the patient's CSF were noted (all, H&E; a, 100X; b, 400X; c, 100X; d, 400X).

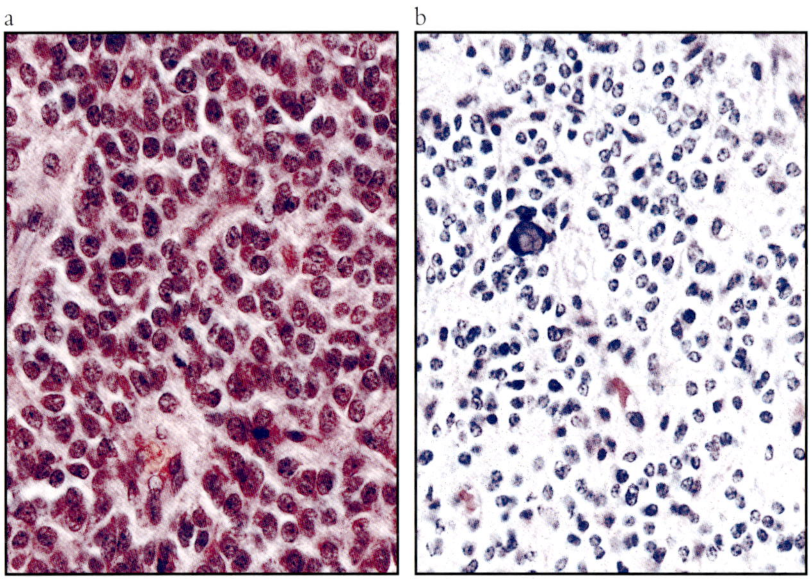

Image 7.11
This oligodendroglioma is composed of sheets of cells with a delicate fibrovascular stroma. On high-power magnification, the round, uniform nuclei and indistinct cytoplasmic borders that are characteristic of this tumor type are apparent (a). Frequently, in paraffin-embedded sections, tumor cells show perinuclear halos that are probably artifacts (b). Focal calcification is frequent (a, H&E, 400X; b, H&E, 250X).

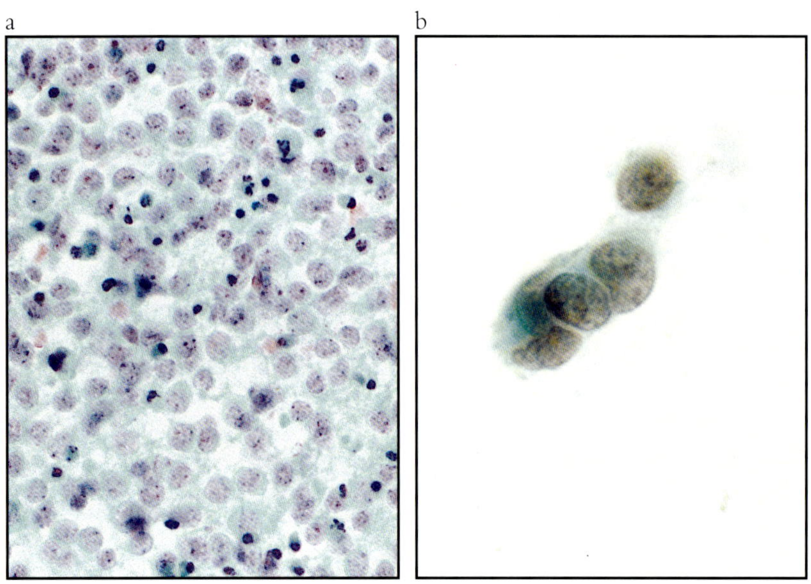

Image 7.12
This imprint of an oligodendroglioma shows uniform cells with round nuclei, delicate chromatin, visible nucleoli, and indistinct cytoplasm (a). Small, undifferentiated malignant cells are from a tumor washing of an anaplastic oligodendroglioma (b) (a, Papanicolaou, 400X; b, Papanicolaou, 1,000X).

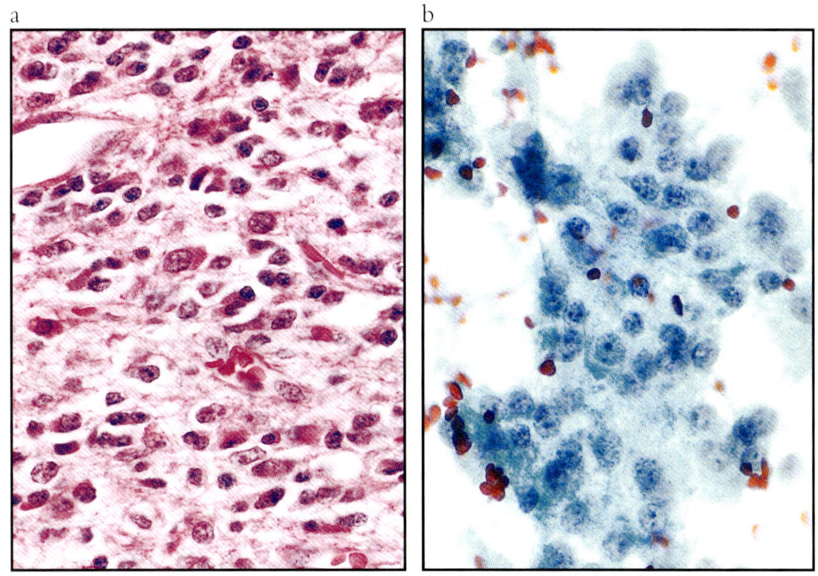

Image 7.13
This mixed glioma contains astrocytes in addition to neoplastic oligodendroglia (a, H&E, 400X; b, Papanicolaou, 400X).

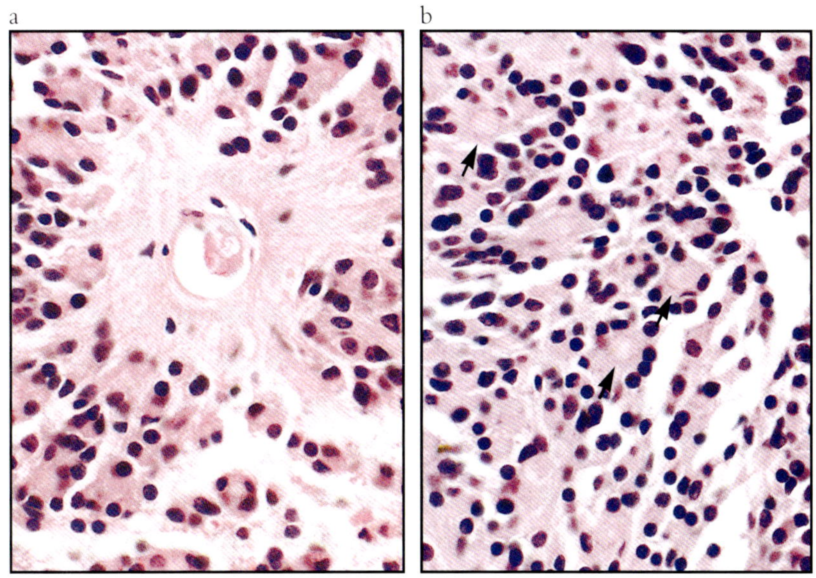

Image 7.14
Ependymomas are composed of small cuboidal to columnar cells with fibrillary processes forming perivascular pseudorosettes (a). Occasional true rosettes with hollow centers are seen as well (arrows) (b) (both, H&E, 400X).

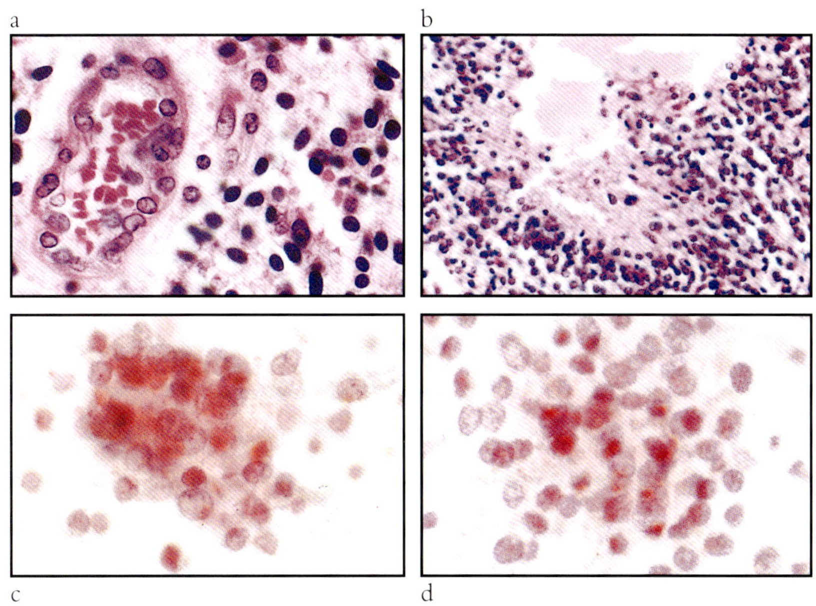

Image 7.15
These sections show an ependymoma from the roof of the fourth ventricle of a 26-year-old man. The lesion had some anaplastic features such as hypercellularity (a) and focal necrosis (b). Cells in a sample of CSF were obtained at autopsy from this patient (c and d). Although some degree of cytoplasmic degeneration is present, the bland, oval nuclei characteristic of ependymal tumors are apparent (a and b, H&E, 200X; c and d, Papanicolaou, 600X).

a b

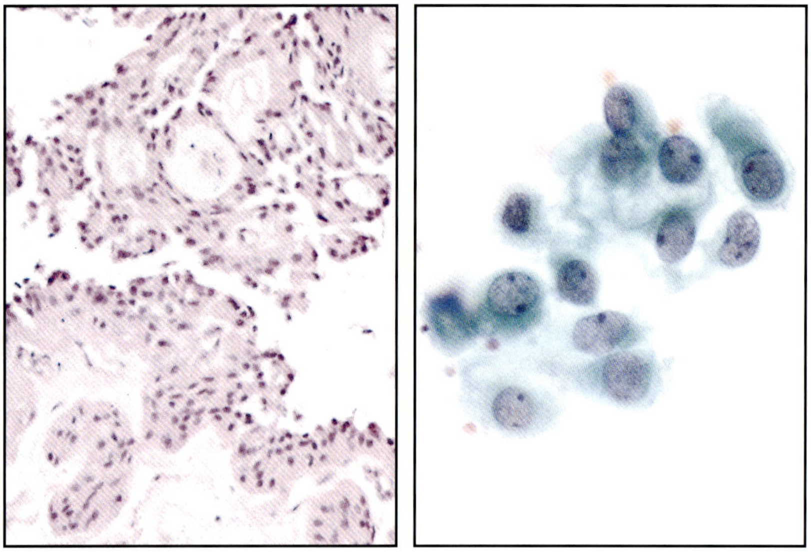

Image 7.16
This section shows the papillary formations and myxoid stroma that are typical of myxopapillary ependymomas (a). This lesion was excised from the filum terminale of a 21-year-old woman. Imprints of this lesion show typical ependymal cells with bland, oval nuclei and a columnar shape (b) (a, H&E, 200X; b, Papanicolaou, 600X).

a b

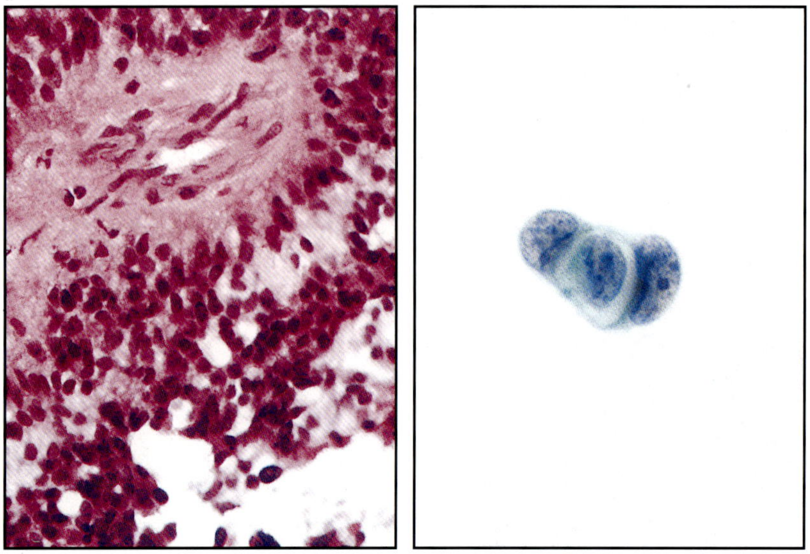

Image 7.17
Anaplastic ependymoma showing sheets of densely packed cells and perivascular pseudorosettes (a). This lesion shed in CSF as tight clusters of small cells with scant cytoplasm (b) (a, H&E, 250X; b, Papanicolaou, 1,000X).

c d

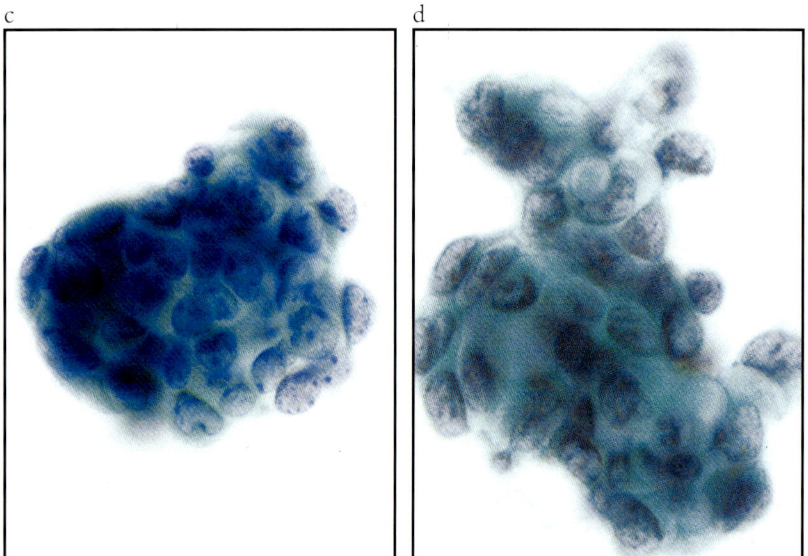

This lesion shed in CSF as tight clusters of small cells with scant cytoplasm (c) or with more columnar-shaped cells (d) (both, Papanicolaou, 1,000X).

Image 7.18
Histologically, the choroid plexus papilloma is composed of abundant benign papillary fronds (a and b) (a, H&E, 200X; b, H&E, 400X).

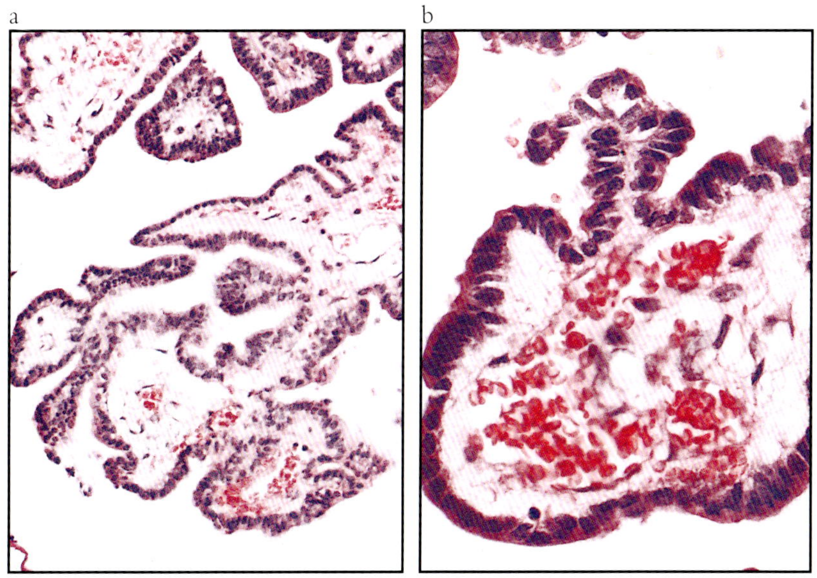

When these papillary fragments shed in CSF, the benign nuclei are readily apparent (c and d) (c, Papanicolaou, 600X; d, Papanicolaou, 1,000X).

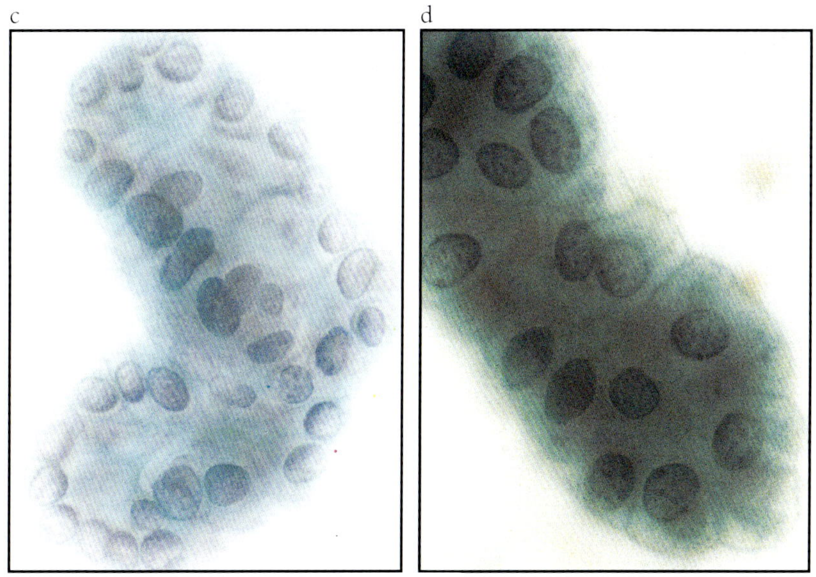

Image 7.19
Malignant choroid plexus papilloma. Histologically, this lesion contains papillary fronds lined by anaplastic cells (a and b) (both, H&E; a, 200X; b, 400X).

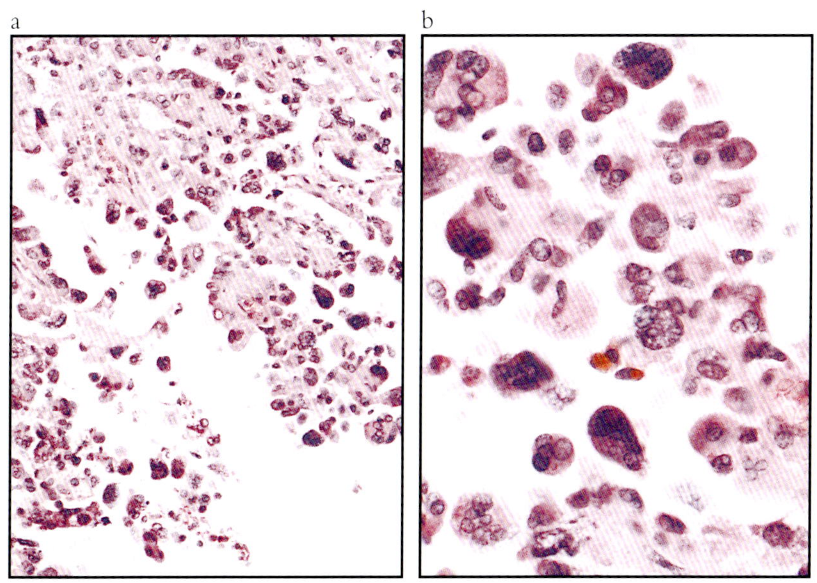

c d

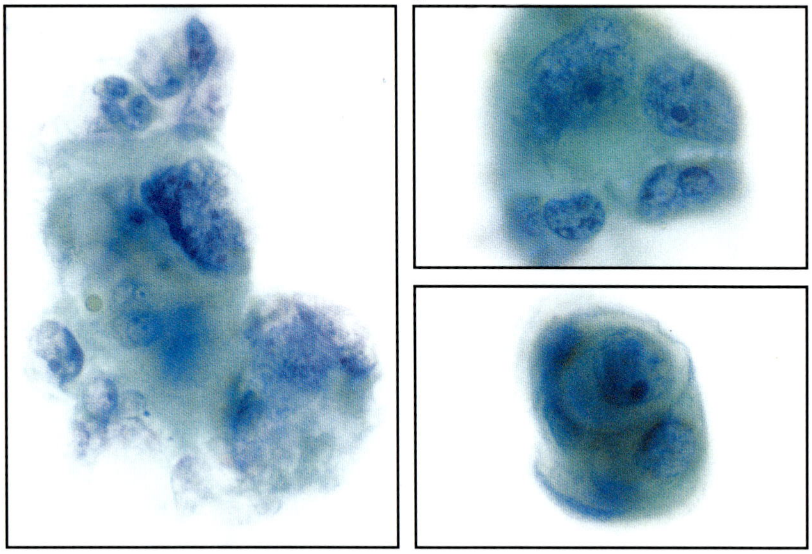

e

This lesion sheds as fragments of malignant cells into CSF (c through e) (all, Papanicolaou, 1,000X).

a b

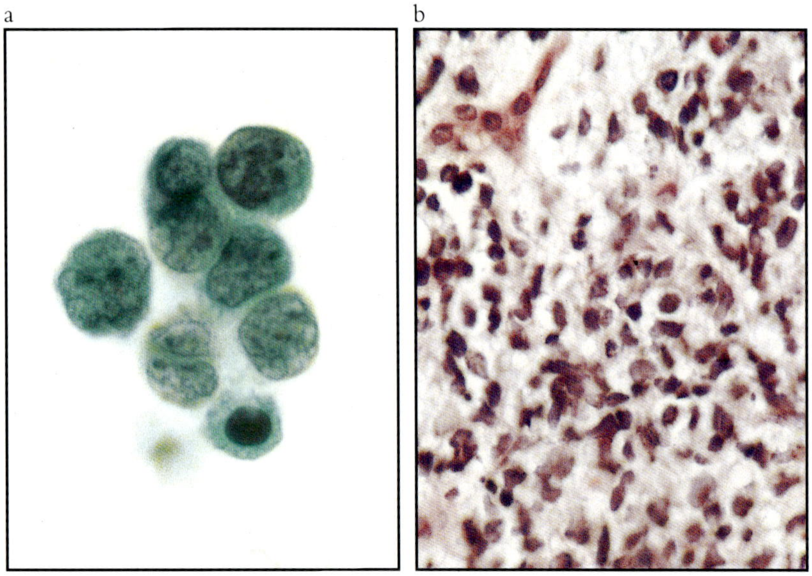

Image 7.20
Small anaplastic cells in CSF of a child with an abdominal neuroblastoma (a). Metastatic neuroblastoma in the liver of the same patient (b) (a, Papanicolaou, 1,000X; b, H&E, 400X).

a b

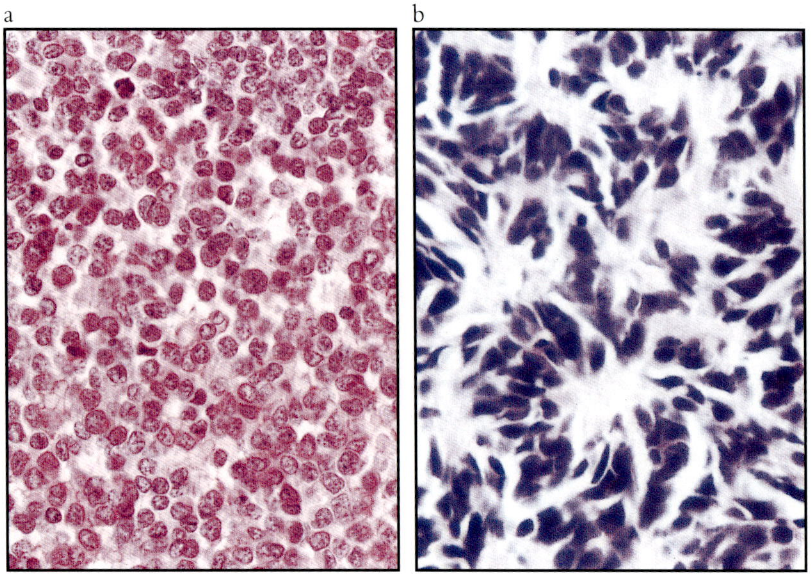

Image 7.21
The medulloblastoma in this histologic section is composed of sheets of anaplastic cells (a). Occasionally, Homer-Wright rosettes are seen in these tumors (b) (both, H&E, 400X).

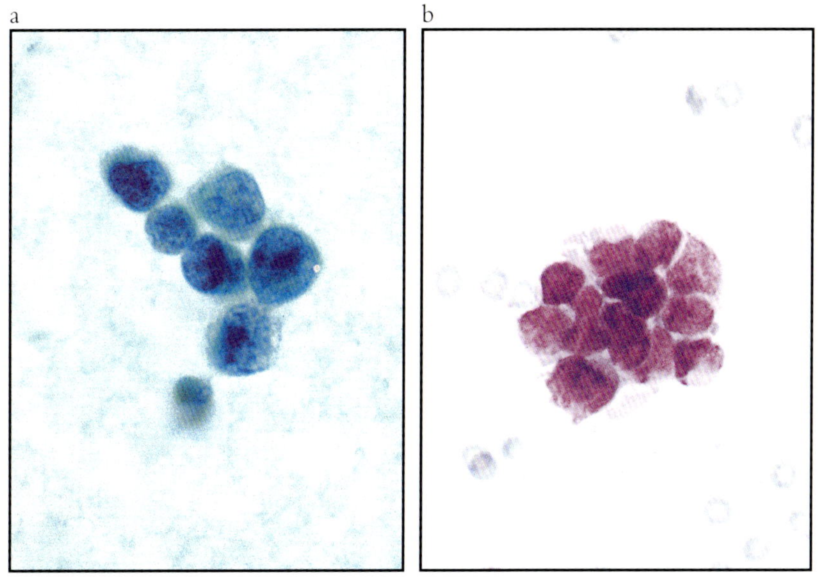

Image 7.22
Medulloblastomas typically present in CSF as small cells with hyperchromatic nuclei and high nuclear/cytoplasmic ratios occurring in loose clusters (a) or in tissue fragments with nuclear molding (b) (a, Papanicolaou, 1,000X; b, Romanowski, 600X).

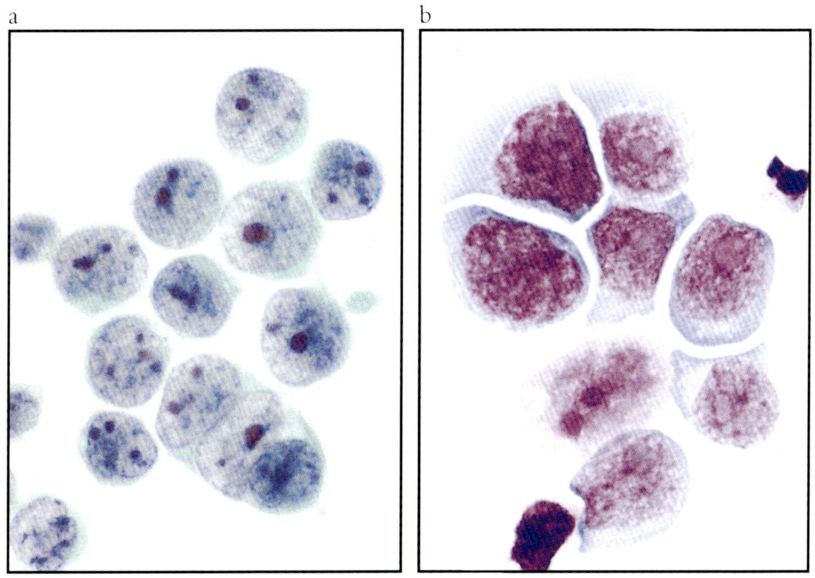

Image 7.23
When cells of medulloblastoma shed in CSF, they occasionally display coarse chromatin and prominent nucleoli. Although these features may signify a poor prognosis, their prognostic significance in CSF has not been demonstrated (a, Papanicolaou, 1,000X; b, Romanowski, 600X).

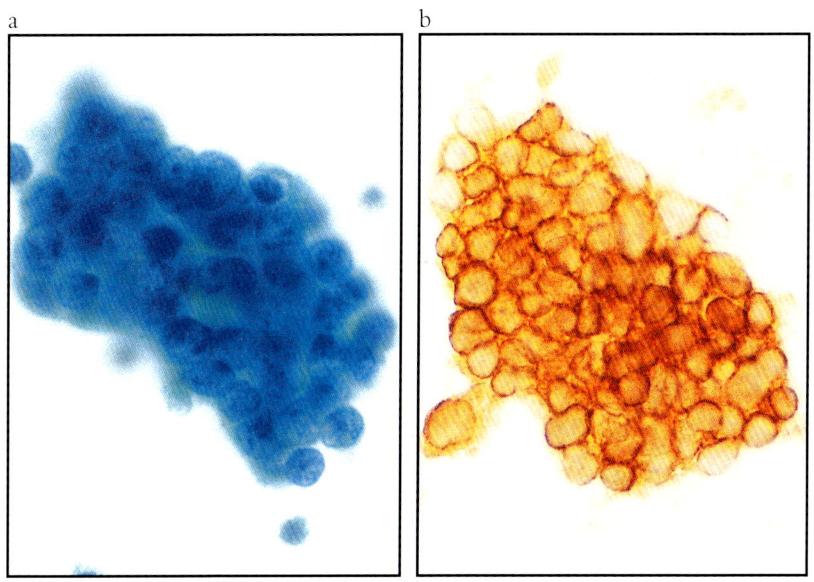

Image 7.24
Medulloblastomas usually express neural cell adhesion molecule (N-CAM) (a, Papanicolaou, 1,000X; b, Immunohistochemistry for N-CAM, 600X).

a b

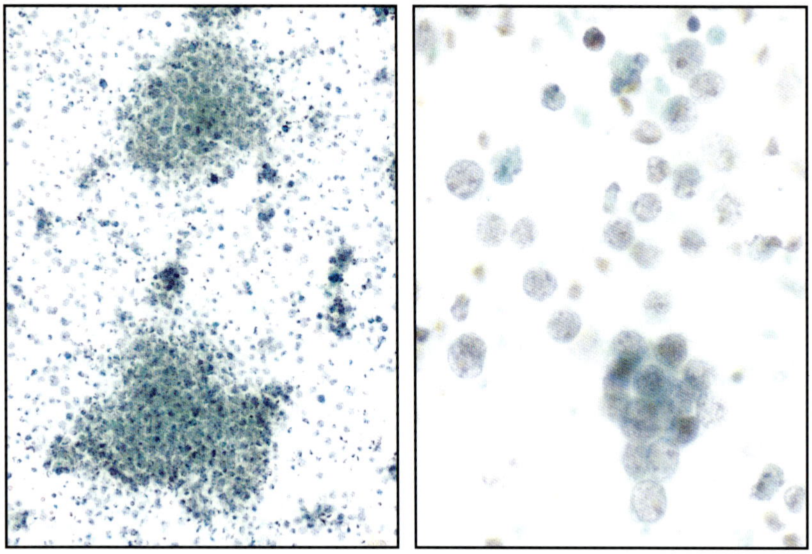

Image 7.25
Small anaplastic cells consistent with metastatic medulloblastoma in a fine needle aspirate from the iliacus muscle of a 2-year-old girl with cerebellar medulloblastoma (both, Papanicolaou; a, 200X; b, 600X).

a b

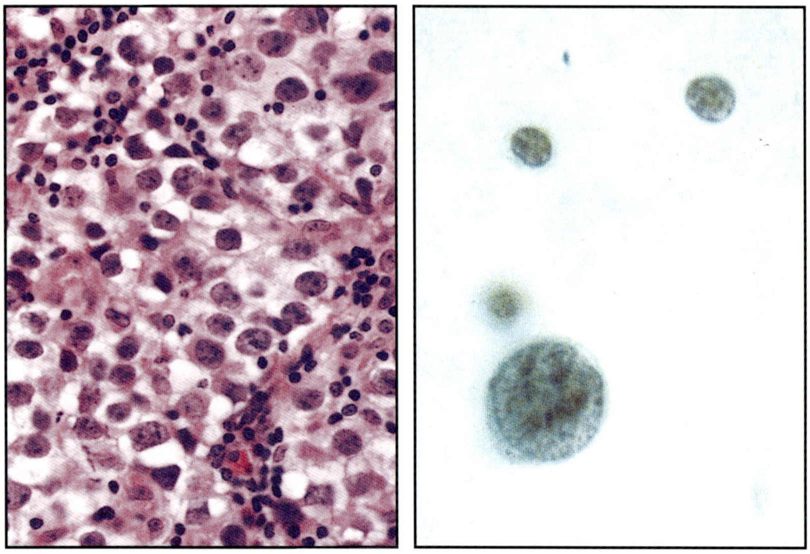

Image 7.26
The pineal germinoma contains two populations: polygonal cells with prominent nucleoli and small mature lymphocytes (a). Single cell from a pineal germinoma in CSF (b) (a, H&E, 400X; b, Papanicolaou, 1,000X).

a b

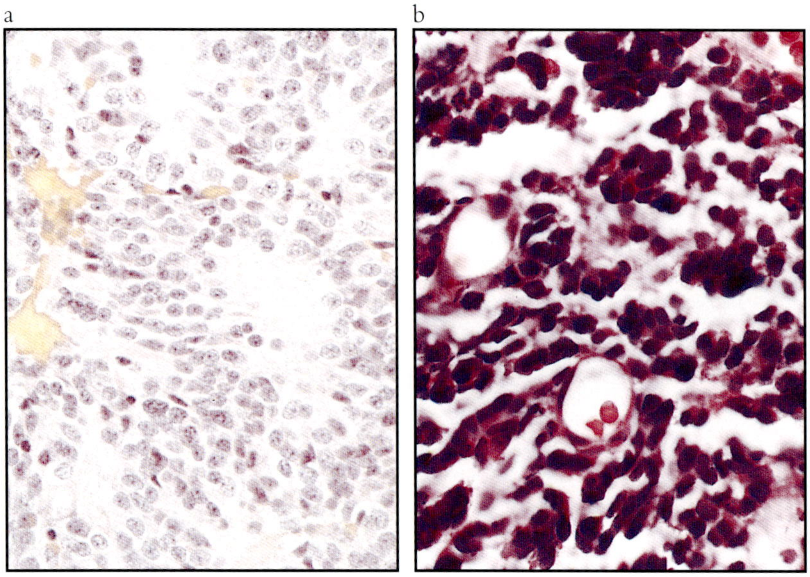

Image 7.27
The pineocytoma is composed of sheets of cuboidal cells forming rosette-like tangles (a). The pineoblastoma is composed of sheets of small anaplastic cells (b) (both, H&E; a, 250X; b, 400X).

Image 7.28
The pineoblastoma often presents in CSF as clusters of small anaplastic cells (a, Papanicolaou, 1,000X; b, Romanowski, 600X).

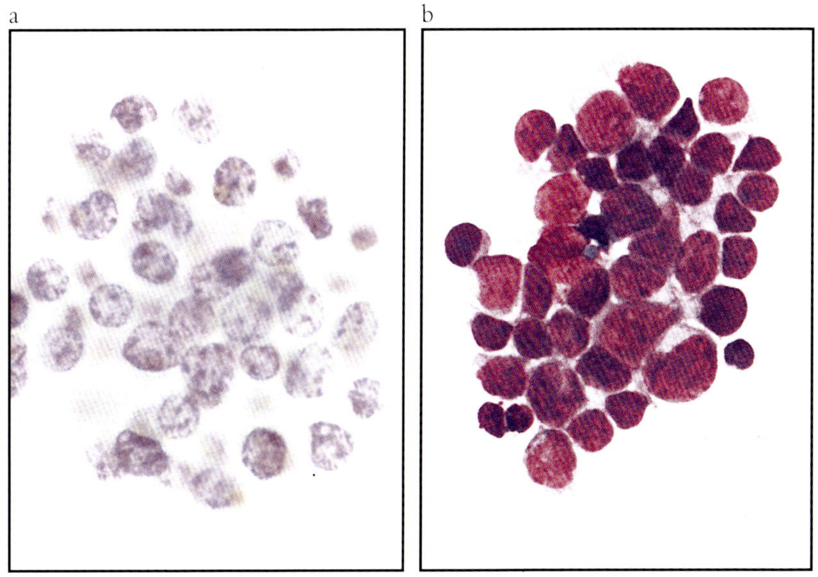

Image 7.29
The pineoblastoma sometimes presents in CSF in cohesive tissue fragments (a) or in rosettes (b) (both, Papanicolaou, 1,000X).

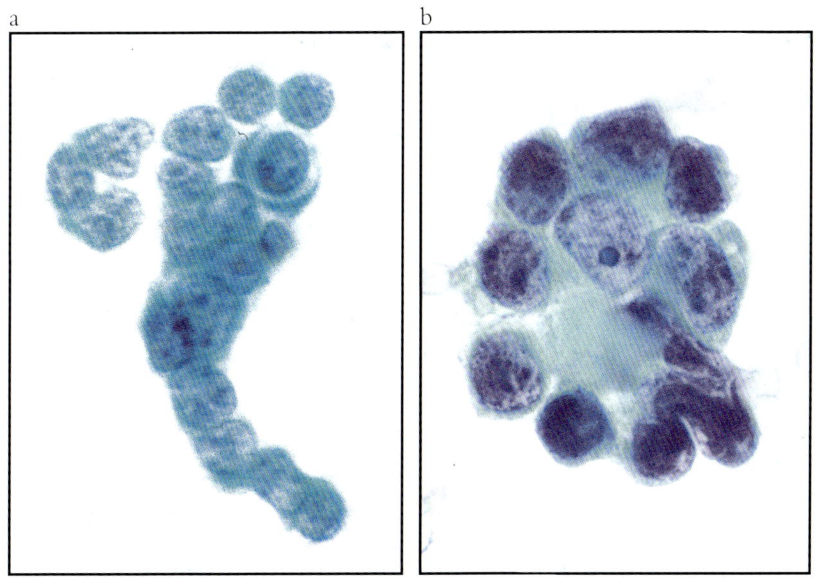

Image 7.30
These histologic sections of a craniopharyngioma show masses of keratin, keratinized squamous cells, and basaloid adamantinomatous cells (a and b). Imprint preparations of this lesion show benign keratinized cells (c) and cuboidal, basaloid cells (d) (a, H&E, 200X; b, H&E, 400X; c and d, Papanicolaou, 1,000X).

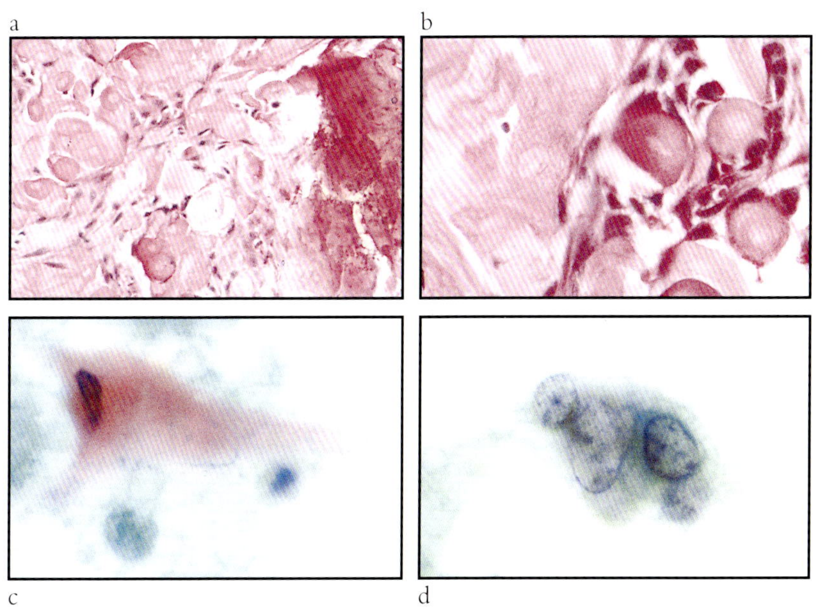

a b

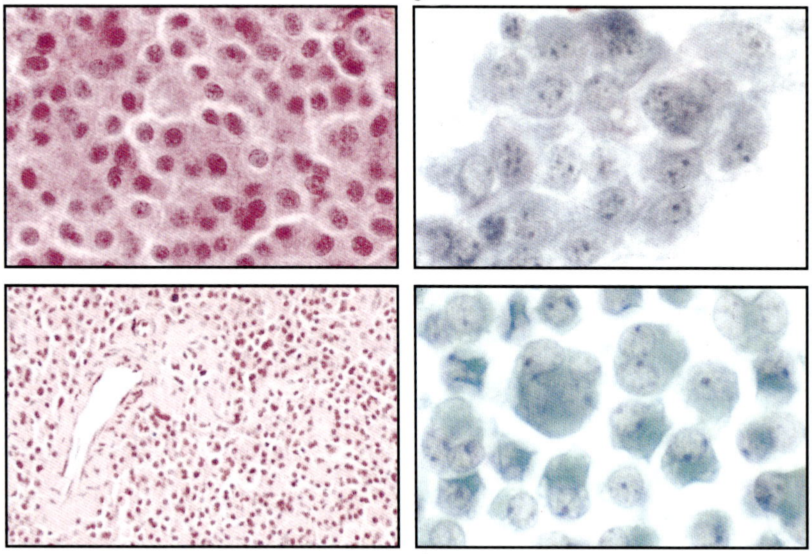

c d

Image 7.31

A pituitary adenoma displays cohesive cuboidal cells with bland nuclei (a and b). A pituitary adenoma in a different patient shows cuboidal cells with round, bland nuclei (c), but these cells shed singly in imprint preparations (d) (a, H&E, 400X; b, Papanicolaou, 600X; c, H&E, 200X; d, Papanicolaou, 600X).

a b

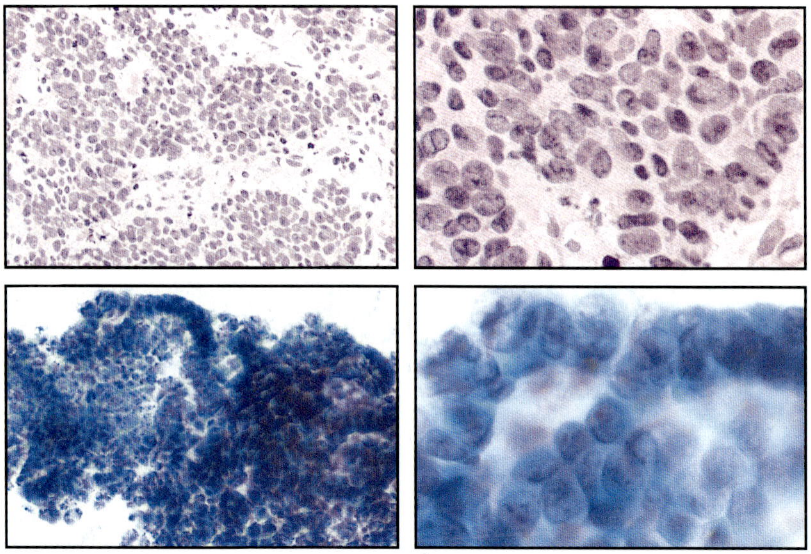

c d

Image 7.32

The histologic presentation of a recurrent pituitary adenoma in a 41-year-old man (a and b). The cells are cuboidal forming a glandlike pattern but are somewhat more crowded with less cytoplasm than the lesions shown in Image 7.31. A fragment of cells with a glandular arrangement is seen in the CSF from this patient (c and d). On high-power magnification (d), the crowded pattern of the cells is apparent (a, H&E, 200X; b, H&E, 400X; c, Papanicolaou, 200X; d, Papanicolaou, 600X).

a b

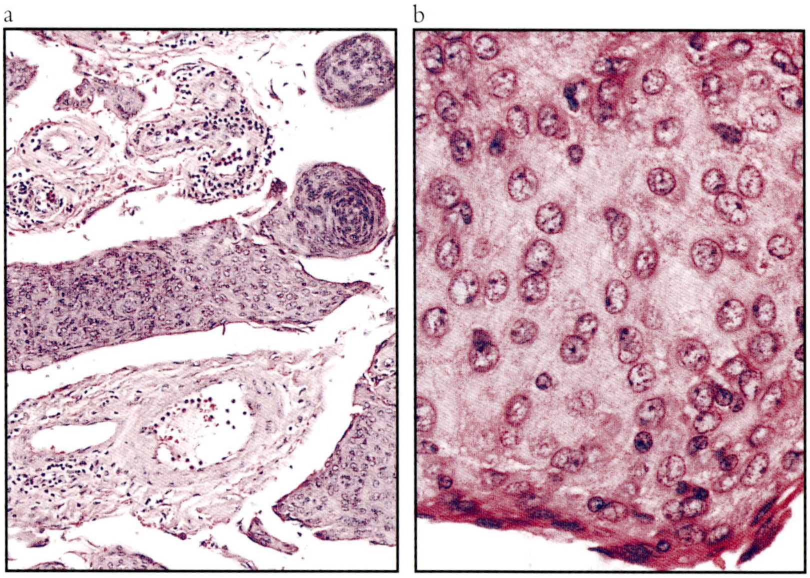

Image 7.33

Histologically, the meningioma is composed of sheets and whorls of bland cells with oval nuclei and indistinct cell borders (a and b) (both, H&E; a, 200X; b, 400X).

Occasional whorls and psammoma bodies may be seen (c and d) (both, H&E, 400X).

c d

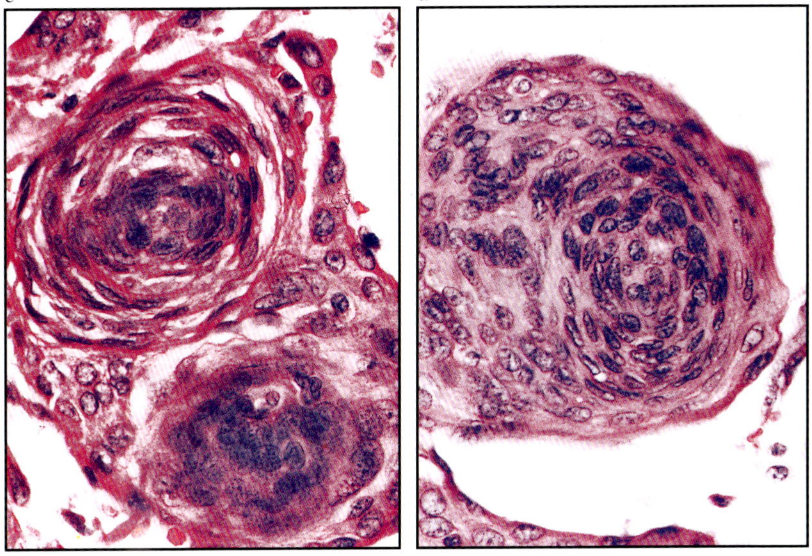

Image 7.34
Imprints of a meningioma reveal a granular chromatin pattern and whorl formation (all, Papanicolaou; a and b, 400X; c and d, 1,000X).

a b

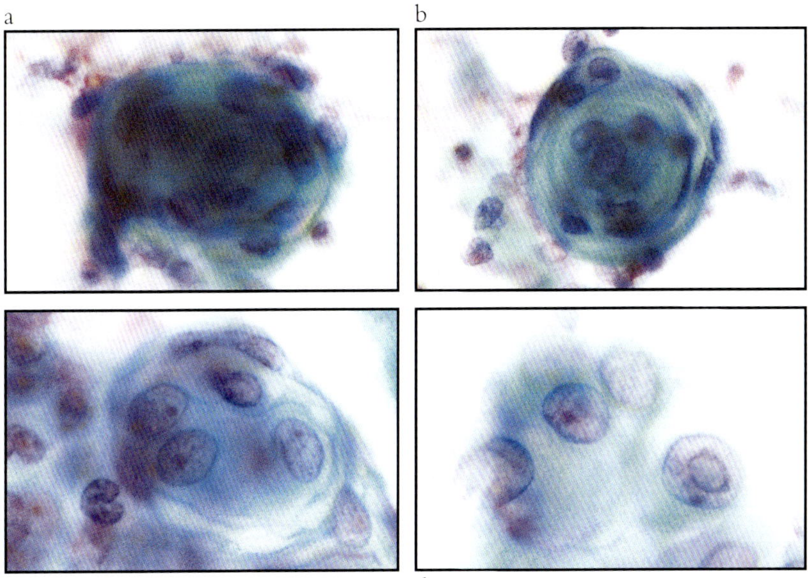

c d

Image 7.35
Histologically, schwannoma is composed of broad sheets of spindle-shaped cells (a). Imprints are sparsely cellular containing only a few spindle-shaped cells with bland nuclei (b) (a, H&E, 200X; b, Papanicolaou, 600X).

a b

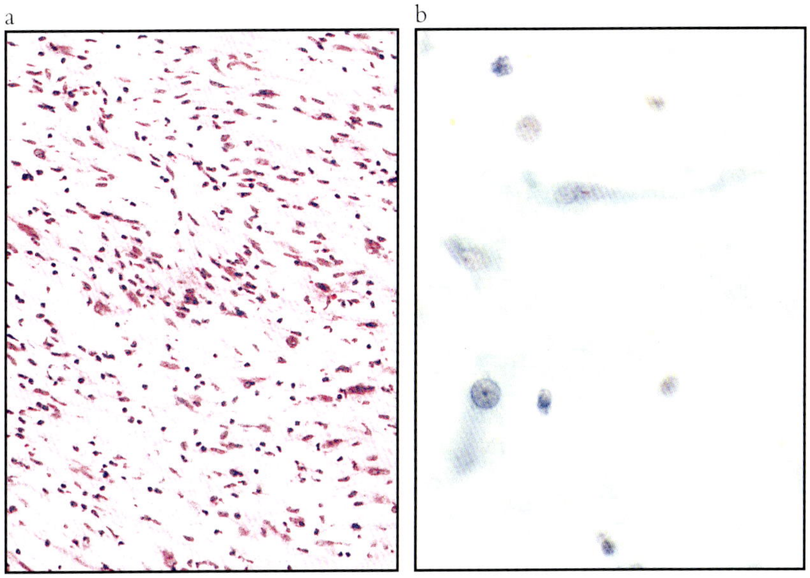

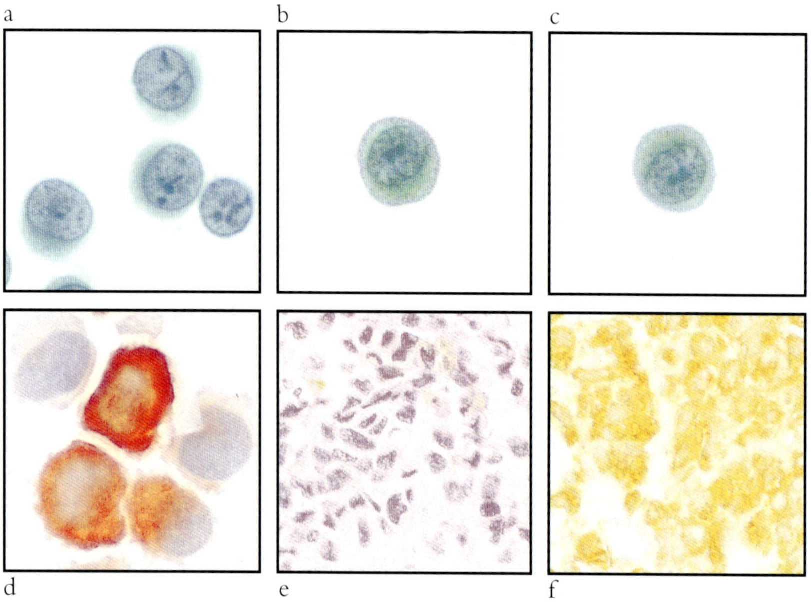

Image 7.36
This CSF specimen from a 10-year-old girl with multiple cutaneous nevi and increased intracranial pressure shows cells with round and sometimes eccentric nuclei (a). The chromatin is bland and nucleoli are visible but not prominent (b and c). Occasional cells contain fine brown cytoplasmic pigment and express HMB-45 (d). A meningeal biopsy specimen reveals sheets of nevoid cells (e) that are positive for HMB-45 (f) (a through c, Papanicolaou, 1,000X; d and f, immunoperoxidase for HMB-45; d, 1,000X; f, 400X; e, H&E, 400X).

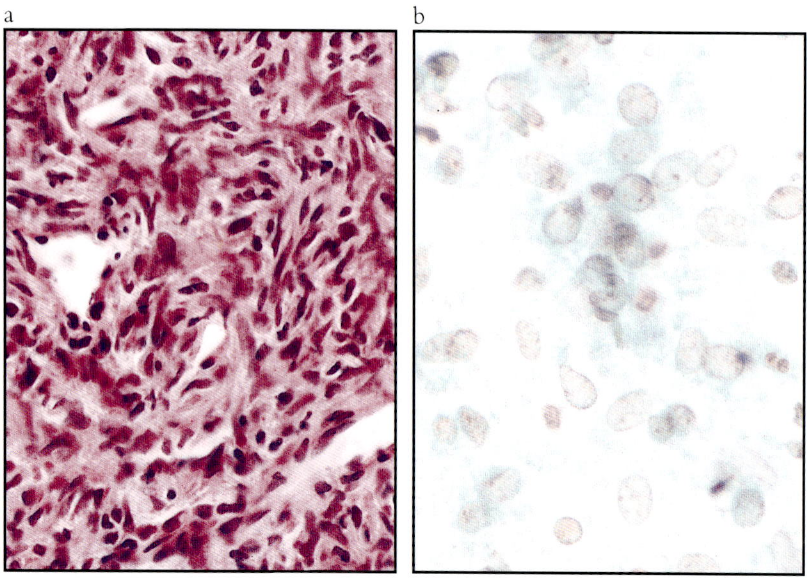

Image 7.37
Histologically, hemangiopericytoma contains sheets of short, spindle-shaped cells and numerous vascular chambers (a). Imprints are cellular, containing clusters of cells with bland ovoid nuclei and indistinct cytoplasmic borders (b) (a, H&E, 400X; b, Papanicolaou, 1,000X).

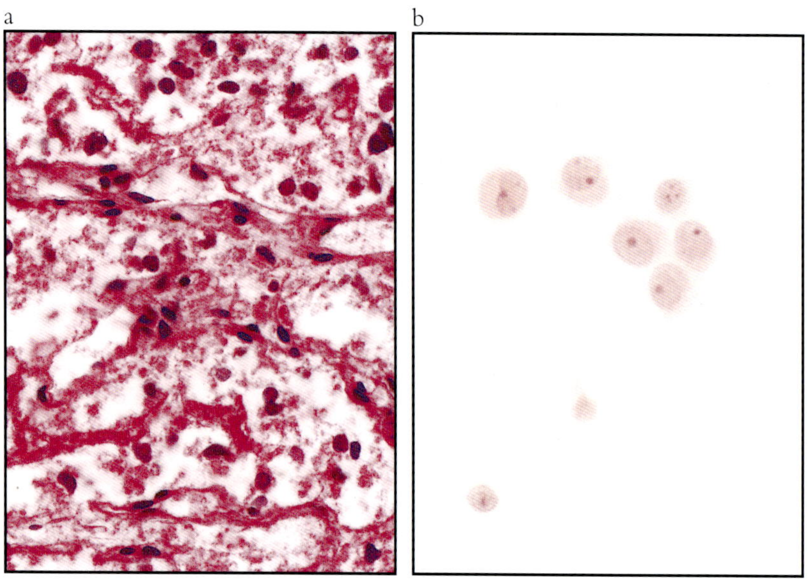

Image 7.38
This hemangioblastoma is composed of numerous vascular channels separated by nests of foamy stromal cells (a). Imprints show numerous cells with round nuclei, granular chromatin, and prominent nucleoli eccentrically placed in moderate amounts of cytoplasm (b) (a, H&E, 400X; b, Papanicolaou, 600X).

Image 7.39
Primary CNS lymphoma is also termed reticulum cell sarcoma, microglioma, histiocytic lymphoma, and immunoblastic sarcoma. This lesion is infiltrative, highly cellular, and characteristically infiltrates massively around blood vessels (a and b). An imprint of this lesion shows single cells with convoluted nuclei, irregular chromatin, and prominent nucleoli, which is the typical presentation of lymphoma in cytologic preparations (c and d) (a, H&E, 200X; b, H&E, 400X; c, Papanicolaou, 600X; d, Papanicolaou, 1,000X).

a b

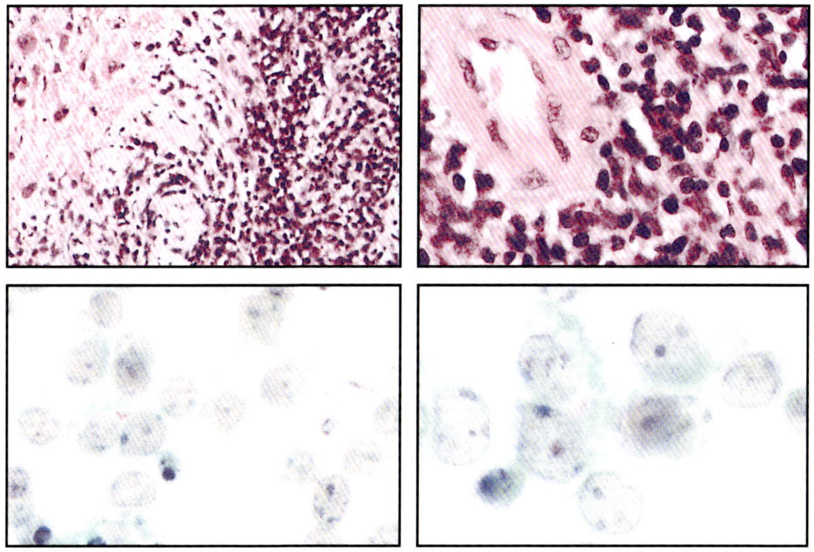

c d

Image 7.40
Primary cerebral lymphoma with meningeal dissemination. Malignant lymphoid cells are apparent with Papanicolaou stain (a). Anti-immunoglobulin antibodies demonstrate a monoclonal B-cell preparation with expression of the kappa light chain (b) (a, Papanicolaou, 600X; b, Immunohistochemistry with anti–kappa light chain antibody, 600X).

a b

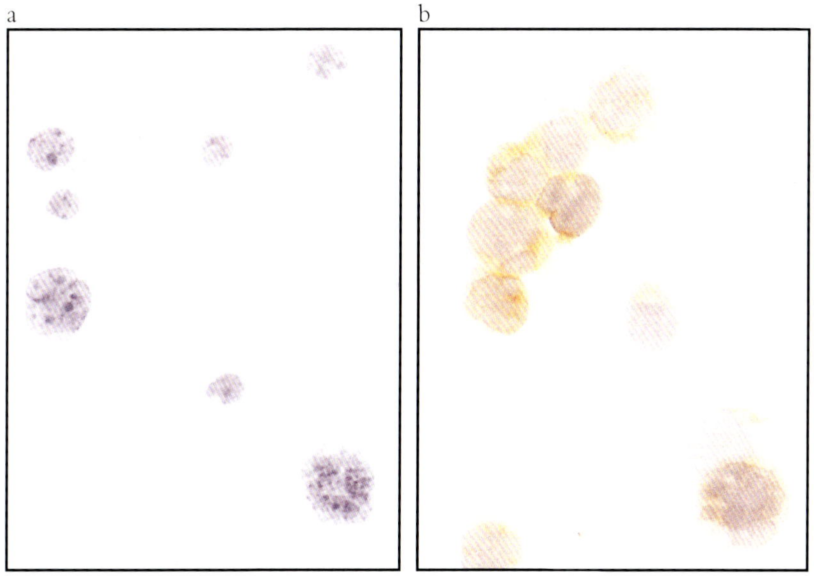

Image 7.41
Bizarre histiocytic cells in the CSF of a 50-year-old woman (a and b). At autopsy, the brain (c) and subarachnoid space (d) were infiltrated by malignant "histiocytes" with moderate amounts of cytoplasm. No tumor was found outside of the CNS. In the older terminology this would be considered "microgliomatosis." The cellular morphology suggests that these cells may be true histiocytes of reticuloendothelial origin (a and b, Papanicolaou, 1,000X; c, H&E, 200X; d, H&E, 400X).

a b

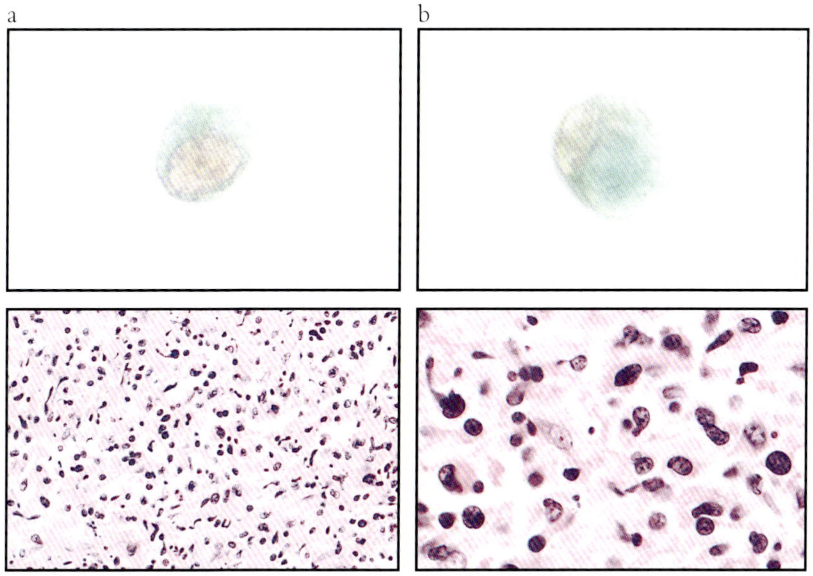

c d

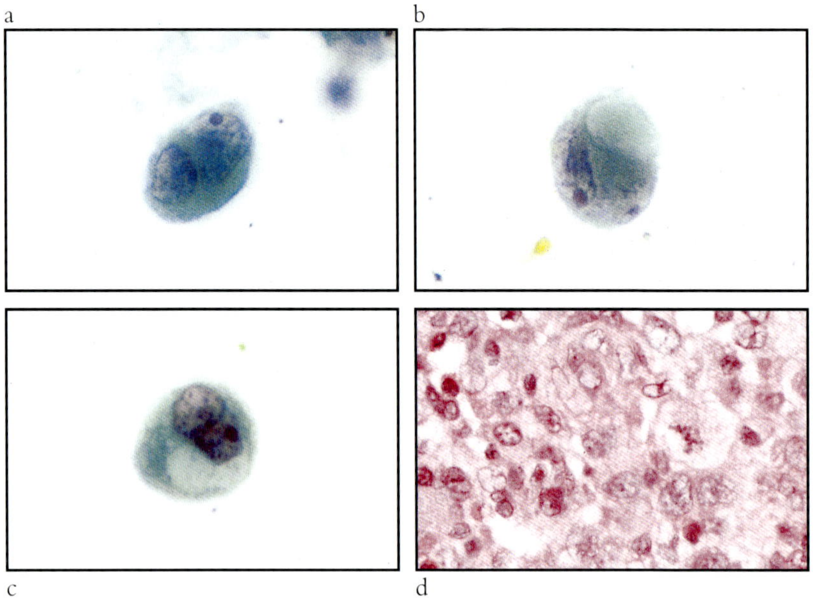

Image 7.42
Bizarre histiocytic cells occurring in CSF of a 7-year-old girl who presented with symptoms of chronic meningitis (a through c). An arachnoid biopsy specimen showed clusters of similar malignant histiocytes (d) (a through c, Papanicolaou, 1,000X; d, H&E, 400X).

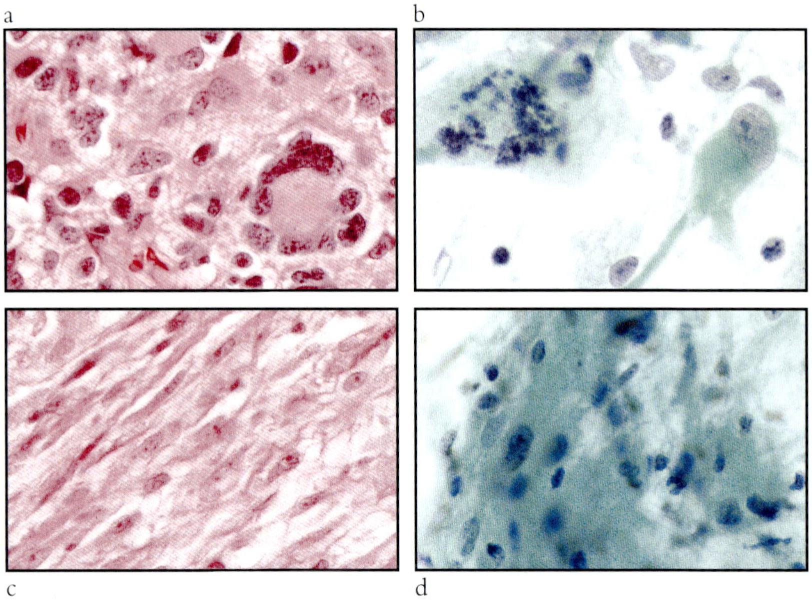

Image 7.43
Mixed cerebral gliosarcoma tumor containing areas of malignant glioma (a and b) and fibrosarcoma (c and d) (a and c, H&E, 400X; b and d, Papanicolaou; b, 600X; d, 400X).

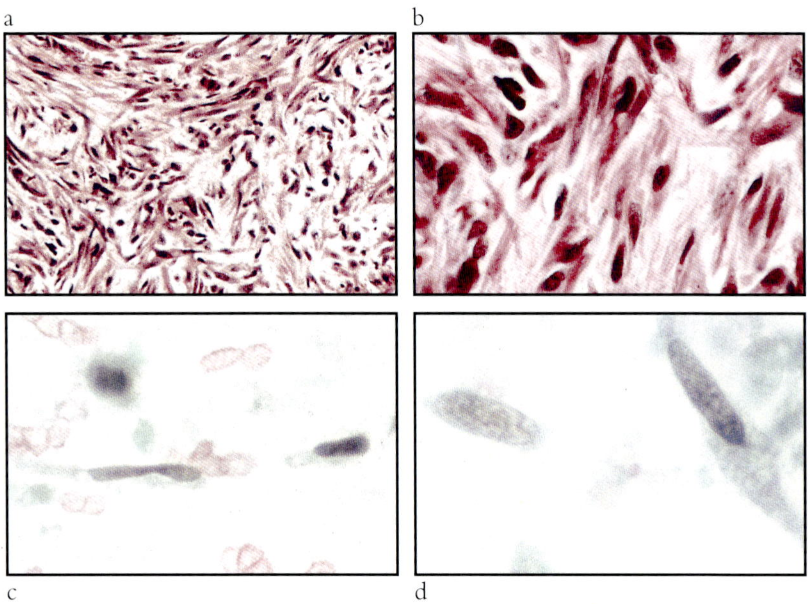

Image 7.44
Primary cerebral fibrosarcoma. Malignant spindle cells are seen in the biopsy specimen (a and b) and imprint (c and d) of the tumor shown in Figure 7.15 (a, H&E, 200X; b, H&E, 400X; c, Papanicolaou, 600X; d, Papanicolaou, 1,000X).

References

1. Bailey P, Cushing H: Medulloblastoma cerebelli, a common type of mid-cerebellar glioma of childhood. *Arch Neurol Psychiatry* 77:192–224, 1925.
2. Bailey P, Cushing H: *A Classification of the Tumors of the Glioma Group on a Histogenetic Basis With a Correlated Study of Prognosis.* Philadelphia, PA, JB Lippincott Co, 1926.
3. Balhuizen JC, Bots GTAM, Schaberg A: The value of cytology in the diagnosis of hypophyseal tumors. *Acta Cytol* 18:370–375, 1974.
4. Balhuizen JC, Bots GTAM, Schaberg A, Bosman FT: Value of cerebrospinal fluid cytology for the diagnosis of malignancies in the central nervous system. *J Neurosurg* 48:747–753, 1978.
5. Bigner SH, Johnston WW: The diagnostic challenge of tumors manifested initially by the shedding of cells into cerebrospinal fluid (CSF). *Acta Cytol* 28:28–36, 1984.
6. Bischoff A: Erfahrungen mit der tumorzelldianostik im liquor cerebrospinalis. *Acta Neurochir* 9:510–524, 1961.
7. Burger PC, Vogel FS, Green SB, Strole TA: Glioblastoma multiforme and anaplastic astrocytoma: pathologic criteria and prognostic implications. *Cancer* 56:1106–1111, 1985.
8. Cairns H, Russell DS: Intracranial and spinal metastases in gliomas of the brain. *Brain* 54:377–420, 1931.
9. DeGirolami U, Schmidek H: Clinicopathological study of 53 tumors of the pineal region. *J Neurosurg* 39:455–462, 1973.
10. Fields WS: *Primary Brain Tumors. A Review of Histologic Classification.* New York, NY, Springer-Verlag, 1989.
11. Firpo A Jr, Watson CW: Cytology of ganglioglioma of the brain: a morphometric study. *Acta Cytol* 25:317–322, 1981.
12. Friedman HS, Oakes WJ, Bigner SH, Wikstrand CJ, Bigner DD: Medulloblastoma tumor: biological and clinical perspectives. *J Neurooncol* 11:1–15, 1991.
13. Gandolfi A: The cytology of cerebral neuroblastoma. *Acta Cytol* 24:344–346, 1979.
14. Garin-Chesa P, Fellinger EJ, Huvos AG, Bereford HR, Melamed MR, Triche TJ, Rettig WJ: Immunohistochemical analysis of neural cell adhesion molecules: differential expression in small round cell tumors of childhood and adolescence. *Am J Pathol* 139:275–286, 1991.
15. Giangsapero F, Rigobello L, Badiali M, Loda M: Large cell medulloblastomas: a distinct variant with highly aggressive behavior. *Am J Surg Pathol* 16:687–693, 1992.
16. Gindhart TD, Tsukahara YC: Cytologic diagnosis of pineal germinoma in cerebrospinal fluid and sputum. *Acta Cytol* 23:341–346, 1979.
17. Gondos B, King EB: Cerebrospinal fluid cytology: diagnostic accuracy and comparison of different technique. *Acta Cytol* 20:542–547, 1976.

18. Gould VE, Jansson DS, Molenaar WM, Rorke LB, Trojanowski JQ, Lee VMY, Packer RJ, Franke WW: Primitive neuroectodermal tumors of the central nervous system: patterns of expression of neuroendocrine markers and all classes of intermediate filament proteins. *Lab Invest* 62:498–509, 1990.

19. Hajdu SI, Ashton PR, Carter D, Lang WR, Sullivan M: Diagnostic cytology seminar. *Acta Cytol* 26:851–882, 1982.

20. Harisiadis L, Chang CH: Medulloblastoma in children: a correlation between staging and results of treatment. *Int J Radiat Oncol Biol Physiol* 2:833–841, 1977.

21. Harper CG, Thomas DGT: Neurocutaneous melanosis. *J Neurol Neurosurg Psychiatry* 37:760–763, 1987.

22. Henry JM, Heffner RR Jr, Dillard SH, Earle KM, Davis RL: Primary malignant lymphomas of the central nervous system. *Cancer* 34:1293–1302, 1974.

23. Ho KL, Hoschner JA, Wolfe DE: Primary leptomeningeal gliomatosis. *Arch Neurol* 38:662–666, 1981.

24. Jellinger K, Radshiewicz TH, Slowik F: Primary malignant lymphoma of the central nervous system in man. *Acta Neuropathol (Berl)* (Suppl) 6:95–102, 1975.

25. Jin L, Hemperly JJ, Lloyd RV: Expression of neural cell adhesion molecule in normal and neoplastic human neuroendocrine tissues. *Am J Pathol* 138:961–969, 1991.

26. Kernohan JW, Mabon RF, Svein HF, Adson AW: A simplified classification of the gliomas. *Proc Staff Meeting Mayo Clin* 24:71–75, 1949.

27. Kernohan JW, Uihlein A: *Sarcomas of the Brain*. Springfield, IL, Charles C Thomas, 1962, pp. 90–98.

28. Kline TS: Cytologic examination of the cerebrospinal fluid. *Cancer* 15:591–597, 1962.

29. Ludwin SK, Conley FK: Malignant meningiomas metastasizing through the cerebrospinal pathways. *J Neurol Neurosurg Psychiatry* 38:136–142, 1975.

30. Lukes RJ, Collins RD: New approaches to the classification of the lymphomata. *Br J Cancer* (Suppl II) 31:1–28, 1975.

31. Miller RR, Lin F, Mallonee MM: Cytologic diagnosis of gliomatosis cerebri. *Acta Cytol* 25:37–39, 1981.

32. Mitsumoto H, Breuer AC, Lederman RJ: Malignant lymphomas of the central nervous system: a case of primary spinal intramedullary involvement. *Cancer* 46:1258–1262, 1980.

33. Naylor B: The cytologic diagnosis of cerebrospinal fluid. *Acta Cytol* 8:141–149, 1964.

34. Pasternak JF: Special problems in pediatric brain tumors. *Semin Neurol* 1:127–136, 1981.

35. Rappaport H: Tumours of the hematopoietic system. In: *Atlas of Tumour Pathology* (section III, fascicle 8). Washington, DC, Armed Forces Institute of Pathology, 1966.

36. Reed WB, Becker SW Sr, Becker SW Jr, Nickel WR: Giant pigmented nevi, melanoma, and leptomeningeal melanocytosis: a clinical and histopathological study. *Arch Dermatol* 91:100–119, 1965.

37. Rorke LB: The cerebellar medulloblastoma and its relationship to primitive neuroectodermal tumors. *J Neuropathol Exp Neurol* 42:1–15, 1983.

38. Rubinstein LJ: Tumors of the central nervous system. In: *Atlas of Tumor Pathology* (second series, fascicle 6). Washington, DC, Armed Forces Institute of Pathology, 1972.

39. Russell DS, Rubinstein LJ: *Pathology Tumours of the Nervous System,* 5th ed. Baltimore, MD, Williams and Wilkins Co, 1989, pp. 83–92, 173, 202, 403, 471, 525.

40. Schmidek HH: *Pineal Tumours.* New York, NY, Masson Publishing USA, Inc, 1977, p. 43.

41. Slaughter JC, Hardman JM, Kempe LG, Earle KM: Neurocutaneous melanosis and leptomeningeal melanomatosis in children. *Arch Pathol* 88:298–304, 1969.

42. Taylor CR, Russell R, Lukes RJ, Davis RL: An immunohistological study of immunoglobulin content of primary central nervous system lymphomas. *Cancer* 41:2197–2205, 1978.

43. Wagner JA, Frost JK, Wisotzkey H Jr: Subarachnoid neoplasia: incidence and problems of diagnosis. *South Med J* 53:1503–1508, 1960.

44. Walt F: A medulloblastoma in an infant with abnormal cells in the cerebrospinal fluid. *Arch Dis Child* 14:84–86, 1939.

45. Willis RA: *The Spread of Tumours in the Human Body,* 3rd ed. London, England, Butterworths, 1973, pp. 259–268.

46. Wolfson WL: Cytopathologic presentation of cerebral histiocytosis. *Acta Cytol* 23:392–398, 1979.

47. World Health Organization: Histological classification of tumors of the central nervous system. *WHO International Histological Classification of Tumors* 23:124, 1979.

48. Zahoropoulos P, Wong JY: Cytology of common primary midline brain tumors. *Acta Cytol* 24:384–390, 1980.

49. Zulch KJ: *Atlas of the Histology of Brain Tumors.* New York, NY, Springer, 1971.

50. Zulch KJ: *Brain Tumors: Their Biology and Pathology,* 2nd ed. New York, NY, Springer, 1965.

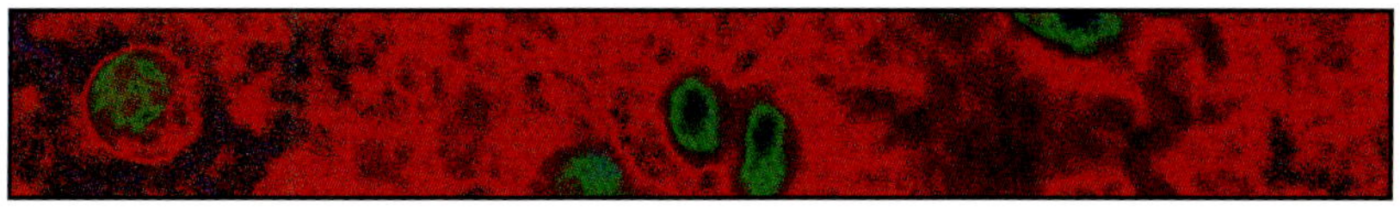

CHAPTER EIGHT

Fine Needle Aspiration Biopsy

Fine needle aspiration (FNA) biopsy of intracranial masses utilizing computed tomography (CT) and stereotactic techniques has recently become recognized in the United States as a useful diagnostic procedure. The procedure utilizes steroids to control edema and CT visualization to detect hemorrhage, resulting in low morbidity and mortality rates.[7,9,11,15] Since it can be performed through a burr hole with local anesthesia, the hospitalization time is short as compared to that of open craniotomy.

This technique is most appropriately applied in clinical settings in which only a diagnosis is required and a large resection is either not possible or not indicated. For example, lesions in the deep cerebrum (Figure 8.1), including the basal ganglia and thalamus, and in the area surrounding the third ventricle are not resectable because they involve vital structures.[6] Similarly, malignant gliomas in the parietal lobe of the dominant hemisphere are generally not excised due to the devastating neurologic deficiencies that result. The pineal area (Figure 8.1) is difficult to approach surgically, and the most common tumor of this location is the pineal germinoma, for which resection is not necessary since it is treated by shunt implantation and radiation.

Optimal use of this technique requires intimate cooperation between the pathologist and the surgeon, since the pathologist is confronted with the task of making a diagnosis from small bits of tissue. As in aspiration procedures from other body sites, the first critical step in correct interpretation of samples obtained stereotactically requires determination of a differential diagnosis based on clinical history, age of the patient, location of the lesion, radiographic appearance, and previous therapeutic intervention. Then, one must be both familiar with the morphologic presen-

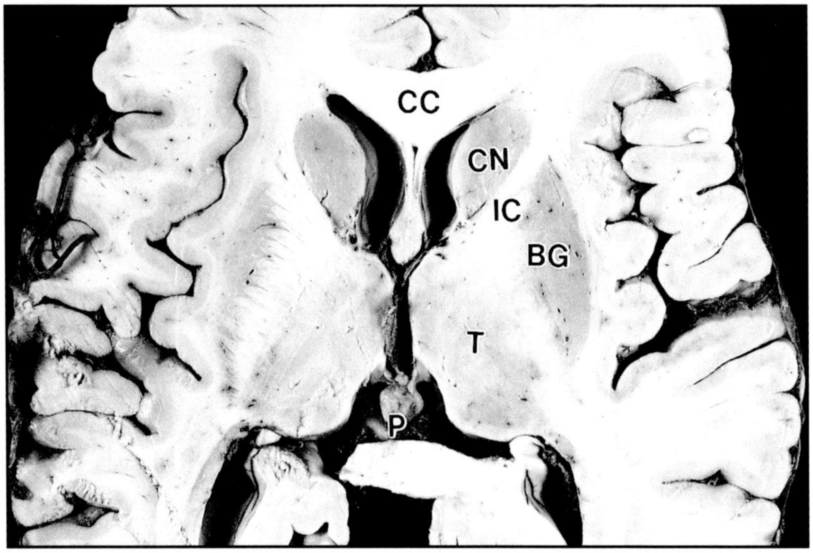

Figure 8.1
Horizontal section of a normal brain demonstrating structures of the deep cerebrum. CN, caudate nucleus; BG, basal ganglia; T, thalamus; IC, internal capsule; CC, corpus callosum; P, pineal glial.

tation of these lesions in samples prepared by different methods and aware of the limitations of each preparatory technique.[3,4,8,10,16] Finally, a close interaction between the surgeon and pathologist provides the opportunity for repeat sampling to ensure that adequate tissue is obtained to permit a definite diagnosis prior to terminating the biopsy procedure.

Close interaction between surgeon and pathologist ensures that adequate tissue is obtained to permit a definite diagnosis

The preparation method for stereotactic biopsy specimens depends on the size and consistency of the sample that is obtained.[2] Solid tissue fragments obtained through a large needle are usually evaluated by frozen section for immediate diagnosis and by formalin fixation and paraffin embedding for final diagnosis. This procedure can be supplemented by imprints of the fragments and by filter and Cytospin® preparations of needle washings to display detailed cellular morphology and to provide material for additional studies such as immunohistochemistry. Smaller fragments obtained through a fine needle are usually smeared or squashed on a slide, while cystic contents are evaluated by Cytospin® or filter methods. Diagnostic material can also be retrieved by cavitron ultrasonic surgical aspiration.[8,16]

The Cerebral Hemispheres

The cerebral hemispheres consist of the cerebral cortex and an underlying fibrillary matrix of white matter (Figure 8.1). The cerebral cortex and nuclei of the basal ganglia and thalamus contain neurons as well as glia. In aspirates, isolated neurons with their prominent nucleoli may be alarming, but the sparsity of these cells in tissue fragments is a useful feature for identification[6] (Image 8.1).

The cytoplasm of individual astrocytes is barely visible in aspirates and histologic sections of normal white matter (Image 8.2). Reactive astrocytes, however, which commonly surround infarcts, abscesses, and

Table 8.1
Common Primary Central Nervous System Neoplasms of the Cerebral Hemispheres

Extracerebral	
Adult	**Children**
Meningioma	Polymorphocellular sarcoma (rare)
Hemangiopericytoma	
Cerebral Hemisphere	
Adult	**Children**
Benign	*Benign*
Astrocytoma	Astrocytoma
Ependymoma	Ependymoma
Oligodendroglioma	
Malignant	*Malignant*
Glioblastoma multiforme	Glioblastoma multiforme
Primary lymphoma	Ependymoblastoma
Ependymoblastoma	Neuroblastoma
Malignant oligodendroglioma	
Gliosarcoma	

metastatic tumors, have obvious cytoplasm (Image 8.3) that is better seen using an immunoperoxidase method for the demonstration of glial fibrillary acidic protein (GFAP). An important pitfall in diagnosis of aspirates from the periphery of cerebral lesions is the incorrect interpretation of these reactive cells as neoplastic astrocytes.

Non-neoplastic lesions that commonly involve the cerebrum include hemorrhage, which is distinguished by red blood cells and hemosiderin-laden macrophages, inflammatory lesions such as abscesses, granulomas, and mycetomas, and cerebral infarcts. Aspirates from inflammatory lesions may contain nonspecific inflammatory cells and necrotic debris, or they may yield a specific etiologic agent. Examples of the infiltrate from staphylococcal and nocardial abscesses are discussed and illustrated in Chapter Three. Figure 8.2 shows the CT scan from a 59-year-old woman who developed a hemiparesis while taking systemic steroids.[1] Image 8.4 shows the broad nonseptate hyphae of a phycomycete demonstrated in an aspirate of this lesion. (This case is also discussed and illustrated in Chapter Three.) Cerebral infarcts present a potential pitfall in the interpretation of fine needle aspirates, since macrophages from the center of these lesions may mimic cells of adenocarcinoma (Image 8.5).

The most common tumors to involve the cerebral hemispheres of adults are astrocytic neoplasms and metastatic tumors

Table 8.1 lists the most common tumors of the cerebral hemispheres for adults and children. The most common tumors to involve the cerebral hemispheres of adults are astrocytic neoplasms and metastatic tumors. In addition to astrocytic tumors, other types of gliomas, lymphomas, and sarcomas may be seen in adults. In some cases, low-grade astrocytomas may be distinguished from normal and reactive astrocytes by their hypercellularity and nuclear hyperchromasia (Image 8.6). In smear and squash preparations, the degree of cellularity may be difficult to determine, and the diagnosis of a low-grade astrocytoma may be limited to those cases that display architectural features distinctive to neoplastic proliferations. For example,

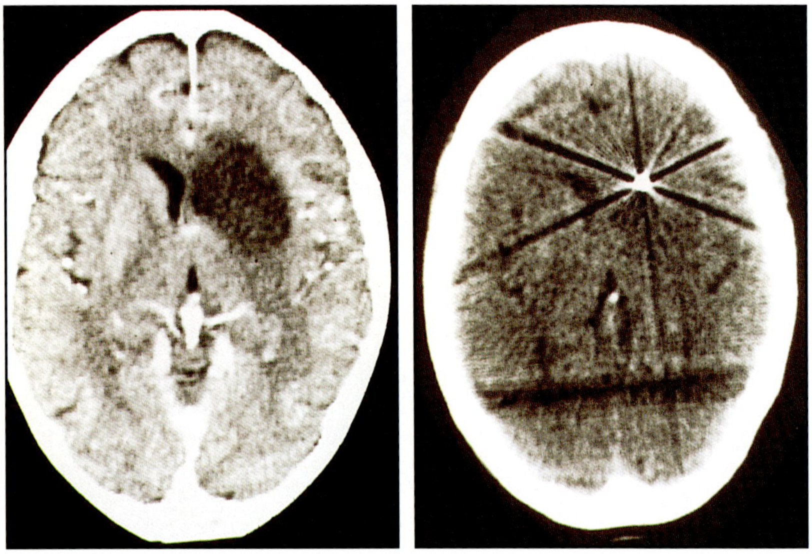

Figure 8.2
a, Computed tomographic scan of a cerebral mass from a 59-year-old woman. The mass was aspirated stereotactically. b, The needle tip can be seen in the lesion.

Image 8.7 shows the cytologic and histologic features of a microcystic astrocytoma; an example of a pilocytic astrocytoma is shown in Chapter Seven. Anaplastic astrocytomas generally retain a fibrillar background and cytoplasmic processes but are more cellular than low-grade astrocytomas (Image 8.8). Glioblastoma multiforme is also hypercellular (Image 8.9), and, in some cases, nuclear and cellular pleomorphism may be seen (Image 8.10). The most reliable feature to distinguish between anaplastic astrocytoma and glioblastoma, however, is the presence or absence of necrosis (Images 8.11 and 8.12). Although this parameter can be identified in core biopsy specimens and cell blocks, it cannot accurately be identified in smear, filter, and Cytospin® preparations. This inability to distinguish between anaplastic astrocytoma and glioblastoma remains a limitation of FNA of brain tumors.

Distinction between anaplastic astrocytoma and glioblastoma depends on the presence or absence of necrosis

Metastases are infrequent in the deep cerebrum, but they are common in the more superficial portions of the cerebral hemispheres. Clumped chromatin, prominent nucleoli, and distinct cell borders generally allow their distinction from primary brain tumors (Images 8.13 and 8.14). Either primary or metastatic lymphomas may occur in the cerebral hemispheres, and they can readily be identified by the single-cell presentation of atypical lymphoid cells (Image 8.15).

Cerebral lesions are frequently cystic, and aspirates of cyst fluid may be obtained either as a closed, CT-guided procedure or at the time of open craniotomy. A variety of non-neoplastic cysts occur in the cerebral hemispheres. Image 8.16 demonstrates ciliated columnar cells from a colloid cyst of the third ventricle. Cysts from low-grade astrocytomas (Image 8.17) generally contain only nonspecific foam cells (Image 8.18), whereas malignant astrocytes may be seen in cystic anaplastic astrocytomas and glioblastomas. Glioblastoma multiforme is likely to present in cyst fluid as isolated pleomorphic cells (Image 8.19), but metastases are more likely to shed as tissue fragments (Image 8.20). This difference in shedding patterns, and the cellular features just described, usually allow their distinction.

Tumors that present in the extracerebral compartment of the hemispheres of adults include the meningioma and hemangiopericytoma. The former lesion, when it occurs along the base of the brain and frontal hemispheres, may protrude into the paranasal sinuses or orbit.[14] Image 8.21 demonstrates an aspirate and subsequent resection of a meningioma that presented as an intraorbital mass in a 70-year-old man with a history of prostatic carcinoma. The aspiration procedure was critical in determining that the lesion was a meningioma rather than a metastasis.

Most supratentorial tumors in children are astrocytic or ependymal in origin

In children, the majority of supratentorial tumors are of astrocytic or ependymal origin, but occasionally neuroblastomas may occur. In addition to the glial tumors, the midline structures may harbor specialized tumors not usually seen elsewhere in the central nervous system (CNS) (Table 8.2). Figure 8.3 demonstrates the region of hypothalamus that surrounds the third ventricle and lies above the pituitary gland and the sella turcica. Craniopharyngiomas, pituitary adenomas, and germ cell tumors may occur in this region[17] (see Images 7.26, 7.31, 7.32, and 7.33; Figures 7.10 and 7.11).

The pineal gland (Figure 8.3) also gives rise to germ cell tumors—most commonly the germinoma. In addition, the pineocytoma and pineoblastoma, which arise from the pineocytes, may be seen. Due to their location in the midline, which is difficult to approach surgically, fine needle aspiration is an appropriate means of establishing a diagnosis.[5,12] The histologic and cytologic presentations of these tumors are demonstrated and discussed in Chapter Seven (Images 7.26 through 7.30 and Figure 7.9).

Table 8.2
Midline Supratentorial Tumors

Hypothalmic and Suprasellar Region

Adults	**Children**
Benign	*Benign*
Pituitary adenoma	Craniopharyngioma
Astrocytoma	Astrocytoma
Ependymoma	Ependymoma
Malignant	*Malignant*
Glioblastoma multiforme	Glioblastoma multiforme
Ependymoblastoma	Ependymoblastoma

Pineal Gland

Germ Cell Tumors
Germinoma (atypical teratoma, pinealoma)
Teratoma
Choriocarcinoma
Embryonal carcinoma
Endodermal sinus tumor

Primary Pineal Tumors
Pineoblastoma
Pineocytoma

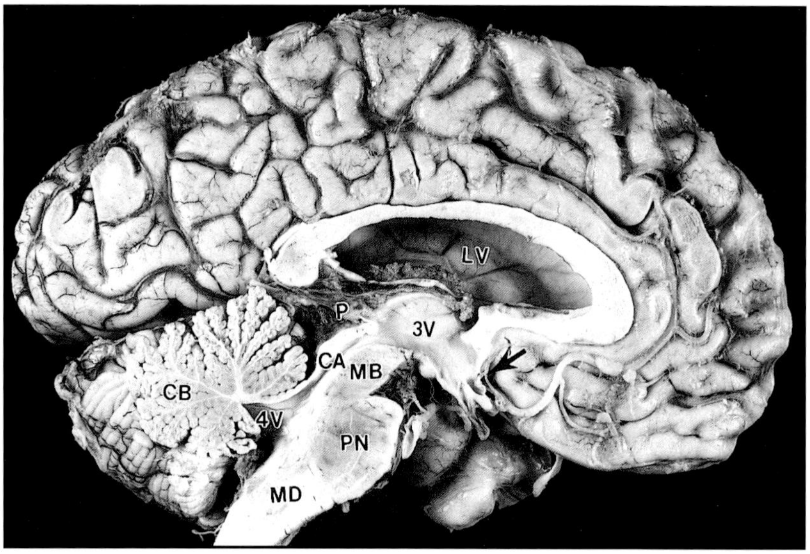

Figure 8.3
Midsagittal brain section demonstrating the locations of the lateral ventricle (LV), the suprasellar area (arrow), the pineal gland (P), the infratentorial compartment that houses the cerebellum (CB), the fourth ventricle (4V), and the brain stem composed of the midbrain (MB), pons (PN), and medulla (MD). The pineal gland (P) is located posterior to the third ventricle (3V) and above the cerebral aqueduct (CA).

The Cerebellum and Brain Stem

The cerebellum and brain stem lie beneath the tentorium in the posterior fossa (Figure 8.3). Metastases are the most common malignant lesions to occur in the cerebellum of adults, whereas glioblastoma is extremely rare in this location. Less common primary malignant tumors are lymphomas, sarcoma, and ependymoblastomas.

Many primary cerebellar tumors in adults are benign

Many primary cerebellar tumors in adults are benign (Table 8.3). They are frequently cystic, but cyst fluid aspirates show only nonspecific foam cells and do not allow distinction between astrocytomas and hemangioblastomas. Imprints of the mural nodules of hemangioblastomas, however, reveal characteristic cells (Image 7.39). In children, medulloblastoma and astrocytoma are the most common tumor types seen in the cerebellum. The former contains abundant small undifferentiated cells; the latter shows the characteristics of low-grade astrocytomas seen elsewhere in the brain. In the brain stem, solitary metastases are rare in all age groups, and the majority of malignant lesions are glioblastomas. Other astrocytic and ependymal tumors are seen, as well as occasional primary lymphomas.

The Spinal Cord

The differential diagnosis of a spinal cord tumor varies with the level of cord at which it occurs and the relationship of the tumor to the meninges (Table 8.4). The meninges include the arachnoid membrane, which forms the outer limit of the subarachnoid space (SAS), and the

Table 8.3
Common Primary Central Nervous System Neoplasms of the Posterior Fossa

EXTRAPARENCHYMAL	
Adults	
Meningioma	
Schwannoma	
CEREBELLUM	
Adults	**Children**
Benign	*Benign*
Hemangioblastoma	Astrocytoma
Ependymoma	Ependymoma
Astrocytoma	
Malignant	*Malignant*
Primary lymphoma	Medulloblastoma
Sarcoma	Ependymoblastoma
BRAIN STEM	
Adults	**Children**
Benign	*Benign*
Astrocytoma	Astrocytoma
Ependymoma	Ependymoma
Malignant	*Malignant*
Glioblastoma multiforme	Glioblastoma multiforme
Primary lymphoma	Ependymoblastoma
Ependymoblastoma	

dense dura (Image 8.22). The latter structure is the outermost covering of the brain and spinal cord, and it lies on the inner aspect of the skull and spinal canal. Lesions may occur extradurally, between the dura and the skull, or subdurally, between the dura and the arachnoid membrane.[13] Trauma may result in extradural or subdural hematomas, while the corresponding inflammatory lesions are extradural or subdural empyemas or abscesses.

Imprint preparations are helpful in distinguishing myeloma, lymphoma, and carcinoma

The most common neoplasms to occupy the extradural space are metastatic tumors, lymphomas, and myelomas (Table 8.4). These tumors frequently involve the bony structures of the skull or the vertebral column and may enter the extradural space directly or travel along perineural spaces from retroperitoneal lymph nodes. Since the extradural compartment does not communicate with the SAS, cells from these lesions do not appear in cerebrospinal fluid (CSF). Although cytologic evaluation of CSF plays little role in diagnosing these lesions, imprint preparations are extremely helpful in distinguishing myeloma, lymphoma, and carcinoma at the time of frozen section.

The intradural, extramedullary compartment contains the subdural and subarachnoid spaces. These extraparenchymal spaces are a favored site for meningiomas and schwannomas. The SAS is the site of CSF spread by lymphoma, leukemia, metastases, and primary CNS tumors.

The most common tumors arising in the spinal cord itself are astrocytic tumors of any grade and ependymomas. The astrocytic tumors are

Table 8.4
Differential Diagnosis of Spinal Cord Tumors

Extradural Space
Metastatic tumors
Lymphoma
Hodgkin's disease
Myeloma
Chordoma
Primary bone tumors
Intradural, Extramedullary
Meningioma: cervical and thoracic
Schwannoma: lumbar
Neurofibroma
Subarachnoid Space
Lymphoma/Leukemia
Meningeal carcinomatosis
Implants from primary brain tumors
Intramedullar
Astrocytoma: cervical and thoracic
Ependymoma: lumbar and cauda equina
Hemangioblastoma

more common in the cervical and thoracic regions and may be associated with cysts. Image 8.17 shows a cystic spinal cord lesion. A cyst fluid aspirate revealed many benign foam cells (Image 8.18a). Histologically, the spinal cord lesion was a low-grade astrocytoma (Image 8.18b), but diagnostic cells were not shed into the cyst cavity. Since foam cells and benign tissue fragments may be exfoliated into non-neoplastic cysts, such as ependymal and arachnoid cysts as well as syringomyelic cavities, cyst fluid aspirates should be interpreted cautiously. Ependymoma is the most common tumor type seen in the lumbosacral cord, especially in the cauda equina. Many of these spinal cord ependymomas are of the myxopapillary type. As the name implies, they histologically and cytologically consist of isolated papillary structures in a myxoid background (see Image 7.16).

The spinal cord is the second most common location for hemangioblastomas. The histologic and cytologic presentations are the same as that seen in the cerebellum. The spinal cord parenchyma is a rare site for metastases. Although occasional cases occur in which the spinal cord is involved as part of widespread CNS metastases, these cases are inevitably discovered at autopsy. Metastases should therefore be very low in the differential diagnosis of lesions involving the spinal cord itself.

The spinal cord parenchyma is a rare site for metastases

Image 8.1
The neuron with its round nucleus, prominent nucleolus, and moderate amount of cytoplasm may be found in needle aspirates from the cerebral cortex and the deep cerebral nuclei, including caudate, putamen, globus pallidus, and thalamus (Papanicolaou, 600X).

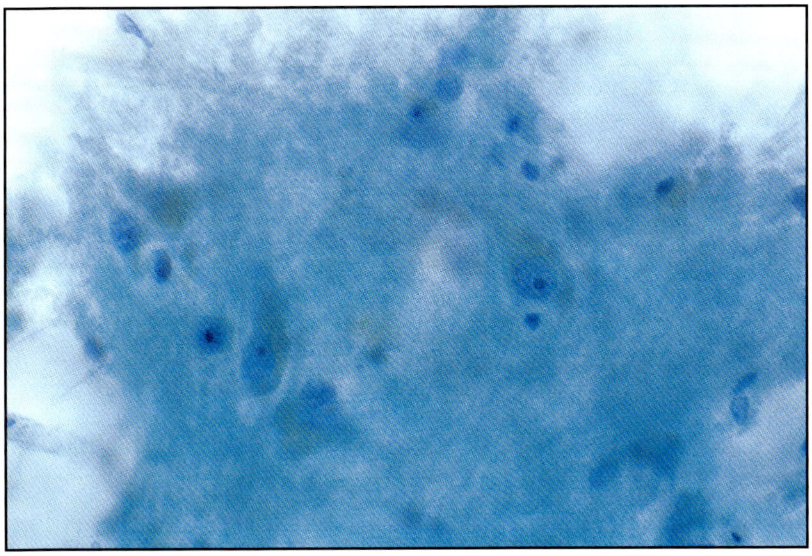

Image 8.2
Astrocytic and oligodendroglial nuclei in an imprint of normal white matter. In routine preparations, the cytoplasm and cytoplasmic processes of individual astrocytes cannot be distinguished from the surrounding neutrophil (Papanicolaou, 1,000X).

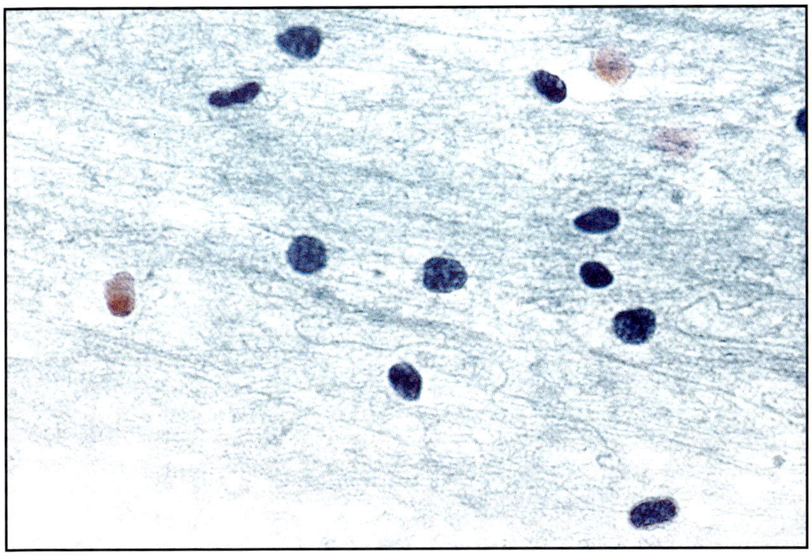

Image 8.3
This histologic section of gliosis demonstrates reactive astrocytes with abundant pink cytoplasm (H&E, 400X).

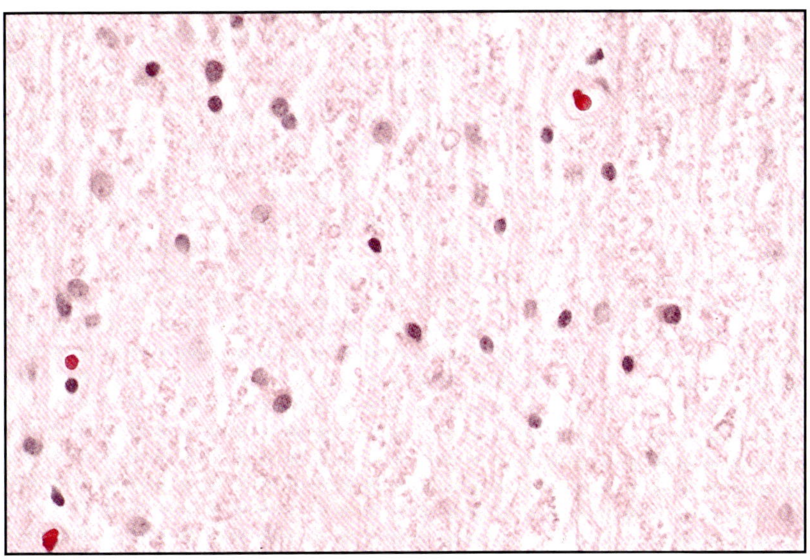

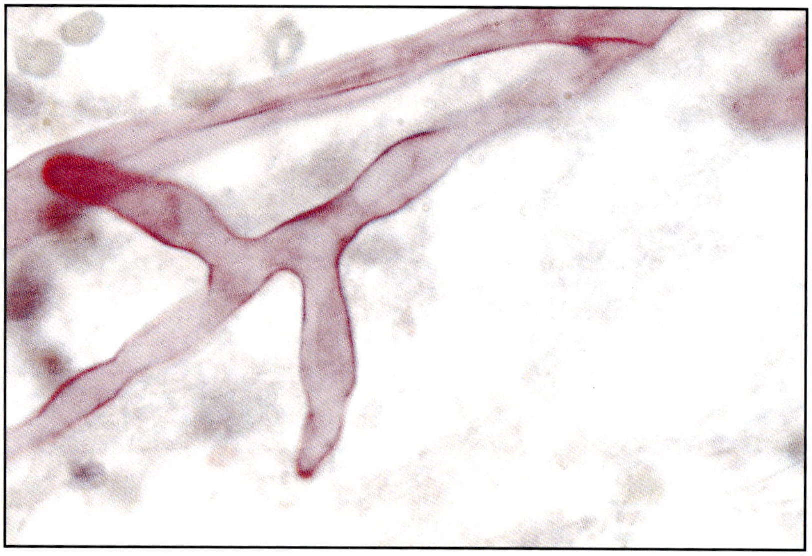

Image 8.4
Broad, nonseptate hyphae of mucormycosis in an aspirate from the patient whose scan is illustrated in Figure 8.2 (Periodic acid-Schiff, 1,000X).

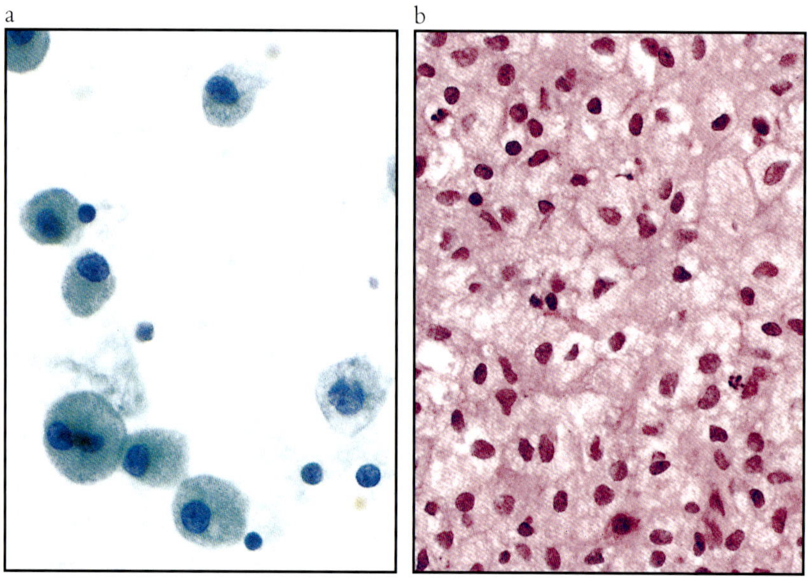

Image 8.5
Aspirate (a) and biopsy specimen (b) of a cerebral infarct show abundant foamy histiocytes that fill the center of these lesions (a, Papanicolaou, 600X; b, H&E, 400X).

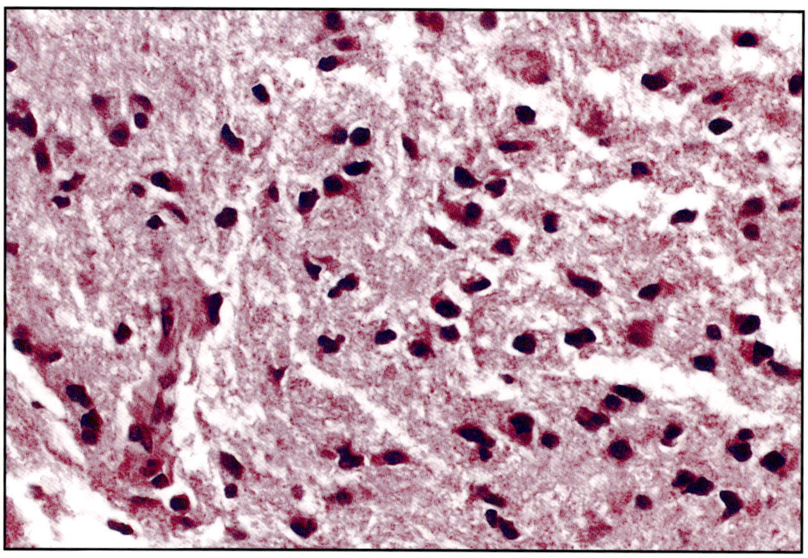

Image 8.6
Core needle biopsy specimen demonstrates the increased number of astrocytes with irregular hyperchromatic nuclei and fibrillar background typical of astrocytomas (H&E, 400X).

Image 8.7
Needle washing (a and b) of a microcystic astrocytoma (both, Papanicolaou, 400X).

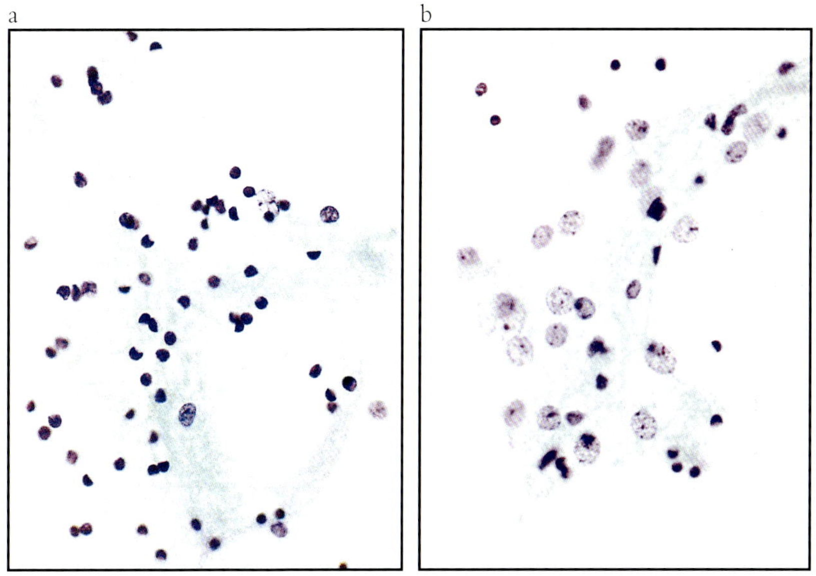

Core biopsy specimen (c and d) of a microcystic astrocytoma. The architecture with microcysts helps distinguish this lesion from gliosis and normal brain tissue (both, H&E; c, 200X; d, 400X).

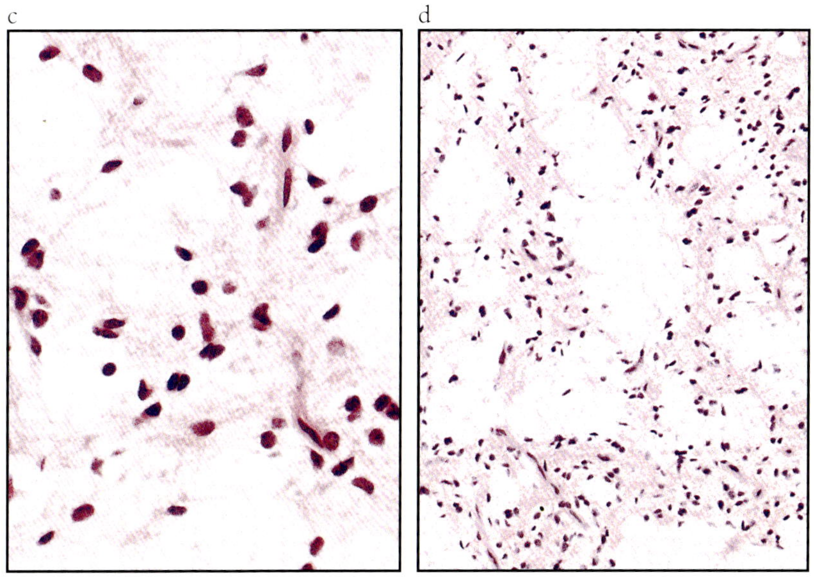

Image 8.8
Imprint (a) and core biopsy specimen (b) of an anaplastic astrocytoma showing the same features as the low-grade astrocytoma, but more nuclear irregularity and hypercellularity are apparent (both, H&E; a, 400X; b, 250X).

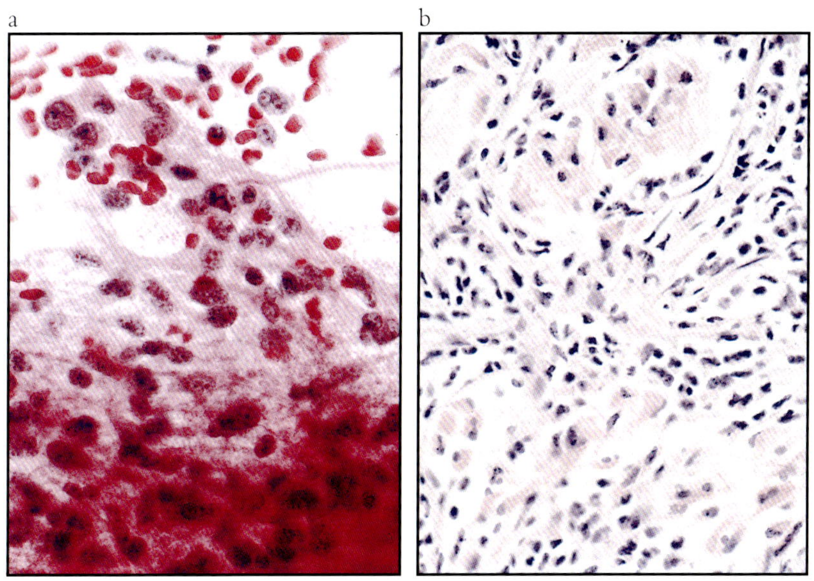

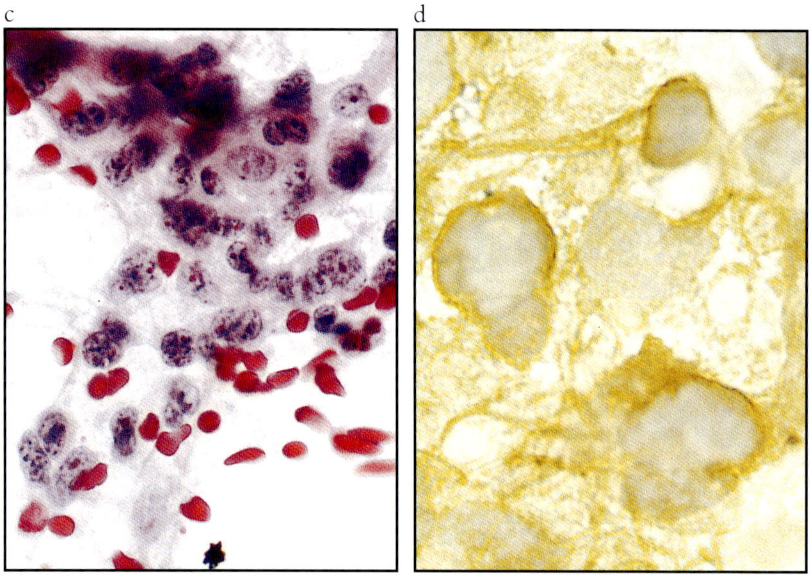

Imprint (c) of anaplastic astrocytoma. Immunoperoxidase for glial fibrillary acid protein (GFAP) readily demonstrates the glial derivation of these cells (d) (c, H&E, 600X; d, Immunoperoxidase, 1,000X).

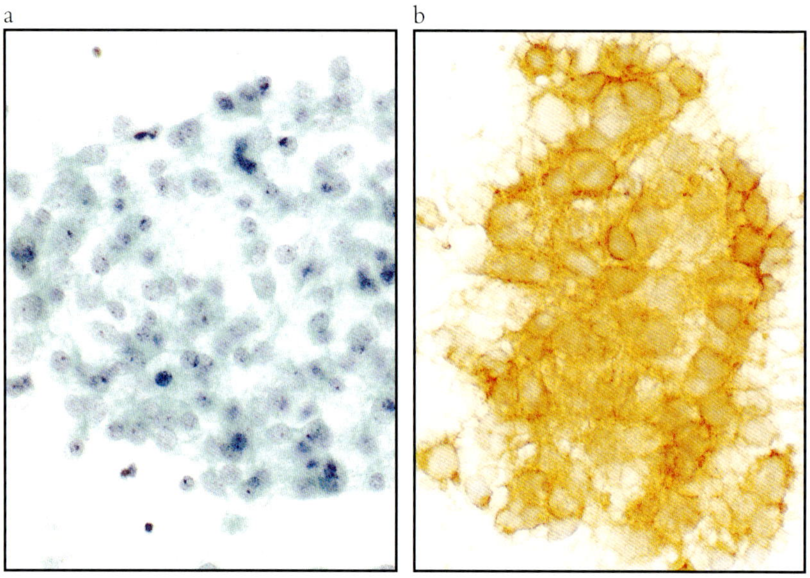

Image 8.9
Needle washings of glioblastoma multiforme show the same hypercellularity and fibrillary background as are seen in anaplastic astrocytomas (a, Papanicolaou, 400X; b, Immunoperoxidase for GFAP, 400X).

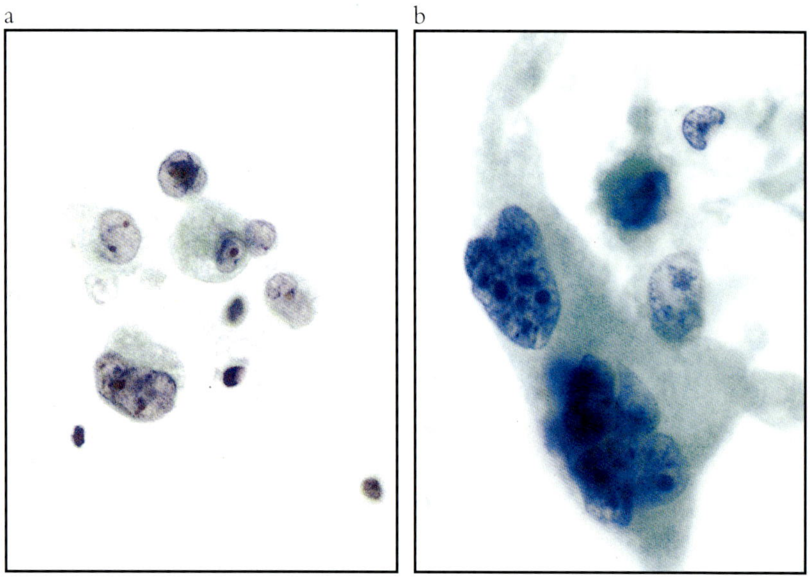

Image 8.10
Some glioblastomas contain pleomorphic forms with indistinct cell borders and fine cytoplasmic processes (Papanicolaou, 600X).

Image 8.11
This hypercellular cluster of malignant astrocytes seen in a needle washing is indistinguishable from cells of anaplastic astrocytomas (a). The accompanying core biopsy specimen, however, contains necrosis, which indicates that this lesion is actually a glioblastoma (b) (a, Papanicolaou, 400X; b, H&E, 200X).

a b

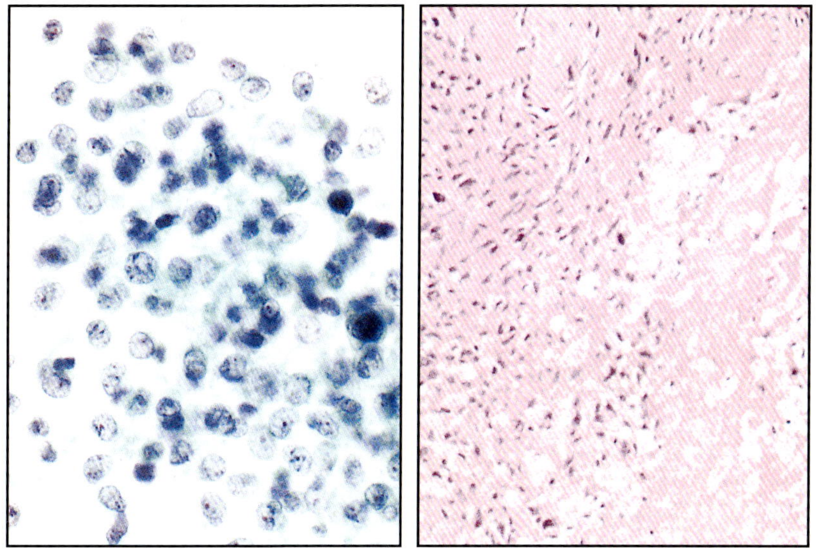

Image 8.12
This needle washing demonstrates neoplastic piloid or spindle-shaped astrocytes (a). An accompanying core biopsy specimen shows that this lesion is a glioblastoma with necrosis rather than a low-grade astrocytoma (b) (a, Papanicolaou, 600X; b, H&E, 400X).

a b

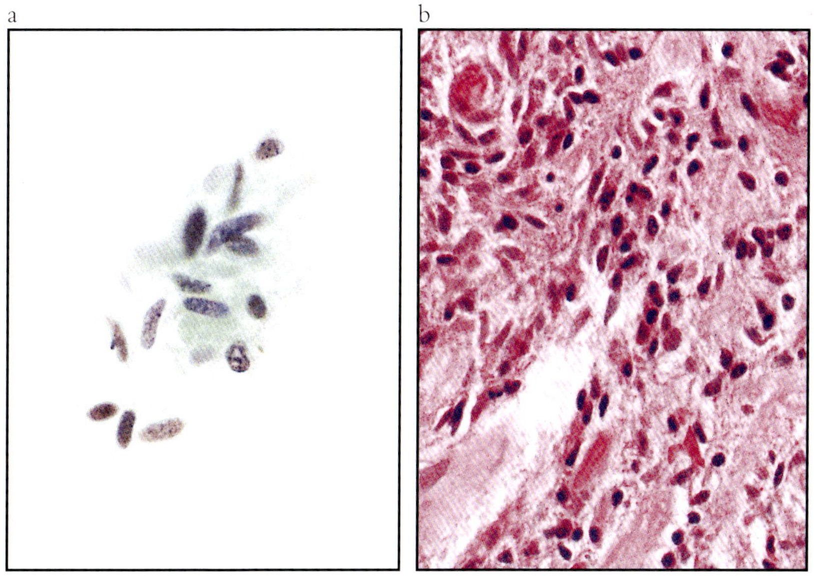

Image 8.13
Undifferentiated carcinoma of intermediate-to-large cell size metastatic to the brain in a needle washing (a) and core biopsy specimen (b) (a, Papanicolaou, 600X; b, H&E, 400X).

a b

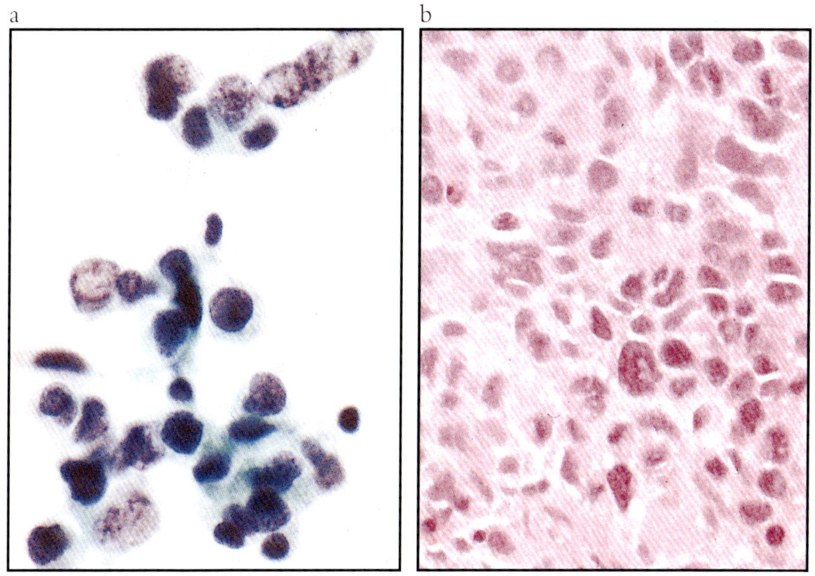

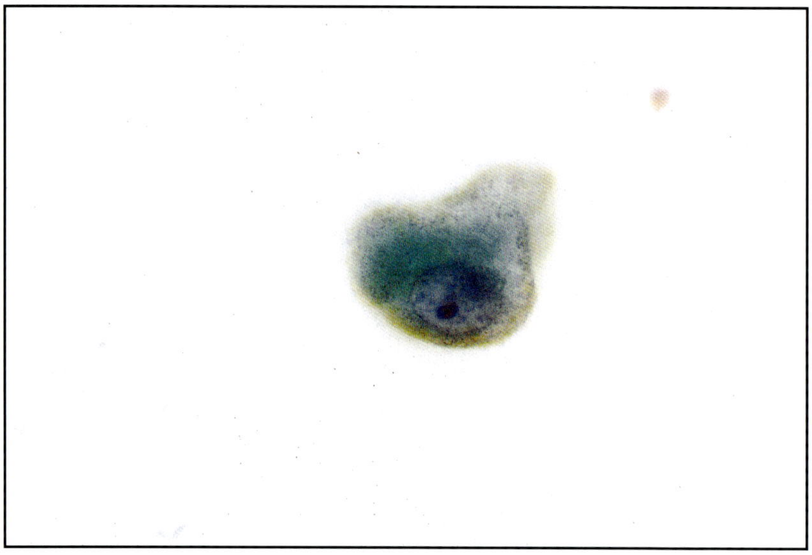

Image 8.14
Malignant cell with discrete cell borders and cytoplasmic melanin in a needle aspirate from melanoma metastatic to the brain (Papanicolaou, 1,000X).

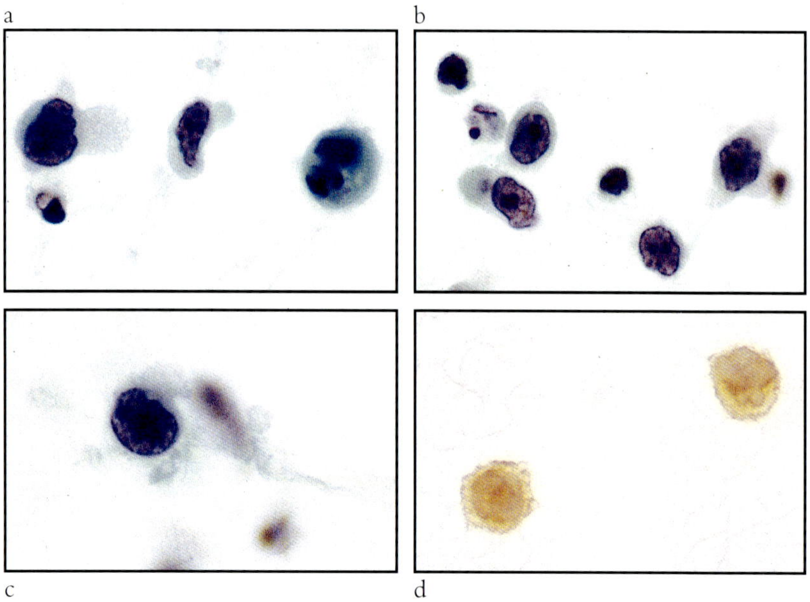

Image 8.15
Atypical lymphoid cells in a brain aspirate from a patient with mycosis fungoides (a through c). Immunoperoxidase confirms the T-cell derivation of these cells (d) (a through c, Papanicolaou; a, 600X; b and c, 1,000X; d, Immunoperoxidase, 600X). (This case is also illustrated in Chapter Five.)

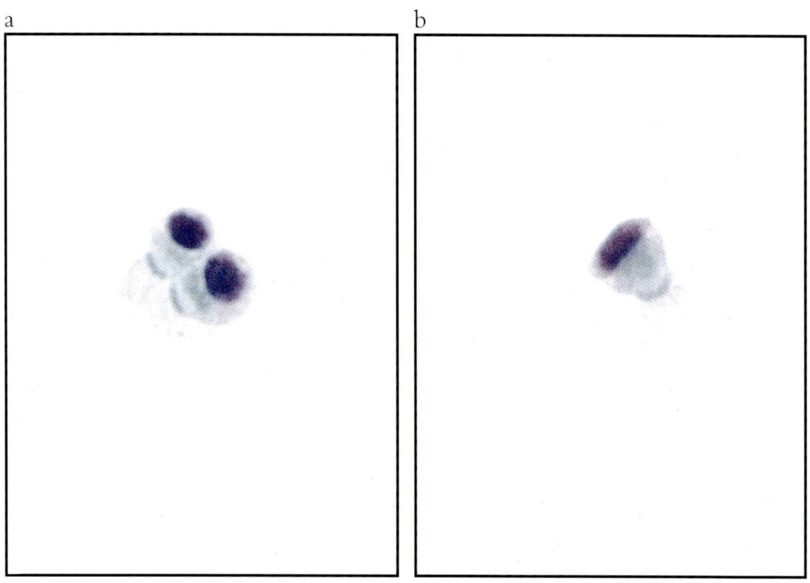

Image 8.16
Ciliated columnar cells in an aspirate from a colloid cyst of the third ventricle (Courtesy of Ed Cibas, MD) (Papanicolaou, 400X).

Image 8.17
Cystic astrocytoma in the thoracic spinal cord specimen of a 15-year-old girl (H&E, Luxol fast blue, 7X).

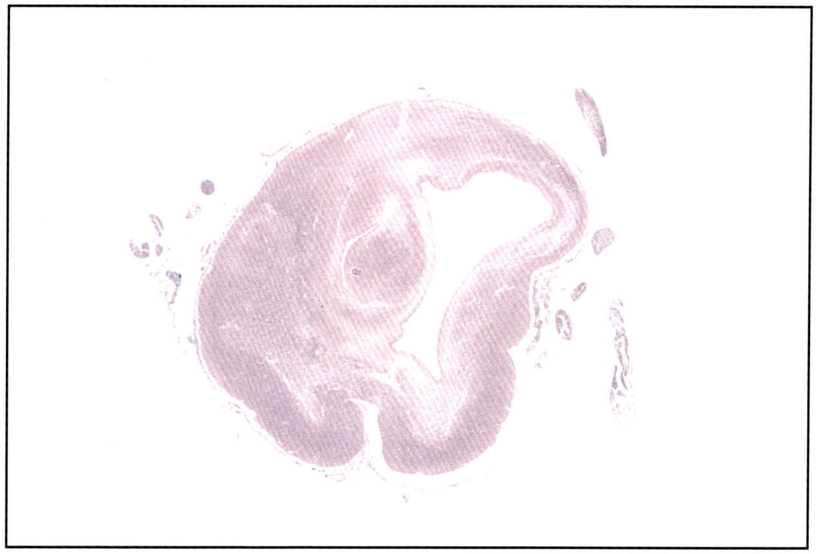

Image 8.18
This benign foam cell was seen in an aspirate from the cystic astrocytoma shown in Image 8.17 (a). This is a non-specific finding, since these cells are found in non-neoplastic cysts as well. At autopsy this lesion was shown to be an astrocytoma (b) (a, Papanicolaou, 1,000X; b, H&E, 200X).

a b

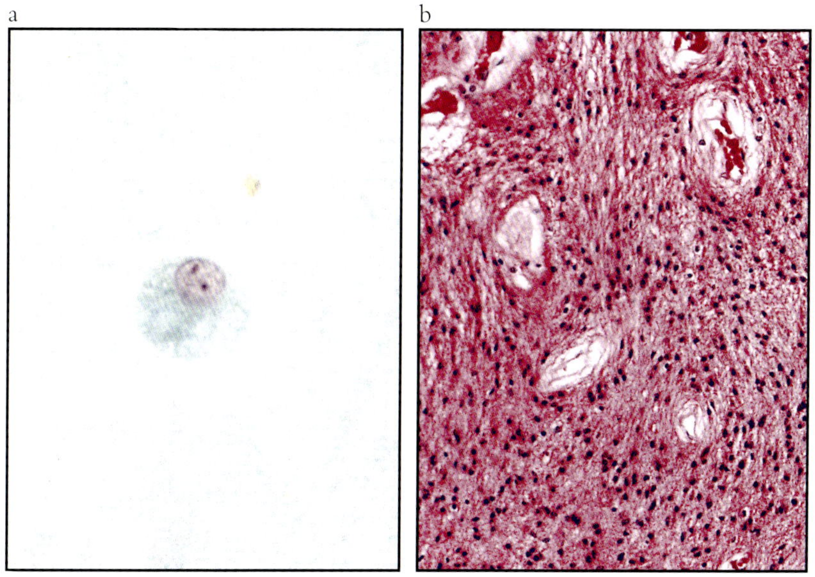

Image 8.19
Pleomorphic cells occurring singly in an aspirate from a cystic glioblastoma multiforme (Papanicolaou, 1,000X).

a b

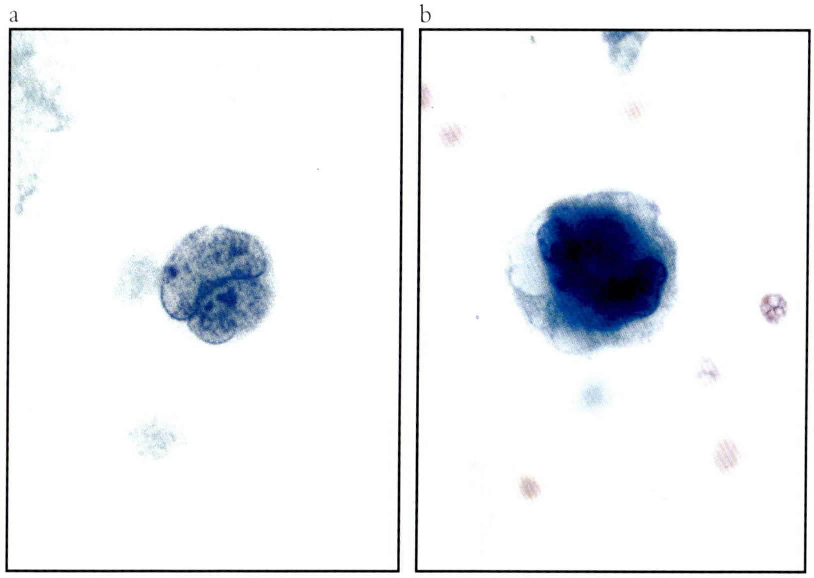

a b

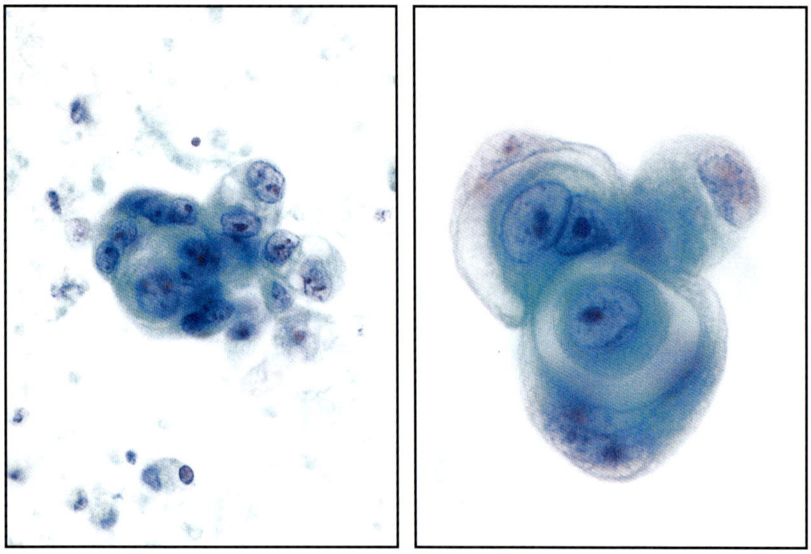

Image 8.20
Cohesive tissue fragments in an aspirate from a cystic metastatic adenocarcinoma (both, Papanicolaou; a, 600X; b, 1,000X).

a b

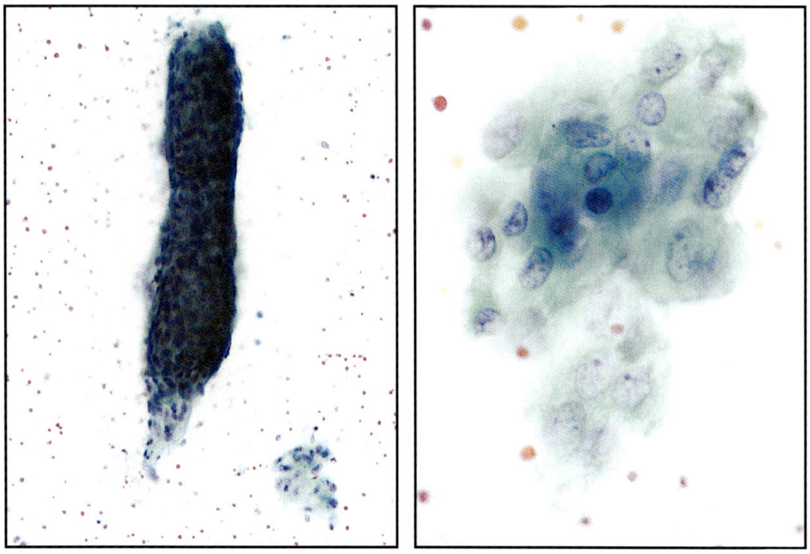

Image 8.21
Needle aspirates (a and b) of an orbital meningioma show whorls and syncytia of bland cells with ovoid nuclei (both, Papanicolaou; a, 200X; b, 400X).

c d

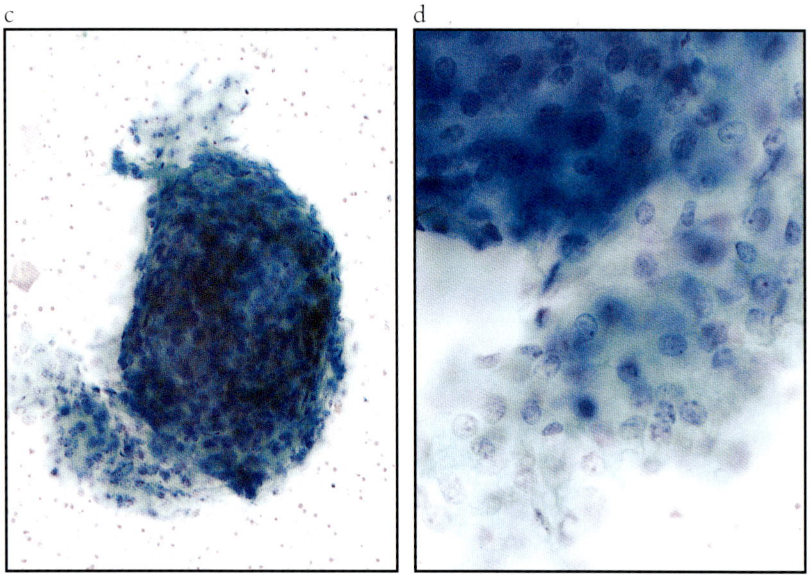

Needle aspirates (c and d) of an orbital meningioma show whorls and syncytia of bland cells with ovoid nuclei (both, Papanicolaou; c, 200X; d, 600X).

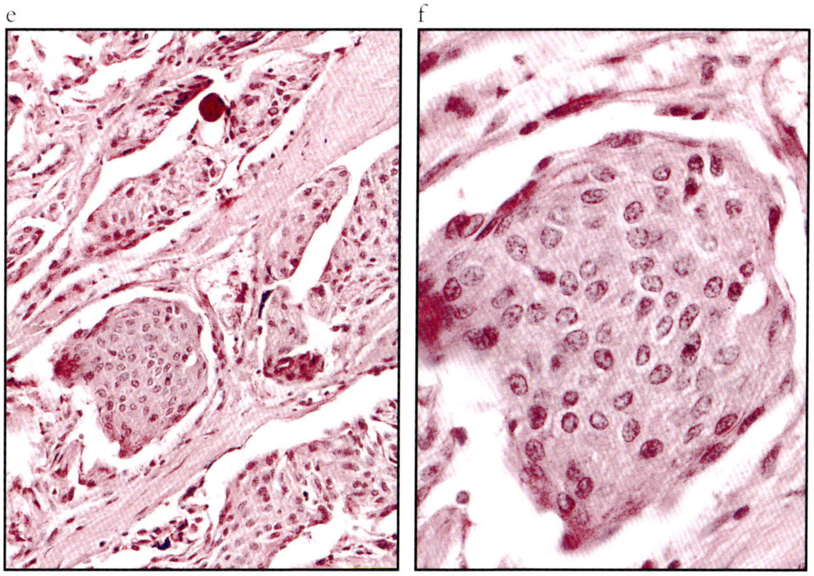

Resection (e and f) of an orbital meningioma (both, H&E; e, 200X; f, 400X).

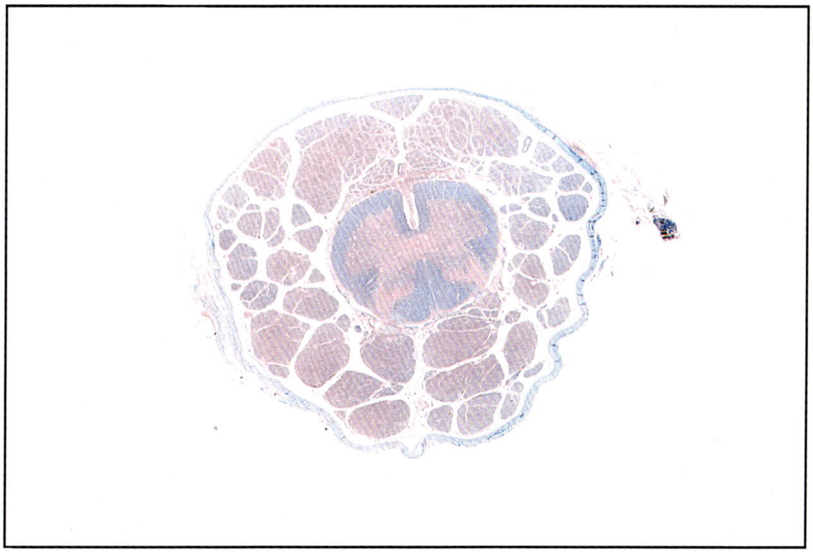

Image 8.22
Cross-section of lumbar spinal cord shows numerous nerve roots within the subarachnoid space (H&E, Luxol fast blue, 7X).

References

1. Bigner SH, Burger PC, Dubois PJ, Nashold BS, Moore JO, Johnston WW: The diagnosis of cerebral mucormycosis by needle aspiration biopsy. *Acta Cytol* 26:699–704, 1982.
2. Bigner SH, Friedman AH, Burger PC: Stereotactic biopsy of the central nervous system. In: Atkinson B, ed. *Atlas of Cytopathology.* Philadelphia, PA, WB Saunders and Co, 1992.
3. Cappabianca P, Spaziante R, Caputi F, Pettinato G, De Caro Del Basso M, Carrabs G, de Divitiis E. Accuracy of the analysis of multiple small fragments of glial tumors obtained by stereotactic biopsy. *Acta Cytol* 35:505–511, 1991.
4. Chandrasoma PT, Apuzzo MLJ: *Stereotactic Brain Biopsy.* Tokyo, Japan, Igaku-Shoin, 1989.
5. Conway LW: Stereotaxic diagnosis and treatment of intracranial tumors including an initial experience with cryosurgery for pinealomas. *J Neurosurg* 38:453–460, 1973.
6. Crain BJ, Bigner SH, Johnston WW: Fine needle aspiration biopsy of deep cerebrum: a comparison between normal and neoplastic morphology. *Acta Cytol* 26:772–778, 1982.
7. Edner G: Stereotaxic brain tumor biopsy: 5 years' experience. *Acta Neurochir* 31:261, 1975.
8. Finley JL, Silverman JF, Dickens MA: Immunocytochemical evaluation of central nervous system tumors obtained by the cavitron ultrasonic surgical aspirator. *Diagn Cytopathol* 6:308–312, 1990.
9. Hahn JF: Letter to the editor. *Neurosurgery* 6:119–120, 1980.
10. Liwnicz BH, Masukawa T, Henderson K: Thin needle aspiration cytology of intracranial lesions: a review of 50 cases. *Acta Cytol* 26:779–786, 1982.
11. Ostertag CB, Mennel HD, Kiessling M: Stereotactic biopsy of brain tumors. *Surg Neurol* 14:275–283, 1980.
12. Pecker J, Scarabin JM, Vallee B, Brucher JM: Treatment in tumours of the pineal region: value of stereotaxic biopsy. *Surg Neurol* 12:341–348, 1979.
13. Quencer RM: Needle aspiration of intramedullary and intradural extramedullary masses of the spinal canal. *Radiology* 124:115–116, 1980.
14. Rorat E, Yang W, DeLaTorre R: Fine needle aspiration cytology of parapharyngeal meningioma. *Acta Cytol* 35:497–500, 1990.
15. Shetter AG, Bertuccini TV, Pittman HW: Closed needle biopsy in the diagnosis of intracranial mass lesions. *Surg Neurol* 8:341–345, 1977.
16. Silverman JF, Jones FD, Unverferth M, Berns L: Cytopathology of neoplasms of the central nervous systems in specimens obtained by the cavitron ultrasonic surgical aspirator. *Acta Cytol* 33:576–582, 1989.
17. Zaharopoulos P, Wong JY: Cytology of common primary midline brain tumors. *Acta Cytol* 24:384–390, 1980.

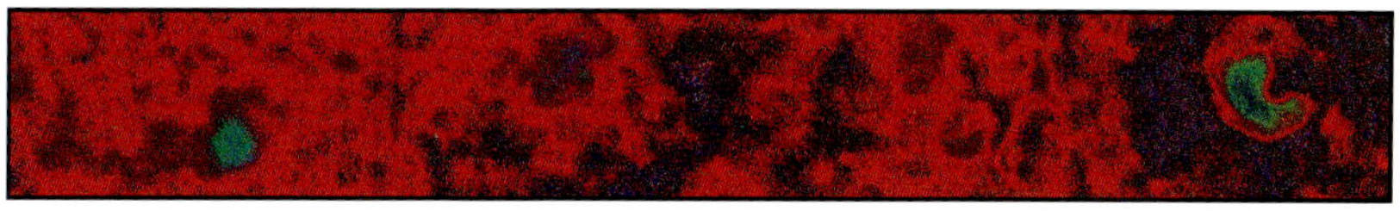

CHAPTER NINE

The Application of Immunohistochemistry to CSF and Brain Aspirates

One of the earliest applications of immunologic methods in tissue sections was the use of polyclonal antisera on renal biopsy specimens by immunofluorescence. In the early 1970s, the development of the Lukes/Collins classification of lymphomas, which was based on a combination of morphologic parameters and immunophenotyping, rapidly led to the extensive use of immunologic and histochemical procedures, such as sheep erythrocyte rosetting in the identification of T cells, nonspecific esterase and lysozyme in the identification of histiocytes, and the production of surface immunoglobulin by B lymphocytes.[10,11] Two important developments in the 1970s dramatically increased the application of immunologic methods to tissue samples: the peroxidase-antiperoxidase method and monoclonal antibodies.

Immunohistochemistry

Although immunofluorescence has the advantages of being rapid and simple, it has the disadvantages of preparations that are not permanent and of individual cellular morphology that cannot be discerned. These two problems were overcome by the use of horseradish peroxidase in the antibody conjugation method developed by Nakane and Kawaoi[13] and the peroxidase-antiperoxidase sandwich method of Sternberger et al.[19] These approaches use a primary antiserum raised against the substance for detection; a secondary antiserum against the species in which the primary antiserum was made; the peroxidase-antiperoxidase complex as a bridge; and diaminobenzidine (DAB) developed with peroxide and a chromogen to stain the cells containing the antigen in question. In the early 1980s, a modification of this concept produced the more sensitive avidin-biotin complex (ABC) method. In this technique, the secondary antibody is conjugated to biotin. Then avidin, which is covalently linked to an enzyme such as horseradish peroxidase, alkaline phosphatase, or a fluorochromosome, is allowed to complex with the biotin.[2] DAB reacts with the avidin, and the reaction is developed with peroxide. Substitution of streptavidin for avidin increases the sensitivity of the reaction and allows a broader spectrum of chromogens to be used. The use of alkaline phosphatase in place of the peroxidase circumvents the interference of endogenous peroxidases, which is a common problem in specimens of CSF.

Monoclonal Antibodies

The usefulness of any antiserum or antibody is dependent on its specificity. In preparing a polyclonal antiserum, specificity is determined by the purity of the immunogen and by the thoroughness of absorptions to remove nonspecific cross-reactivity. Major disadvantages of polyclonal antisera are that each batch is limited in quantity and that each new batch has an entirely different titer and characteristics. Thus, each batch must be individually titrated and its patterns of reactivity assessed. This problem has been overcome by the development of monoclonal antibody technology.[8] In this procedure, a mouse is immunized with the antigen. When an antibody response is detected against the immunogen, the immunized mouse spleen cells are harvested and fused in vitro with a mouse myeloma cell line (Figure 9.1). The resultant hybrids are plated as individual cells, and single-cell clones are developed, each of which produces a single antibody that reacts with a single epitope. The majority of these epitopes are not specific for the immunizing substance but are shared among many molecules. Thus, an important step in preparing these reagents is to screen hundreds or thousands of the hybridomas to select the few that are specific for the immunogen. An additional problem with hybridomas is instability. Many of these clones shut down antibody production, an occurrence that can often be prevented by early and repeated cloning. However, once a stable hybridoma that produces a specific monoclonal antibody is obtained, it provides a perpetual source for the reagent. Antibody is obtained by growing the cells in culture and harvesting the supernatant or by growing the cells intraperitoneally in mice and harvesting the ascites.

Monoclonal antibody technology has expanded the application of immunohistochemistry to tissue samples

The development of monoclonal antibody technology has contributed to the rapid expansion in the application of immunohistochemistry to tissue samples, because large quantities of antibodies specific for a vast variety of substances can be produced and are readily available through commercial laboratories. In addition to antibodies produced against defined products, hybridomas have been made using whole cells or tissue homogenates as immunogens. These approaches have yielded operationally useful reagents for detecting specific cell types in the absence of knowledge of the nature of the epitope-bearing molecule. These antibodies have not only been applied in tumor diagnosis and classification, but they

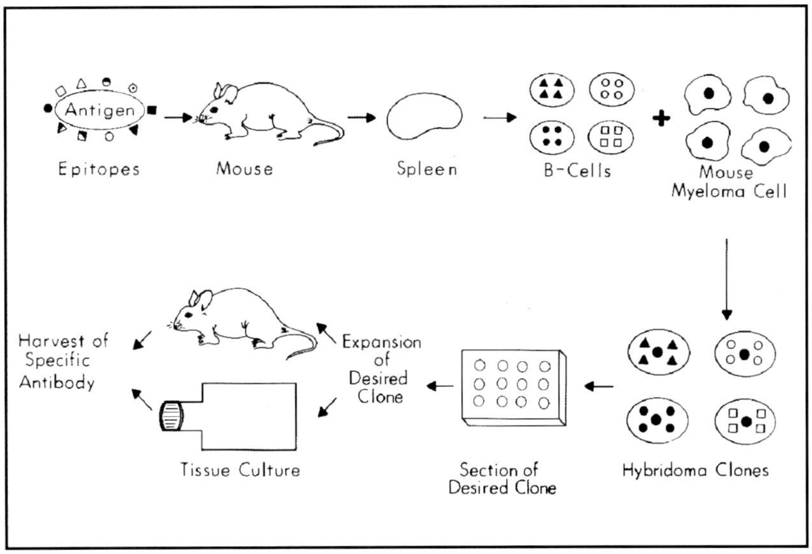

Figure 9.1
To produce a mouse monoclonal antibody, the antigen in question is injected into a mouse. The spleen is removed, and B cells, each producing an antibody against a single epitope, are harvested. Then, B cells are fused with a mouse myeloma cell line, and the resultant hybridoma cells are cloned. Each clone produces an antibody against a different epitope. These clones are screened to select those producing antibodies of the desired specificities; the selected clones are expanded; and their antibodies are harvested.

have been used to isolate the epitope-bearing molecules, leading to the discovery of new proteins important in tumor biology.

Chimeric Antibodies

Although the end product of monoclonal antibody technology is a unique and useful immunologic reagent, the generation of these tools is tedious, time consuming, and expensive. Recent advances in molecular cloning techniques have resulted in precise and specific chimeric antibodies that are generated in vitro.[14] The variable regions of the immunoglobulin light-chain and heavy-chain genes—VH and VL—confer specificity. The rest of the molecule is termed the constant region and, although species specific, is the same among immunoglobulin genes. This fact has led to the generation of vectors that contain these conserved portions of the immunoglobulin genes. To produce a chimeric antibody, one can then clone specific cDNA sequences that code for the variable region (VH and VL) that detects the epitope of choice from murine hybridoma cells (Figure 9.2). These exons are then spliced into expression vectors that contain the human constant region genes for the heavy and light immunoglobulin chains. These two vectors are cotransfected into a nonproducing myeloma cell line that produces the desired chimeric antibody in vitro. Not only are specific reagents produced, but the conserved portion of the resultant antibody is of human rather than rodent or rabbit origin. These reagents are thus better suited for therapeutic administration than rabbit antisera or mouse monoclonal antibodies, which can elicit toxicity due to the species differences.

The conserved portion of a chimeric antibody is of human origin, and thus is better suited for therapeutic administration

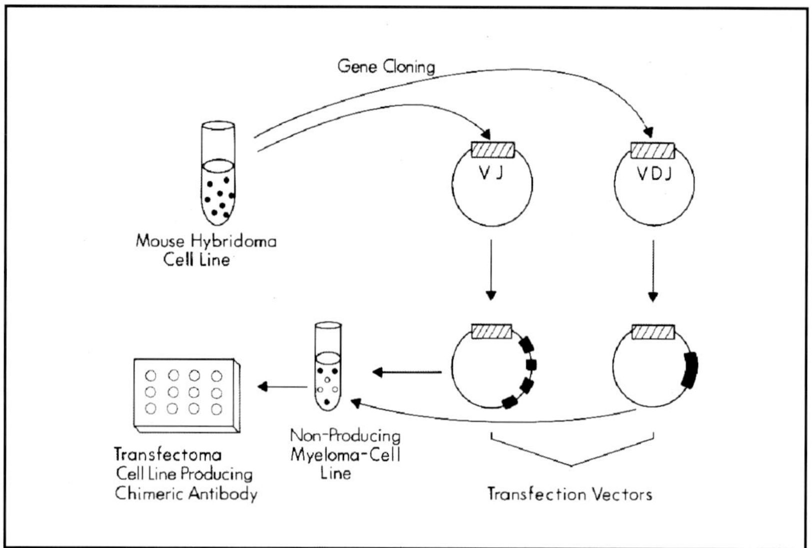

Figure 9.2
To produce a chimeric antibody, the light- (VJ) and heavy- (VDJ) chain variable regions are cloned from a mouse hybridoma cell line that produces the target antibody. These sequences are spliced into transfection vectors that contain the constant regions for the human light- and heavy-chain genes. These vectors are cotransfected into a nonproducing myeloma cell line, and clones are derived that produce a human/mouse chimeric antibody molecule.

Pitfalls in Immunohistochemistry

The basic steps in carrying out an immunohistochemical procedure are relatively simple and straightforward; the methods used in our laboratory are given in detail in the Cytologic Techniques section of Chapter One. The major areas leading to problems in performing and interpreting these preparations are antibody specificity, antibody concentration, controls, and fixation.

Antibody Specificity

A common misconception concerning monoclonal antibodies is that they are uniformly specific. Even after careful selection of monoclonal antibodies for specific reactivity, the presence of the detected epitope on a related or unrelated molecule remains a possibility. One useful means of excluding this possibility is to test the antibody against a panel of purified, structurally related proteins that are potential sources of cross-reactivity. Image 9.1 shows an immunoblot of monoclonal antibodies made against purified bovine glial fibrillary acid protein (GFAP).[17] One antibody detects an epitope that is specific for GFAP. The other antibody, although it detects GFAP, also detects another intermediate filament protein, vimentin, because the epitope it detects is shared among these closely related proteins. This approach is useful in detecting potential cross-reactivity among structurally related molecules, but it does not exclude cross-reactivity with molecules whose overall structure is grossly not related but that nevertheless bear the same epitope. Testing for this possibility is best performed on a series of cases of known diagnoses rep-

Testing for antibody specificity should be performed on cases of known diagnoses

resenting the following: cell types with which the antibody is expected to react; cell types expected to be negative for the antigen; and cell types that potentially could be distinguished using the antibody in a diagnostic setting. Table 9.1 illustrates such an approach using a panel of antibodies on specimens derived from the central nervous system (CNS).

Antibody Concentration

Any antibody will react with a given cell if it is used in a high-enough concentration

A simple but often-overlooked principle in using antibodies is that any antibody will react with a given cell if it is used in a high-enough concentration and, conversely, that the same antibody will fail to react with the same cell if it is diluted sufficiently. The best working concentration for each antibody is the point at which it can discriminate the cell types under investigation. The best way to determine this point is to titrate the antibody on replicate cell samples known to express the antigen and cell samples known not to express the antigen. At the same time, an irrelevant antibody of the same isotype should be used at similar concentrations. Image 9.2 shows the results of such a titration in which an antibody against GFAP stains a glioma cell line but is negative for a sarcoma line at the same concentration. The negative control antibody when used at the same concentration is negative for both cell types. When antibodies are purchased from companies, the reagents are often supplied diluted to a concentration near the recommended working dilution. In these cases, one should still perform a limited titration rather than simply using the concentration recommended by the distributor.

Controls

The most important control that should be applied to each sample tested is an irrelevant antibody of the same isotype as the primary antibody used at the same concentration. For polyclonal antisera, the corresponding control is ideally pre-immune serum from the animal in which

Table 9.1
Summary of Antibody Reactivity Patterns

	UJ13A	α-GFAP	B72.3	Cytokeratin	2D1	S-100	Mel-14	HMB-45
Gliomas	+	+	–	–	±	+	+	Unknown
Normal Brain Fragment	+	+	–	–	–	+	+	Unknown
Nonglial Primary CNS Tumors	+	–	–	–	–	+	+	Unknown
Small-Cell Undifferentiated Carcinoma and Embryonal Rhabdomyosarcoma	+	–	–	±	–	–	–	–
Non–Small-Cell Carcinoma	–	–	+	+	–	±	–	–
Melanoma	–	–	–	–	–	+	+	+
Lymphoma, Leukemia	–	–	–	–	+	–	–	–
Inflammation	–	–	–	–	+	–	–	–

the antiserum was made. If this preparation is not available, normal serum from an animal of the same species can be substituted. A broadly reactive antibody, such as one reactive with all human cells, should be included to ensure that the sample retains antigen expression. In addition, a known-positive and known-negative case should each be included to check the general integrity of the procedure.

Fixation

Some fixatives destroy some antigens, making the choice of fixative an important consideration in designing immunohistochemical studies. Many of the antilymphocyte monoclonal antibodies only work on air-dried cells with a brief exposure to acetone. In contrast, some reagents have been specifically designed and selected to react with fixed cells. The best approach is to test each monoclonal antibody on replicate samples prepared with a spectrum of fixatives to determine optimal conditions for its application. The method of slide preparation is particularly critical for CSF where only limited cellular material may be available. In our laboratory, replicate Cytospin® samples are made in all cases where sufficient volume is present. These slides are air-dried, stored at –70 °C, and can thus be retrieved and postfixed in the fixative of choice for applying appropriate antibodies.

Test each monoclonal antibody on replicate samples prepared with a spectrum of fixatives

Antibodies Useful for CSF and CNS Aspirates

Antibodies that are helpful in evaluating samples of CSF and brain aspirates can be divided into three categories. First, as discussed in Chapters Three and Five, immunophenotyping panels can be applied to these samples, just as they can be to lymph node aspirates and body cavity fluids, to distinguish between reactive lymphocytosis and lymphoma (Image 9.3). A second application is the use of antibodies to distinguish primary brain tumors from metastatic carcinoma, melanoma, and lymphoma, a problem commonly encountered in examining CSF and needle aspirates of brain lesions when cytologically malignant cells of undetermined derivation are identified. Table 9.1 lists a selection of antibodies that have proved useful in evaluating malignant CNS specimens in our laboratory.[18,20] Most gliomas, including all grades of astrocytomas, ependymomas, and oligodendrogliomas, react with GFAP antibodies (Image 9.4) and pan-neuroectodermal antibody UJ13A, which detects neural cell adhesion molecule (N-CAM).[1,16] These tumors fail to react with antibodies against cytokeratin and B72.3, an anticarcinoma antibody. Although the majority of these tumors are negative with panleukocyte antibody 2D1, occasional tumors are positive with this antibody. Thus, this pattern of reactivity can be used to distinguish gliomas as a group. Nonglial primary brain tumors, including medulloblastomas, neuroblastomas, retinoblastomas, pineoblastomas, and meningiomas, differ from gliomas only in that they are negative for GFAP. Small-cell carcinoma of the lung reacts identically with nonglial primary brain tumors, making this panel ineffective in distinguishing this type of carcinoma from other small-cell neoplasms.

Non–small-cell carcinomas, including large-cell undifferentiated carcinomas, adenocarcinomas from a variety of organs, and squamous cell carcinoma, show an entirely different pattern of reactivity, with negative reactions with GFAP, UJ13A, and 2D1 and positive reactions with anticytokeratins (Image 9.5). In addition, most adenocarcinomas and some large-cell carcinomas stain with B72.3 (Image 9.6). Melanomas react with S-100 protein antibodies and antimelanoma monoclonal antibodies such as HMB-45 and Mel-14 (Images 9.7 and 9.8).[15] Since normal brain tissue and primary CNS tumors also stain with these reagents, negative reactivity with UJ13A and GFAP are also important factors in distinguishing among melanomas and these cell types. Additionally, S-100 reacts with about one third of carcinomas, making it unwise to use this reagent alone in distinguishing melanoma from other types of metastases.[3,4,7,9] Lymphomas demonstrate a unique pattern, staining only with 2D1.

Although we have found the panel shown in Table 9.1 to be useful in categorizing the majority of cases of malignant cells in CSF, observations of immunohistochemical reactions in tissue sections of brain tumors raise the possibility of several pitfalls. Franke et al[5] described sporadic examples of cross-reactivity of some desmin and cytokeratin antibodies with glia and of occasional staining of neurofilament and keratin antibodies with examples of anaplastic gliomas. Gould et al[6] demonstrated GFAP positivity in bipotential cells in medulloblastomas. Immunohistochemical studies of cells in CSF using these antibodies on additional cases will be necessary to determine if these potential pitfalls present diagnostic difficulties when applied to cells in CSF.

Although antibody panels are useful in evaluating many types of cells in CSF, there are pitfalls and limitations

The major limitations of this panel are its inability to subclassify gliomas, to distinguish among most of the small round-cell tumors of childhood, and to distinguish neoplastic from non-neoplastic cells within the CNS. No antibodies have been developed to date that have been conclusively shown to differentiate among gliomas. β-Galactosidase selectively stains normal oligodendroglia, but these antibodies do not reliably distinguish oligodendrogliomas from other types of glial neoplasms. Synaptophysin, N-CAM, and neurofilament protein are expressed by most small, round cell central and peripheral nervous system tumors of neurogenic origin, including neuroblastoma, retinoblastoma, pineoblastoma, and medulloblastoma, but antibodies are not available that distinguish these tumors from one another[6,12,21] (Table 9.2). GFAP and UJ13A stain normal and reactive brain tissues, negating their usefulness in distinguishing glial neoplasms from these tissues. The panleukocyte reagent used in the panel, 2D1, was chosen for its broad reactivity with a spectrum of types of lymphomas, although it is negative for the majority of nonlymphoid neoplasms. It does, however, stain most types of non-neoplastic leukocytes, making it useless in distinguishing lymphoma from reactive lymphocytoses. For this specific problem, a panel of antilymphocytic-subtype antibodies can be used as discussed previously.

The third type of useful antibodies is the small group of cell type–specific reagents, such as: antibodies against prostatic-specific antigen (PSA) and prostatic acid phosphatase (PAP) to detect neoplastic and non-neoplastic cells of prostatic origin; anticalcitonin antibodies to detect medullary thyroid carcinoma and other calcitonin-secreting neoplasms; and antibodies against the pituitary hormones. Although these reagents are exquisitely precise, clinical settings where they can be applied to CNS

Table 9.2
Antibody Reactivity of Small-Cell Childhood Tumors

	Synaptophysin	N-CAM	Neurofilament Protein	GFAP	Vimentin	Desmin	p30/32 MIC2
Neuroblastoma, Pineoblastoma, Retinoblastoma	±	+	+	–	–	±	–
Medulloblastoma	+	+	+	±	+	–	–
Ewing's Sarcoma	–	–	–	–	+	–	+
Embryonal Rhabdomyosarcoma	–	+	–	–	+	+	±
Lymphoma	–	–	–	–	–	–	–

samples occur only infrequently. Image 9.9 shows metastatic prostatic carcinoma in a needle biopsy specimen of a brain lesion, the origin of which was confirmed by its positivity for PSA and PAP.

Current Developments and Future Applications

This chapter has focused on the immunohistochemical application of antibodies to CNS specimens for diagnosis and tumor classification. In the nervous system, as well as other body sites, antibodies conjugated to toxins or isotopes are being used therapeutically in some clinical settings. Since these applications require demonstration that the tumor cells react with the antibody being applied therapeutically, an increasingly important role of the cytopathologist and cytotechnologist is to carry out these immunohistochemical reactions on cytologic preparations from the CNS. For meningeal carcinomatosis and meningeal spread of primary brain tumors, antibodies bearing high doses of isotopes can be injected directly into the intrathecal compartment by way of the ventricles or subarachnoid space, and treatment within this enclosed area minimizes exposure of the bone marrow, liver, and kidneys. This type of treatment is completely dependent on the ability of the cytopathology laboratory to demonstrate reactivity of the tumor cells in CSF with the therapeutic antibody. Another example of closed-compartment therapy is the injection of radiolabelled antibodies into the cystic cavities that occur in a subgroup of malignant gliomas. Although in cases where one is unable to isolate tumor cells from the cyst fluid itself, needle aspiration of the cyst wall is a viable means for obtaining tumor cells for testing of antibody reactivity. This step is important in a large proportion of these patients, since their initial tumor resection may have been performed without preparation of tissue samples for immunohistology. As more tumor-specific antibodies become available, particularly using the molecular approaches that will be discussed in Chapter Ten, the cytopathology laboratory will increasingly become involved as part of these therapeutic teams.

An important role of the cytopathologist and cytotechnologist is to carry out these immunohistochemical reactions on cytologic preparations from the CNS

Image 9.1
Transblots of cytoskeletal proteins from primary cultures of rat astrocytes stained with monoclonal antibodies to bovine glial fibrillary acid protein (GFAP) and polyvalent antivimentin. Antibody 2B11A4 shows only one band by immunoblot analysis. This band exhibits the same mobility as GFAP and confirms the specificity of this reagent. Antibody 4A12H5, in contrast, shows bands similar to both GFAP and vimentin, which demonstrates that the epitope it detects is common to these two molecules.

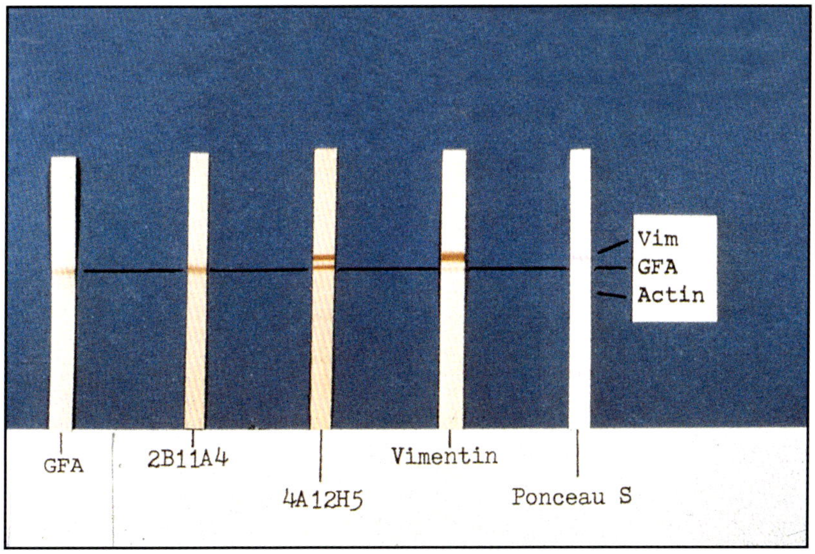

Image 9.2
The optimal concentration for applying a GFAP monoclonal antibody is the highest concentration at which the positive control glioma cells are positive (a), while the negative control antibody at the same concentration is negative (b). At this same concentration, both the GFAP antibody (c) and negative control antibody (d) are negative for sarcoma cells (all, Immunohistochemistry using GFAP antibody, 1,000X).

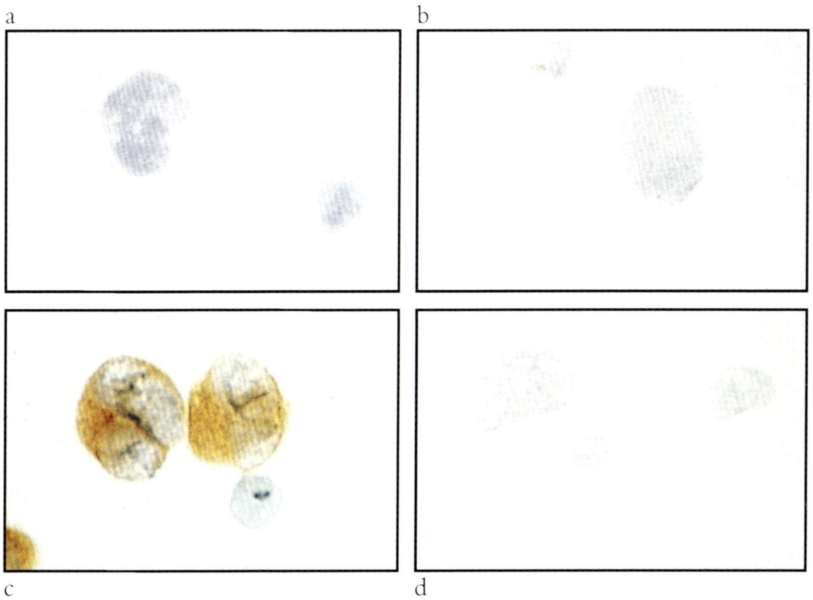

Image 9.3
B-cell lymphoma in CSF shows a monoclonal IgM lambda population (a, Romanowski, 1,000X; Immunoperoxidase for kappa (b) and lambda chain (c), 600X).

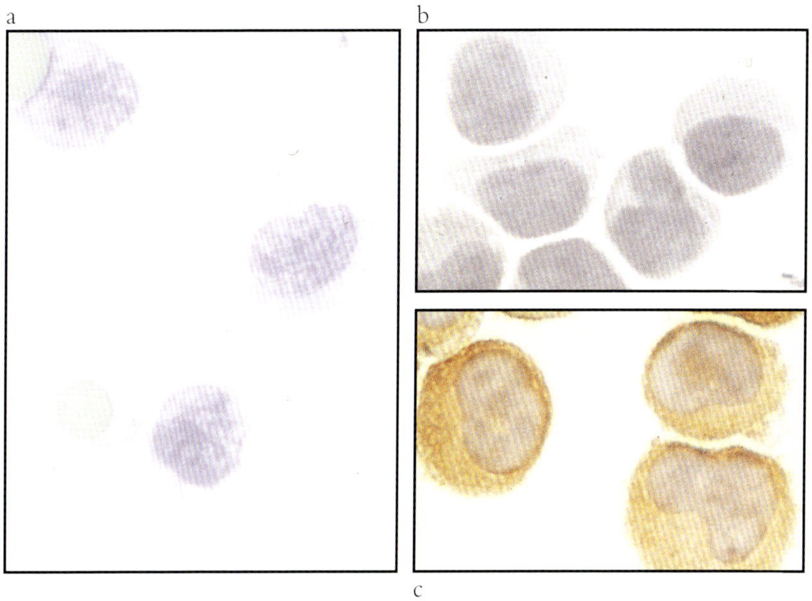

a b

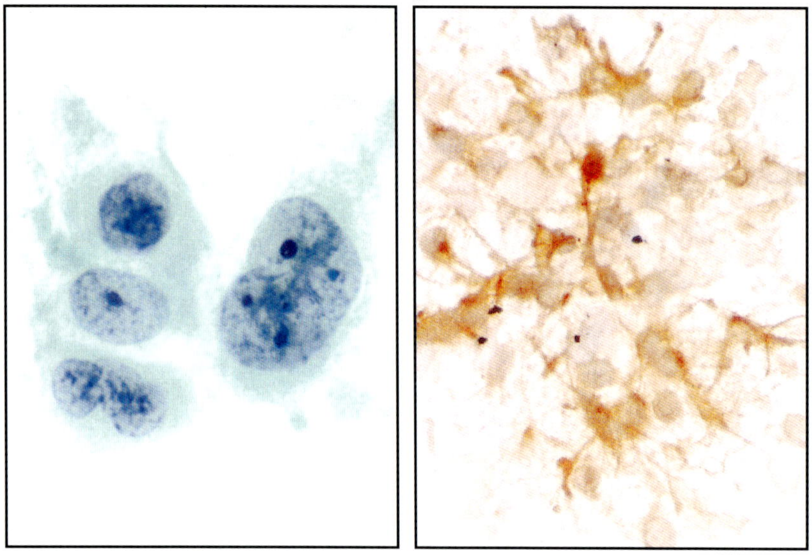

Image 9.4
Glioblastoma in a needle aspirate of a brain lesion expresses GFAP (a, Papanicolaou, 600X; b, Immunoperoxidase for GFAP, 400X).

a b

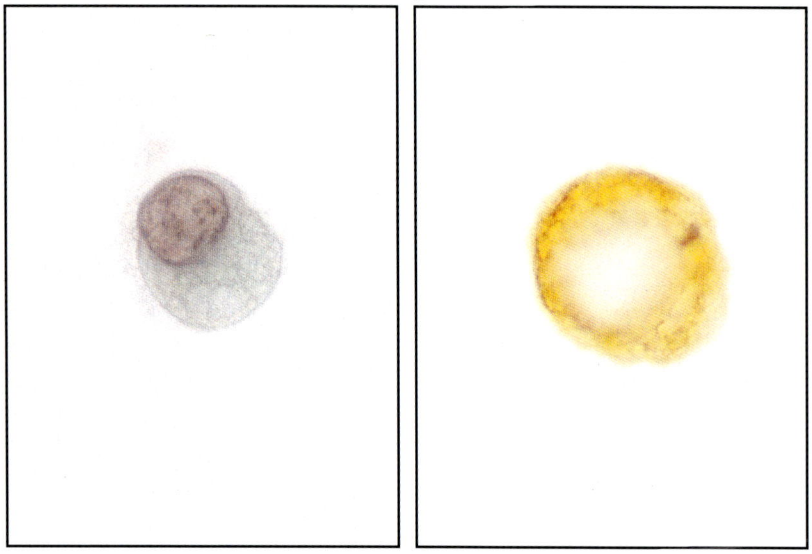

Image 9.5
Adenocarcinoma from the lung in CSF expresses cytokeratin (a, Papanicolaou, 1,000X; b, Immunoperoxidase for cytokeratin AE13, 1,000X).

a b

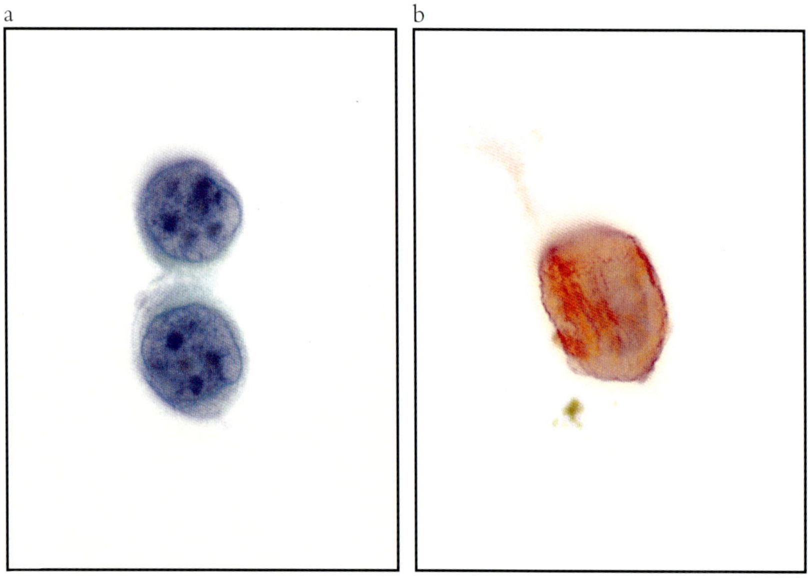

Image 9.6
Large-cell undifferentiated carcinoma from the lung in CSF expresses B72.3 (a, Papanicolaou, 1,000X; b, Immunoperoxidase for B72.3, 1,000X).

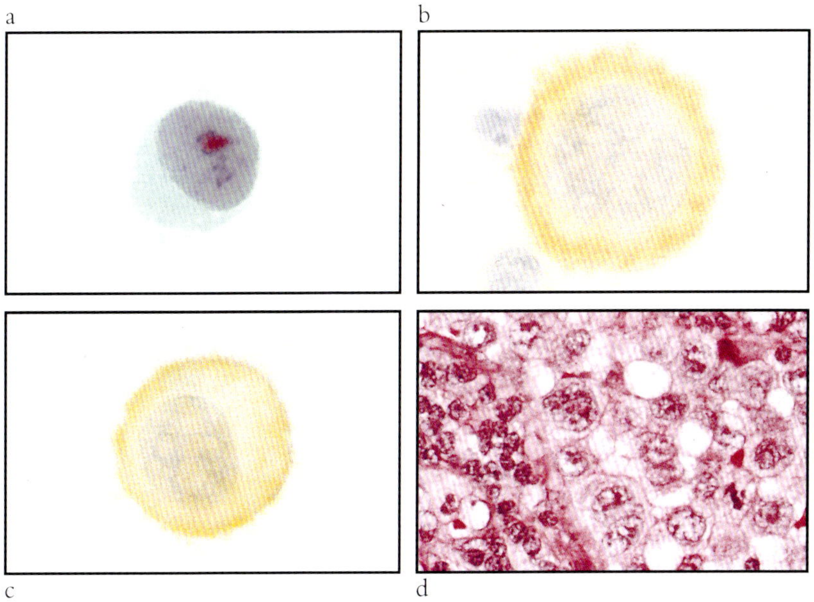

Image 9.7
Melanoma in CSF expresses S-100 protein (b) and antimelanoma antibody Mel-14 (c). Histologic section of this patient's melanoma metastatic to a lymph node (d) (a, Papanicolaou, 1,000X; b, Immunoperoxidase for S-100 protein, 1,000X; c, Immunoperoxidase for Mel-14, 1,000X; d, H&E, 400X).

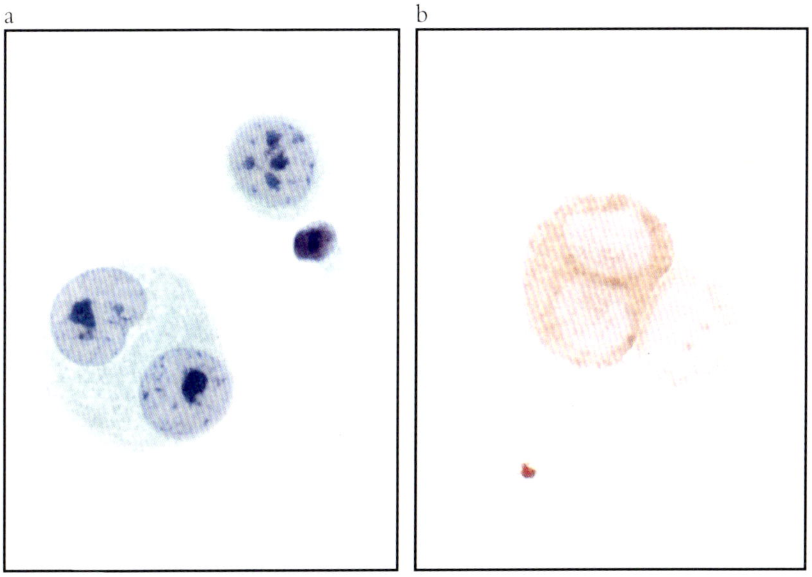

Image 9.8
Melanoma in CSF expresses HMB-45 (a, Papanicolaou, 1,000X; b, Immunoperoxidase for HMB-45, 1,000X).

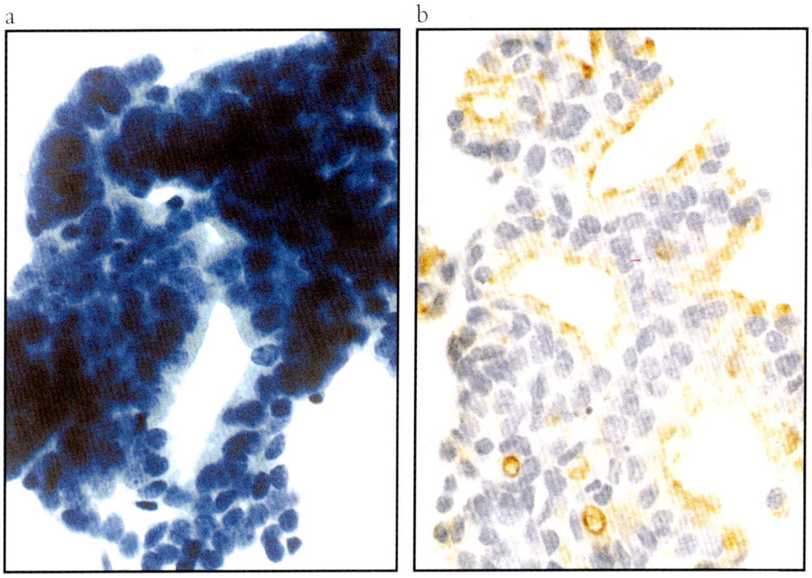

Image 9.9
Needle aspirate (a and b) of metastatic prostatic adenocarcinoma of the brain (a, Papanicolaou, 400X; b, Immunoperoxidase for prostatic-specific antigen, 400X).

c d

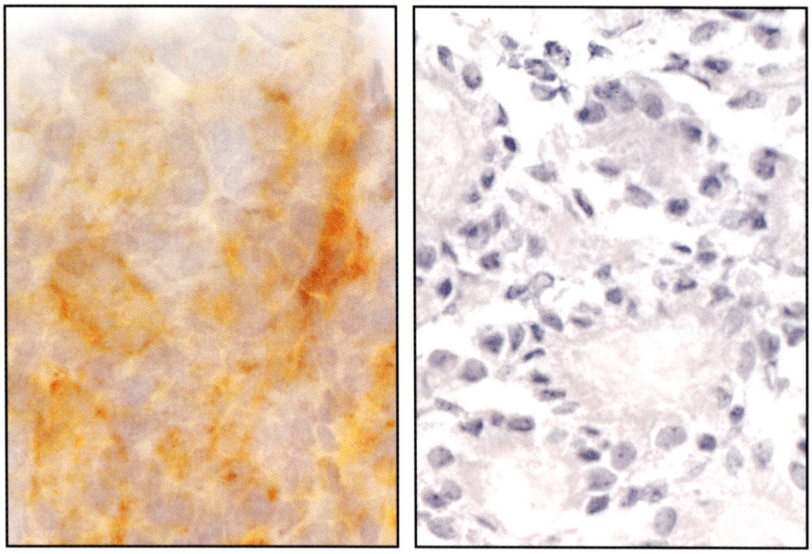

Needle aspirate (c) and biopsy specimen (d) of metastatic prostatic adenocarcinoma of the brain (c, Immunoperoxidase for prostatic acid phosphatase, 400X; d, H&E, 400X).

References

1. Allan PM, Garson JA, Harper EI, Asser U, Coakham HB, Brownell B, Kemshead JT: Biological characterization and clinical applications of a monoclonal antibody recognizing an antigen restricted to neuroectodermal tissues. *Int J Cancer* 31:591–598, 1983.
2. Bayer EA, Wilchek M: The use of avidin-biotin complex as a tool in molecular biology. *Methods Biochem Anal* 26:1–45, 1980.
3. Bonetti F, Pea M, Martignoni G, Mombello A, Colombari R, Zamboni G, Scarpa A, Piubello Q, Bacchi CE, Gown A: False-positive immunostaining of normal epithelia and carcinomas with ascites fluid preparations of antimelanoma monoclonal antibody HMB-45. *Am J Clin Pathol* 95:454–459, 1991.
4. Drier JK, Swanson PE, Cherwitz DL, Wick MR: S-100 Protein immunoreactivity in poorly differentiated carcinomas. *Arch Pathol Lab Med* 111:447–452, 1987.
5. Franke FE, Schachenmayr W, Osborn M, Altmannsberger M: Unexpected immunoreactivities of intermediate filament antibodies in human brain and brain tumors. *Am J Pathol* 139:67–79, 1991.
6. Gould VE, Jansson DS, Molenaar WM, Rorke LB, Trojanowski JQ, Lee VMY, Packer RJ, Franke WW: Primitive neuroectodermal tumors of the central nervous system: patterns of expression of neuroendocrine markers and all classes of intermediate filament proteins. *Lab Invest* 62:498–508, 1990.
7. Gullermo HA, Turbat-Herrera EA, Lott RL: S-100 Protein expression by primary and metastatic adenocarcinomas. *Am J Clin Pathol* 89:168–176, 1988.
8. Koprowski H, Steplewski Z, Herlyn D, Herlyn M: Study of antibodies against human melanomas produced by somatic cell hybrids. *Proc Natl Acad Sci USA* 75:3405–3409, 1978.
9. Lee AK, Dwarkanath S, DeLellis RA: S-100 Protein positivity in breast carcinoma. *Lab Invest* 54:35A, 1986.
10. Lukes RJ: The immunologic approach to the pathology of malignant lymphomas. *Am J Clin Pathol* 72:657–669, 1979.
11. Lukes RJ, Collins RD: Immunologic characterization of human malignant lymphomas. *Cancer* 34:1488–1503, 1974.
12. Miller DC, Koslow M, Budzilovich G, Burstein D: Synaptophysin: a sensitive and specific marker for ganglion cells in central nervous system neoplasms. *Hum Pathol* 21:271–276, 1990.
13. Nakane PK, Kawaoi A: A peroxidase-labeled antibody: a new method of conjugation. *J Histochem Cytochem* 22:1084–1091, 1974.
14. Oi VT, Morrison SL: Overview: chimeric antibodies. *Biotechniques* 4:214–221, 1986.
15. Ordonez NG, Sneige N, Hickey RC, Brooks TE: Use of monoclonal antibody HMB-45 in the cytologic diagnosis of melanoma. *Acta Cytol* 32:684–688, 1988.
16. Patel K, Rossell RJ, Bourne S, Moore SE, Walsh FS, Kemshead JT: Monoclonal antibody UJ13A recognizes the neural cell adhesion molecule (NCAM). *Int J Cancer* 44:1062–1068, 1989.

17. Pegram CN, Eng LF, Wikstrand CJ, McComb RD, Lee Y-L, Bigner DD: Monoclonal antibodies reactive with epitopes restricted to glial fibrillary acidic proteins of several species. *Neurochem Pathol* 3:119–138, 1983.

18. Shoup SA, Johnston WW, Seigler HF, Tello JW, Schlom J, Bigner DD, Bigner SH: A panel of antibodies useful in the cytologic diagnosis of metastatic melanoma. *Acta Cytol* 34:385–392, 1990.

19. Sternberger LA, Hardy PH Jr, Cuculis JJ, Meyer HG: The unlabeled antibody enzyme method of immunohistochemistry: preparation and properties of soluble antigen-antibody complex (horseradish peroxidase-antihorseradish peroxidase) and its use in identification of spirochetes. *J Histochem Cytochem* 18:315–333, 1970.

20. Vick WW, Bigner SH, Wikstrand CJ, Bullard DE, Kemshead J, Coakham H, Schlom J, Johnston WW, Bigner DD: The use of a panel of monoclonal antibodies in the evaluation of cytologic specimens from the central nervous system. *Acta Cytol* 31:815–824, 1987.

21. Zeltzer PM, Bodey B, Marlin A, Kemshead J: Immunophenotype profile of childhood medulloblastomas and supratentorial primitive neuroectodermal tumors using 16 monoclonal antibodies. *Cancer* 66:273–283, 1990.

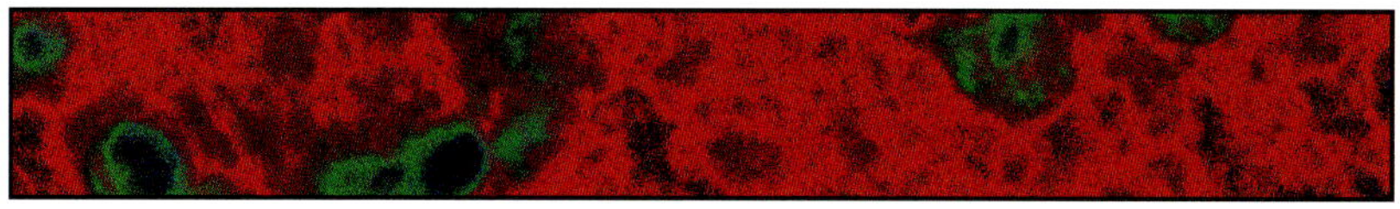

CHAPTER TEN

Cytogenetic and Molecular Genetic Aspects of Nervous System Tumors

The earliest specific chromosomal changes identified in human neoplasia was the 9;22 translocation of chronic myelogenous leukemia (CML), which was termed the Philadelphia chromosome (Figure 10.1). This initial observation was followed by other specific translocations in acute promyelocytic leukemia (APML) and Burkitt's lymphoma and other types of leukemia and lymphoma (Figure 10.2).[2] The development of molecular techniques in the 1980s has led to an understanding of the molecular events that are reflected in cytogenetic changes, such as the translocation of the c-*abl* gene into the breakpoint cluster region (BCR) of chromosome 22 in CML, the juxtaposition of the c-*MYC* and immunoglobulin genes in Burkitt's lymphoma, and the alteration of the retinoic acid receptor gene in APML.[6,12]

With the exception of soft tissue tumors,[8] the majority of solid tumors differ from leukemia and lymphoma in that specific balanced translocations are rare. Alterations in these tumors, instead, consist of gains and losses of chromosomes and chromosomal regions, often through deletions and unbalanced translocations, and gene amplification. Neurogenic tumors in particular are among the prototypes for these genetic aberrations.

Gene Amplification

Gene amplification is the selective duplication of a small (less than 1,000 kilobase) region of chromosome. This change is manifested at the cytoge-

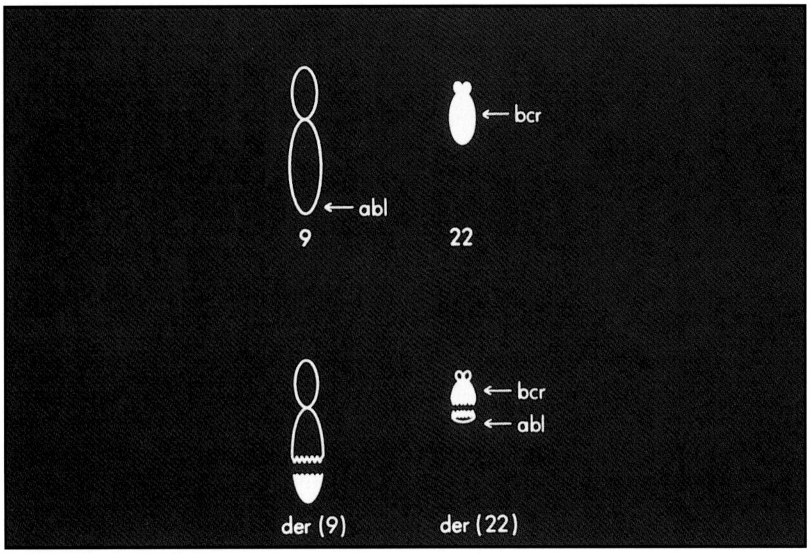

Figure 10.1
The Philadelphia chromosome translocation is a reciprocal 9;22 translocation in which the c-*abl* oncogene moves from chromosome 9 to the breakpoint cluster region (BCR) of chromosome 22q.

netic level as double-minute chromosomes (DMs) (Figure 10.3), homogeneously staining regions (HSRs), or abnormally banded regions (ABRs). Gene amplification is demonstrated by Southern blot or slot blot analysis in

Gene amplification is demonstrated by Southern blot or slot blot analysis

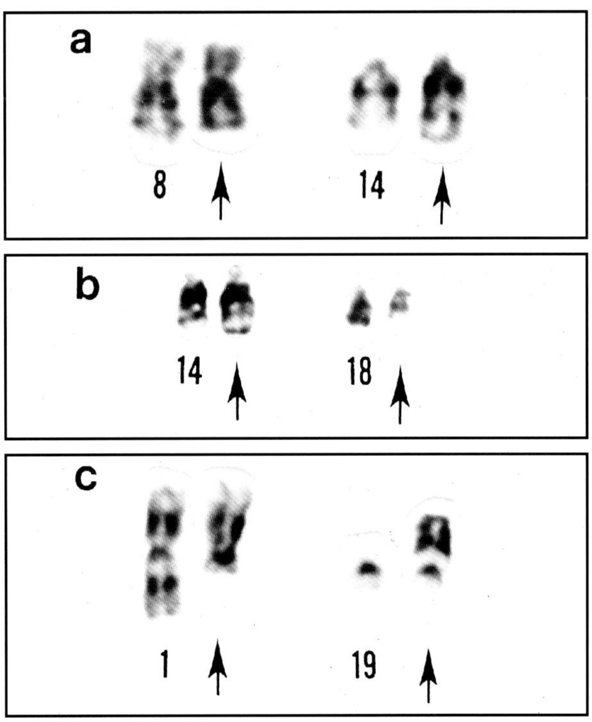

Figure 10.2
8;14 translocation of Burkitt's lymphoma (a). 14;18 translocation of follicular lymphoma (b). 1;19 translocation of pre–B-cell leukemia (c) (arrows indicate the abnormal chromosome).

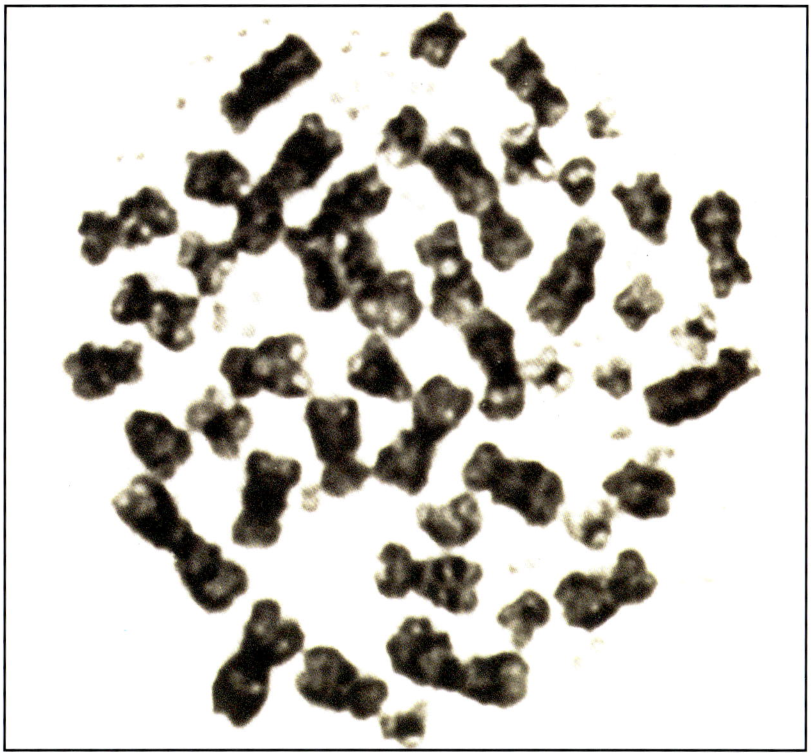

Figure 10.3
This chromosome spread from a glioblastoma multiforme with amplification of the *gli* gene contains numerous double-minute chromosomes (D-259MG direct).

which an increased copy number of the gene in question is demonstrated through the use of a specific probe (Figure 10.4). Amplification is inevitably accompanied by high-level expression of the gene as manifested by high levels of mRNA and demonstrated by Northern blot analysis or in situ hybridization. The protein product of the gene is generally increased as well, as can be seen by immunoblot or immunohistochemistry.

Gene amplification has been demonstrated in subsets of most solid tumors

Gene amplification has been demonstrated in subsets of most types of solid tumors. The highest incidences include amplification of the N-*myc* gene in about one third of neuroblastomas and amplification of the epidermal growth factor receptor (EGFR) gene in 30% to 40% of malignant gliomas.[9] Gene amplification is less prevalent in other tumors, such as amplification of the HER2/NEU or c-*MYC* genes in 23% and 20% of breast carcinomas[1] and of the N-*MYC* or c-*MYC* genes in 3% to 5% of retinoblastomas and medulloblastomas.

In neuroblastoma, a significant relationship exists between advanced tumor stage and N-*myc* gene amplification.[5,19] Although most instances of the amplified gene occur in late-stage tumors, a poor prognosis can be predicted in the occasional patient with a localized tumor and this genetic property. A similar relationship has been described in malignant gliomas in which the majority of cases of EGFR gene amplification occur in the most advanced histologic stage—glioblastoma multiforme.[9] Although this genetic property is thus associated with histologic progression rather than prognosis, the identification of the occasional case of gene amplification in a lower-grade tumor delineates patients more likely to have rapid disease progression.

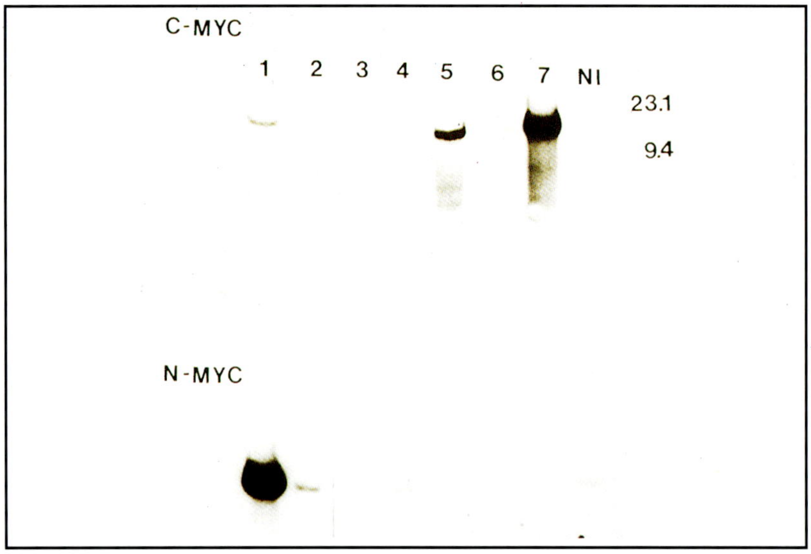

Figure 10.4
This Southern blot analysis of multiple medulloblastoma cell lines and xenografts (lanes 2–7) shows amplification of the c-*myc* gene in the cases in lanes 5 and 7 (a). The same blot rehybridized with an N-*myc* probe shows gene amplification only in the control neuroblastoma cell line in lane 1 (b).

Epidermal Growth Factor Receptor (EGFR)

Approximately one third of gliomas with amplification of the EGFR gene undergo rearrangement of the gene as well.[9] The rearrangement results in deletion of a portion of the gene that codes for the extracellular domain of the receptor protein. Not only do these deletions result in altered properties of the receptor, but they produce new and unique polypeptides at the junction sites. These amino acid sequences provide targets for the production of antibodies that show great promise of being tumor specific. As these reagents continue to be produced and purified, their usefulness in the diagnosis, classification, and immunotherapy of brain tumors will be determined.

Suppressor Genes

In the 1970s, a subgroup of patients with familial retinoblastoma were observed to have deletions of chromosome band 13q14 in one copy of this chromosome in their germline cells. This finding led Knudson to hypothesize the existence of genes (suppressor genes) that, when functioning normally, suppress the growth of tumor cells. For patients with loss of one copy of a suppressor gene on 13q14 through chromosomal deletion in their somatic cells, a second insult (mutation, deletion, or chromosomal loss) involving the remaining gene copy in retinal cells leads to inactivation of the gene and could produce retinoblastoma. This hypothesis was substantiated in the late 1980s when the retinoblastoma gene, which functions precisely in this manner, was isolated.[14] Since that time, not only has the retinoblastoma gene been shown to be altered in additional types of solid human tumors, but other tumor suppressor genes have also been isolated, such as the p53, DCC, MCC genes.[7,13] Furthermore, through cytogenetic and molecular approaches, such as restriction fragment length polymorphism (RFLP) analysis, sites of regional chromosomal loss that are likely to contain additional tumor suppressor genes have been identified. For neuroblastoma, the most frequently deleted region is 1p36[20] and for medulloblastoma it is 17p[3] (Figure 10.5). Although 17p is the location of the p53 gene, this gene is rarely altered in these tumors, suggesting that another previously undescribed gene may be the target for 17p loss in these tumors.[4]

Sites of regional chromosomal loss likely to contain tumor suppressor genes have been identified

The most common cytogenetic alterations in malignant gliomas are gains of chromosome 7 and losses of chromosome 10 (Figure 10.6).[3,17] By adding RFLP analysis, the chromosome 10 loss has been confirmed and the region narrowed to 10q24–26.[18] In addition, loss of 17p occurs in about one third of cases in RFLP studies, and point mutations of the p53 gene can be demonstrated in most of these tumors. Another frequent site of chromosomal loss is 9p. The region on 9p has been narrowly localized due to the demonstration of homozygous deletions of the interferon genes that are in the same general area.[11,15] As these efforts to identify the relevant genes on 9p and 10q are successful, it is likely that genes directly involved in the genesis and progression of human gliomas will be identified.

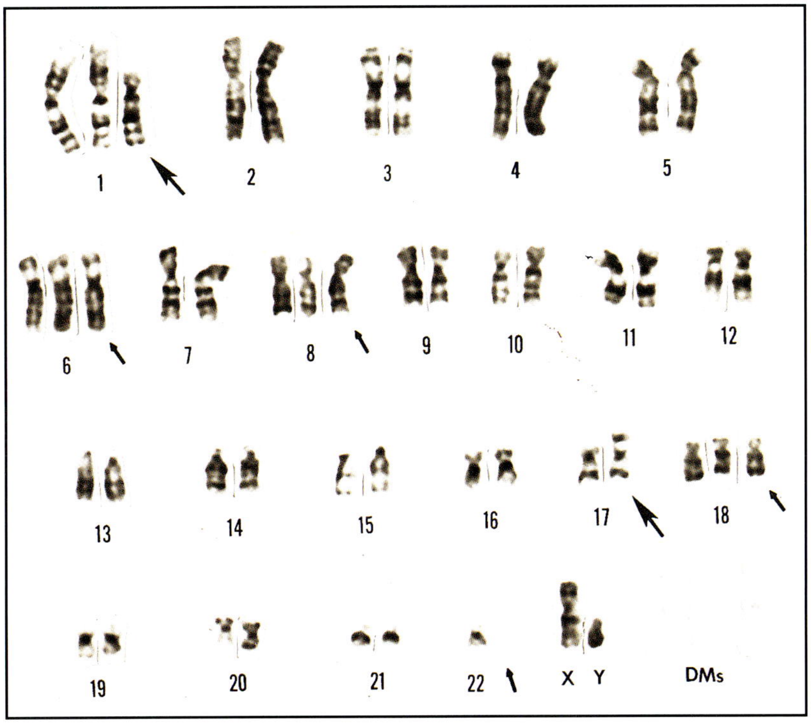

Figure 10.5
This medulloblastoma karyotype shows loss of 17p through the formation of isochromosome 17q. Other changes are also seen, including the presence of double-minute chromosomes (DMs) (arrows indicate the extra, missing, and structurally abnormal chromosomes).

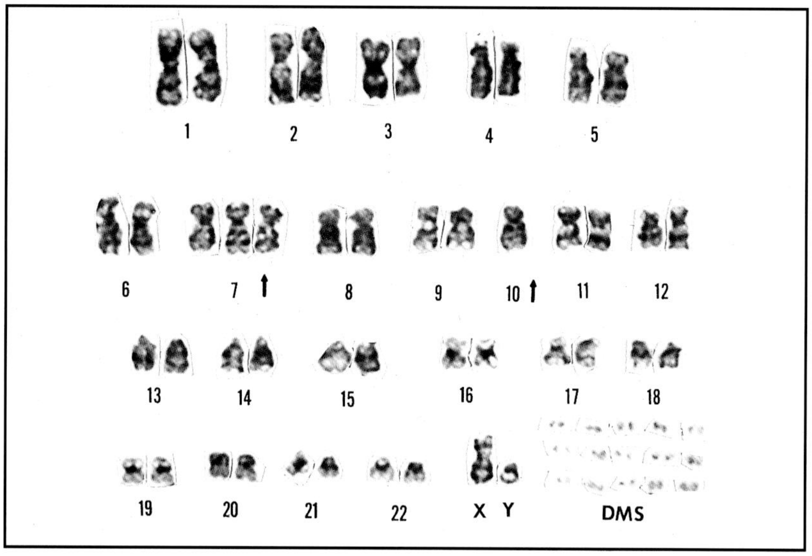

Figure 10.6
This glioblastoma karyotype shows the most common cytogenetic changes of this tumor type—gains of chromosome 7, loss of chromosome 10, and the presence of double-minute chromosomes (DMs).

Technical Advances[10]

In the late 1980s, a method for precisely amplifying small regions of DNA was devised. This approach uses specific primers that flank the region of interest. By using repeated cycles of Taq polymerase, the region of interest can be copied numerous times, producing sufficient quantities of the target region to allow cloning and sequencing. This method is termed polymerase chain reaction (PCR), and it has been applied widely to many aspects of molecular biology including the streamlining of cloning procedures. PCR is the primary approach now used to demonstrate gene mutations. It is critical for the determination of p53 gene mutations in gliomas and other types of solid tumors. Since this approach can use limited quantities of DNA isolated from a small number of cells, these techniques are of great potential usefulness in examining cytologic specimens, including those derived from cerebrospinal fluid (CSF).

In situ hybridization is a procedure by which specific gene or cDNA sequences can be detected in intact cells using specific gene probes and displayed by autoradiography or by fluorescence. This method can be altered to identify genes and gene amplification or to detect mRNA. Pinkel and associates[16] have pioneered a method of in situ hybridization in which chromosome-specific probes that localize to the centromere are labelled with biotin and are detected by fluorescence. This method—termed "FISH" for fluorescence in situ hybridization—detects copy number of individual chromosomes in interphase nuclei as well as in metaphase spreads. By using biotin-labelled chromosome-specific libraries, the entire chromosome can be seen. This method, termed "chromosome painting," is helpful in metaphase spreads to identify translocations and is of potential use in identifying translocations in interphase nuclei. Although the primary

The adaptation of these new methods to cytologic preparations makes them potentially applicable to clinical situations

applications of these methods remain in the research setting today, their ready adaptation to cytologic specimens makes them potentially applicable to a wide range of clinical situations as well.

References

1. Berns Els MJJ, Klijn JGM, van Putten WLJ, van Staveren IL, Portengen H, Foekens JA: C-*myc* amplification is a better prognostic factor than *HER2/neu* amplification in primary breast cancer. *Cancer Res* 52:1107–1113, 1992.
2. Bigner SH: Cytogenetics of human neoplasia. In: Schmidt WA, ed. *Cytopathology Annual 1992.* Baltimore, MD, Williams and Wilkins Co, 1992, pp. 1–21.
3. Bigner SH, Mark J, Bigner DD: Cytogenetics of human brain tumors. *Cancer Genet Cytogenet* 47:141–154, 1990.
4. Biegel JA, Burk CD, Barr FG, Emanuel BS: Evidence for a 17p tumor-related locus distinct from p53 in pediatric primitive neuroectodermal tumors. *Cancer Res* 52:3391–3395, 1992.
5. Brodeur GM, Seeger RC, Schwab M, Varmus HE, Bishop JM: Amplification of N-*myc* in untreated human neuroblastomas correlates with advanced disease stage. *Science* 224:1121–1124, 1984.
6. de Thé H, Lavau C, Marchio A, Chomienne C, Degos L, Dejean A: The PML-RARα fusion mRNA generated by the t(15;17) translocation in acute promyelocytic leukemia encodes a functionally altered RAR. *Cell* 66:675–684, 1991.
7. Fearon ER, Vogelstein B: A genetic model for colorectal tumorigenesis. *Cell* 61:759–767, 1990.
8. Fletcher JA, Kozakewich HP, Hoffer FA, Lage JM, Weidner N, Tepper R, Pinkus GS, Morton CC, Corson JM: Diagnostic relevance of clonal cytogenetic aberrations in malignant soft tissue tumors. *N Engl J Med* 324:436–442, 1991.
9. Fuller GN, Bigner SH: Amplified cellular oncogenes in neoplasms of the human central nervous system. *Mutat Res* 276:299–306, 1992.
10. Hilborne LH, Grody WW: Diagnostic applications of recombinant nucleic acid technology: basic techniques. *Lab Med* 22:849–856, 1991.
11. James CD, He J, Carlbom E, Nordenskjold M, Cavenee WK, Collins VP: Chromosome 9 deletion mapping reveals interferon α and interferon β-1 gene deletions in human glial tumors. *Cancer Res* 51:1684–1688, 1991.
12. Kakizuka A, Miller WH, Umesono K, Warrell RP, Frankel SR, Murty VVVS, Dmitrovsky E, Evans RM: Chromosomal translocation t(15;17) in human acute promyelocytic leukemia fuses RARα with a novel putative transcription factor, PML. *Cell* 66:663–674, 1991.
13. Kinzler KW, Nilbert MC, Vogelstein B, Bryan TM, Levy DB, Smith KJ, Preisinger AC, Hamilton SR, Hedge P, Markham A, Carlson M,

Joslyn G, Groden J, White R, Miki Y, Miyoshi Y, Nishisho I, Nakamura Y: Identification of a gene located at chromosome 5q21 that is mutated in colorectal cancers. *Science* 251:1366–1370, 1991.

14. Lee W-H, Bookstein R, Hong F, Young L-J, Shew J-Y, Lee E: Human retinoblastoma susceptibility gene: cloning, identification, and sequence. *Science* 235:1394-1399, 1987.
15. Olopade OI, Jenkins RB, Ransom DT, Malik K, Pomykala H, Nobori T, Cowan JM, Rowley JD, Diaz MO: Molecular analysis of deletions of the short arm of chromosome 9 in human gliomas. *Cancer Res* 52:2523–2529, 1992.
16. Pinkel D, Straume T, Gray JW: Cytogenetic analysis using quantitative, high-sensitivity, fluorescence hybridization. *Proc Natl Acad Sci USA* 83:2934–2938, 1986.
17. Rasheed ABK, Bigner SH: Genetic alterations in glioma and medulloblastoma. *Cancer Metastasis Rev* 10:289–299, 1991.
18. Rasheed ABK, Fuller GN, Friedman AH, Bigner DD, Bigner SH: Loss of heterozygosity for 10q loci in human gliomas. *Genes Chromo Cancer* 5:75–82, 1992.
19. Seeger RC, Brodeur GM, Sather H, Dalton A, Siegel SE, Wong KY, Hammond D: Association of multiple copies of the N-*myc* oncogene with rapid progression of neuroblastomas. *N Engl J Med* 313:1111–1116, 1985.
20. Weith A, Martinsson T, Cziepluch C, Bruderlein S, Amler LC, Berthold F, Schwab M: Neuroblastoma consensus deletion maps to 1p36.1-2. *Genes Chromo Cancer* 1:1–8, 1989.

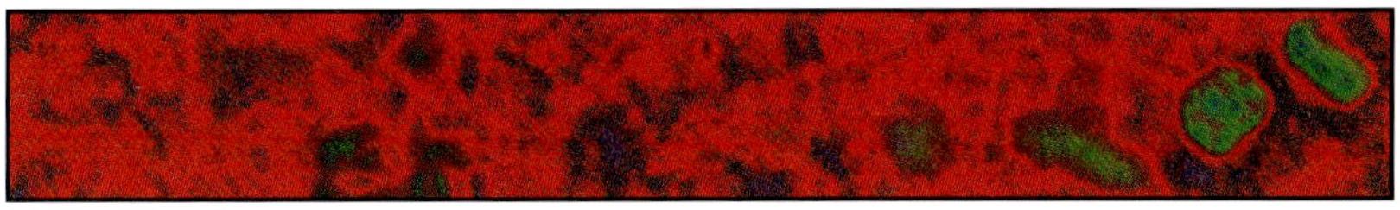

Index

Numbers in **boldface** refer to pages on which images, tables, and figures appear.

B

C

N

O

P